IMMUNOLOGY AND IMMUNE SYSTEM DISORDERS

IGG4 RELATED DISEASE

ILLUSTRATED PATHOLOGY OF NOVEL SYSTEMIC DISEASE

IMMUNOLOGY AND IMMUNE SYSTEM DISORDERS

Additional books and e-books in this series can be found on Nova's website under the Series tab.

IMMUNOLOGY AND IMMUNE SYSTEM DISORDERS

IGG4 RELATED DISEASE

ILLUSTRATED PATHOLOGY OF NOVEL SYSTEMIC DISEASE

SYUICHI KOARADA
EDITOR

nova
Medicine & Health
New York

NOTICE TO THE READER

Library of Congress Cataloging-in-Publication Data

Names: Koarada, Syuichi, editor.
Title: IgG4 related disease : illustrated pathology of novel systemic disease / Syuichi Koarada, editor.
Description: New York : Nova Science Publishers, [2020] | Series: Immunology and immune system disorders | Includes bibliographical references and index. |
Identifiers: LCCN 2020022897 (print) | LCCN 2020022898 (ebook) | ISBN 9781536180503 (hardcover) | ISBN 9781536180510 (adobe pdf)
Subjects: LCSH: Autoimmune diseases. | Immunoglobulin G.--Pathophysiology.
Classification: LCC RC600 .I34 2020 (print) | LCC RC600 (ebook) | DDC 616.97/8--dc23
LC record available at https://lccn.loc.gov/2020022897
LC ebook record available at https://lccn.loc.gov/2020022898

Published by Nova Science Publishers, Inc. † New York

CONTENTS

PREFACE

IgG4-related disease (IgG4-RD) is an increasingly recognized rare and novel systemic inflammatory disorder characterized by tumefactive lesions with infiltrating IgG4-positive plasma cells.

The disease affects virtually every organ system. Immunologically, serum levels of IgG4, plasmablasts and plasma cells increase in patients with IgG4-RD in which activation and dysregulation of B cells may be involved.

However, serum IgG4 levels are elevated only in about two-thirds of the patients with IgG4-RD.

It is a well-known fact that serum IgG4 is not necessarily elevated in serum in significant patients even before treatment, despite the presence of the histopathologic finding in involved tissue.

Consequently, accurate characterization by a method using various modalities and immunological evaluation including plain radiography, ultrasound, CT, scintigraphy, MRI, PET-CT and flow cytometry should be required. Comprehensively, we review and illustrate the systemic and organ-specific findings of IgG4-RD. This book shows immunological and radiological findings for general practitioners. Moreover, the book is also interesting for the subspecialists including rheumatologists, dermatologists, otologists, respiratory physicians, and radiologists because patients with IgG4-RD visit every subspecialist by the tremendous various clinical symptoms and findings.

The study included 147 patients with IgG4-RD who visited Saga University Hospital from January 1, 2001 to March 31, 2020. Although the number of patients studied in this monograph was very small, the cases that could be comprehensively evaluated at a single institution were considered clinically significantly valuable.

In this book, we will focus on the most recent advances in immunological background and imaging in IgG4-RD.

The spring sun rises through the cherry blossoms in Saga Castle, old moated big castle in Saga, and the sun's light shimmers in the wind.

Syuichi Koarada

ACKNOWLEDGMENTS

The authors thank the reviewers and editors of NOVA Science Publishers for their excellent work and giving us the opportunity to publish this valuable book. We would like to express our deep appreciation to our patients who provided valuable data and images.

I would like to show my greatest appreciation to colleagues whose enormous support and insightful comments were invaluable during my study. I also owe a very important debt to assistants Kimiko Eguchi who provided technical help and sincere encouragement. I would also like to express my gratitude to my family, my parents, my wife (Miwako; beautiful harmony), and my daughter (Sakura; cherry blossom), for their warm support and encouragements.

In: IgG4 Related Disease
Editor: Syuichi Koarada
ISBN: 978-1-53618-050-3

Chapter 1

INTRODUCTION OF IGG4-RELATED DISEASE

Syuichi Koarada**, Nobuyuki Ono and Yoshifumi Tada
Division of Rheumatology, Faculty of Medicine,
Saga University, Nabeshima, Saga, Japan

ABSTRACT

IgG4-related disease has been a relatively recently established systemic disease that causes organ infiltration by IgG4 positive plasma cells and fibroinflammatory tissues and mimics other inflammatory or neoplastic diseases. Many organs have various lesions and symptoms, and the images show various findings. In this book, head and neck, thorax, urinary system, cardiovascular system, musculoskeletal system, abdomen, and other lesions are described comprehensively. In the final chapter, we review the position of IgG4-related disease among autoimmune diseases from the immunological background. IgG4-related disease is a disorder that causes systematic space-occupying lesions targeting the lumens of multiple organs accompanied by immunological abnormalities of B cells, particularly plasmablasts. The targeted lumens are various such as blood vessels, lymphatic vessels, respiratory tract, digestive tract, biliary tract, and secretory glands.

---

* Corresponding Author's Email: koarada@cc.saga-u.ac.jp.

INTRODUCTION

IgG4-related disease has been a relatively recently established systemic disorder that causes organ infiltration by fibroinflammatory tissue and mimics other inflammatory or neoplastic diseases.

In 2001, Hamano et al., reported that serum IgG4 is a useful marker for the diagnosis of autoimmune pancreatitis (Hamano H., 2001). After that, not only autoimmune pancreatitis but also sclerosing cholangitis, retroperitoneal fibrosis, inflammatory pseudotumor, Küttner's tumor, and interstitial nephritis were found to be characterized by high serum IgG4 levels, tissue infiltration of IgG4-positive plasma cells, tumor formation, and fibrosis.

This condition has become known as an IgG4-related disease.

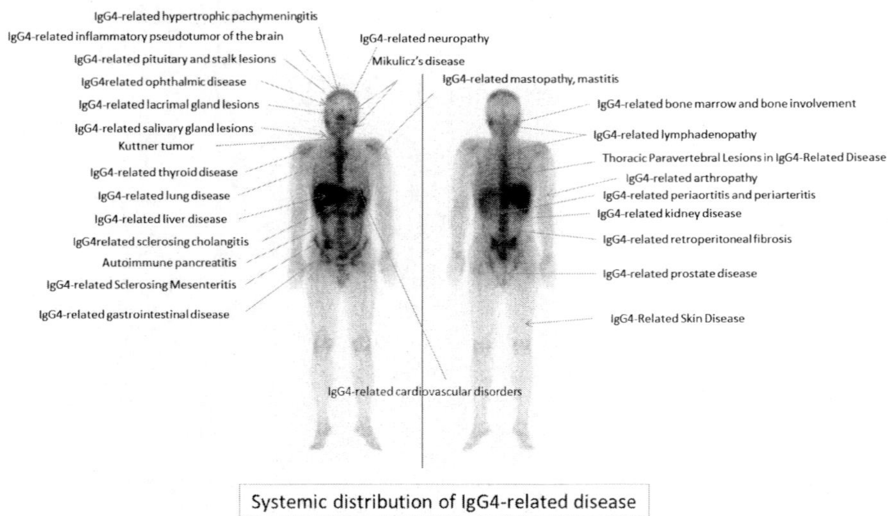

Figure 1. Systemic distribution o IgG4-related disease.

IgG4-related disease has the following clinical features. 1) generally systemic distribution, 2) imaging findings of swelling, nodules, and/or wall thickening, 3) high levels of serum IgG4, 4) IgG4-positive plasma cell infiltration and fibrosis in affected organs, 5) good response to corticosteroid therapy, and 6) simultaneous or metachronous co-existence with other IgG4-related disease.

IgG4-related disease is a disorder that causes systematic space-occupying lesions targeting the lumens of multiple organs accompanied by immunological abnormalities of B cells, particularly plasmablasts. The targeted lumens are various such as blood vessels, lymphatic vessels, respiratory tract, digestive tract, biliary tract, and secretory glands.

LABORATORY FINDINGS

Electrophoresis of Serum

Gel protein electrophoresis of sera of patients with IgG4-related disease shows β-γ bridging. This bridge is a polyclonal band of the rapidly migrating fraction of γ-globulins.

This abnormal band was confirmed by immunoelectrophoresis with elevated serum IgG4.

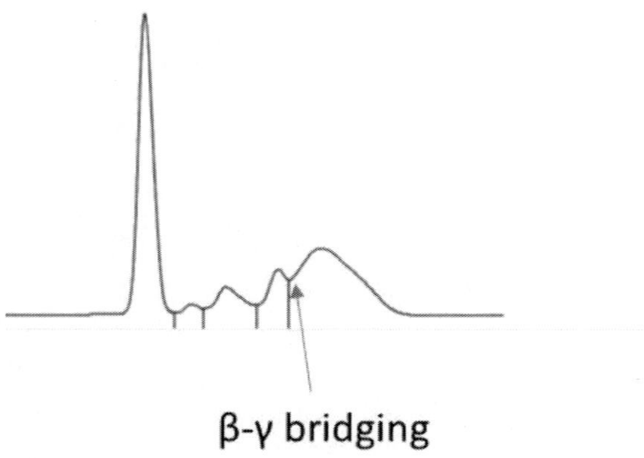

Figure 2. Gel electrophoresis of serum of a patient with IgG4 related disease reveals β-γ globulin bridging.

Serum IgG4 Levels

Elevated IgG4 levels are observed in 90% of patients with autoimmune pancreatitis, but rarely in other diseases. Therefore, IgG4 can be a sensitive and specific marker for autoimmune pancreatitis and IgG4-related disease. However, not all patients have elevated IgG4, and patients with other disorders may be positive.

Reference

Hamano H., K. S. (2001). High serum IgG4 concentrations in patients with sclerosing pancreatitis. *N Engl J Med., 344*, 732-738.

In: IgG4 Related Disease
Editor: Syuichi Koarada
ISBN: 978-1-53618-050-3

Chapter 2

IgG4-Related Disease in Head and Neck

Syuichi Koarada* and Mariko Sakai
Division of Rheumatology, Faculty of Medicine,
Saga University, Nabeshima, Saga, Japan

Abstract

The lesions in the head and neck of IgG4-related disease are very diverse. Various lesions can occur, including lacrimal and salivary gland lesions. Lacrimal and submandibular gland lesions are often found in patients with IgG4-related disease. In addition to cervical lymphadenopathy, intraorbital lesions, sinusitis, and mastoid cellulitis may occur. Moreover, thyroid lesions, pituitary lesions, and nerve lesions may sometimes occur, and rarely, inflammatory pseudotumors in the brain or hypertrophic pachymeningitis may occur.

---

* Corresponding Author's Email: koarada@cc.saga-u.ac.jp.

INTRODUCTION

The head and neck are sites that are involved in IgG4-related disease. Symptoms can occur anywhere in the head and neck. However, IgG4-related disease often involves the salivary glands, the lacrimal glands, the orbits, the thyroid gland, the lymph nodes, sinonasal cavities, and the pituitary stalk (Table 1). Other areas such as the larynx are less common.

Table 1. IgG4-Related disease in the head and neck

Salivary glands
Mikulicz's disease
Küttner tumor, chronic sialadenitis
Orbits
Lacrimal glands
Mikulicz's disease
Chronic dacryoadenitis
Idiopathic orbital inflammation
Pseudotumor
Lymphoid hyperplasia
Perineural spread
Trigeminal nerve branches
Dilatation of the ophthalmic veins
Pituitary gland
Hypophysitis, pituitary stalk/gland
Sinonasal cavities
Paranasal sinusitis
Mastoid sinuses
Mastoiditis
Thyroid gland
Hashimoto thyroiditis
Riedel thyroiditis
Larynx
Submucosal lesion
Lymph nodes
Lymphadenopathy
Pachymeninges
Hypertrophic Pachymeningitis

Salivary Gland Involvement

IgG4-related sialadenitis is characterized by bilateral and painless swelling of the glands (Hamano H 2006). Involvement of major salivary glands (the parotid or the submandibular) is a common feature of IgG4-related disease. This condition was previously thought to be a subcategory of Sjögren's syndrome, but its clinical entity is different from that of Sjögren's syndrome (Geyer JT 2010) (Masaki Y 2010) (Himi T 2012). Patients may present with lacrimal and parotid gland hypertrophy, a condition previously known as Mikulicz's disease. Patients may also present with the submandibular gland hypertrophy, formerly called Kuttner's tumor.

IgG4-related disease is characterized by no or mild keratoconjunctivitis sicca caused by decreased lacrimal gland secretion, and by mild xerostomia. Regarding the salivary glands, the parotid glands are enlarged in Sjögren's syndrome; however, the submandibular glands are enlarged in IgG4-related disease. Patients with IgG4-related sialadenitis are negative for anti-SS-A and anti-SS-B antibodies. Histopathological specimens show marked infiltration of IgG4-positive plasma cells in the salivary glands. Patients with IgG4-related sialadenitis respond well to corticosteroid treatment. Salivary gland lesions are mostly symmetric and bilateral, but sometimes unilateral.

Imaging of IgG4-Related Sialadenitis

Various types of imaging modalities, including ultrasonography, sialography, CT, MRI, and PET/CT, are important for differential diagnosis from Sjögren's syndrome and malignancy, and for evaluation of lesions such as site and time course.

CT

Non-Contrast Enhanced CT (NCECT) Images

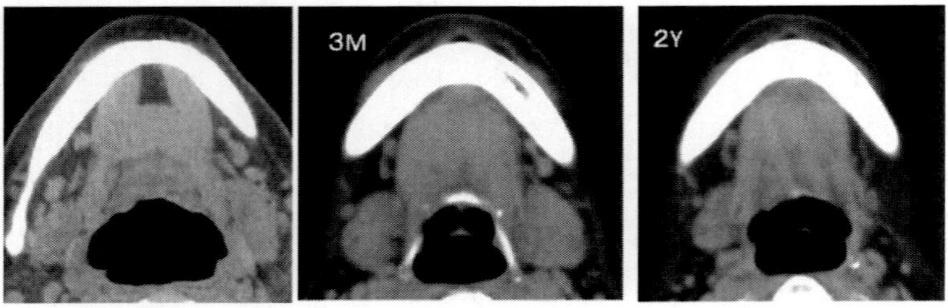

Figure 1. IgG4-related sialadenitis in a 75-year-old woman. Axial non-contrast enhanced CT (NCECT) images. At the first consultation, CT image (left panel) shows enlargement of the submandibular glands. Three months later (middle panel), the swelling increased, and infiltration of IgG4-positive cells were confirmed by resection of the left submandibular gland for biopsy. Two years later, CT image (right panel) shows that salivary gland swelling resolved spontaneously without treatment.

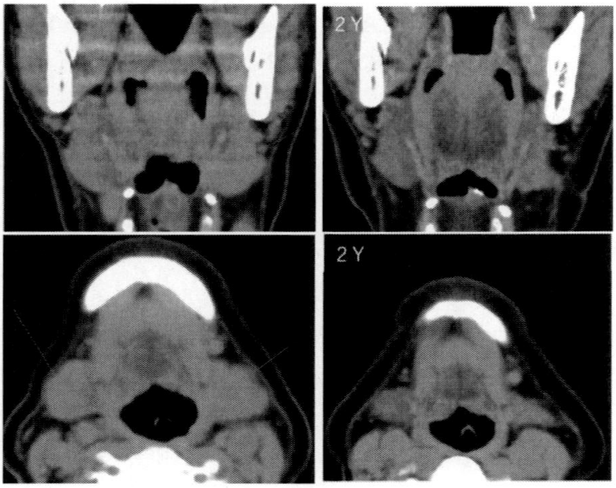

Figure 2. IgG4-related sialadenitis in a 76-year-old man. Coronal (left upper panel) and axial non-contrast enhanced CT (NCECT) (left lower panel) images show bilateral submandibular gland enlargement (arrows). Two years after corticosteroid treatment, CT images (right panels) show reduced submandibular gland swelling.

On CT images, the enlarged salivary glands in IgG4-related disease basically have chronic inflammatory changes. In addition, the lesions may have homogenous attenuation and abundant blood flow, and then may have findings such as a slightly homogenous contrast enhanced effect. On the other hand, Sjögren's syndrome often exhibits a salt and pepper pattern due to fatty degeneration.

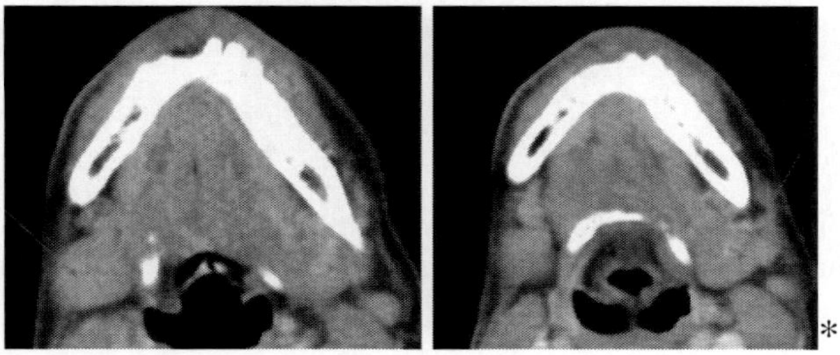

Figure 3. IgG4-related sialadenitis in a 38-year-old man. Axial non-contrast enhanced CT images show mild submandibular gland enlargement (arrows).

Contrast Enhanced CT Images (CECT)

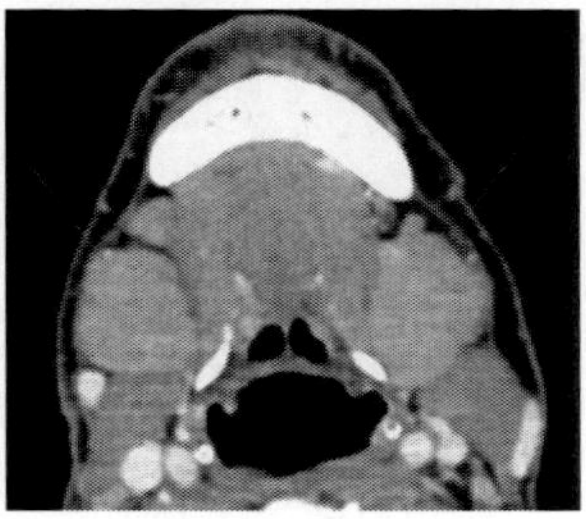

Figure 4. IgG4-related sialadenitis in a 67-year-old man. Axial contrast enhanced neck CT image shows severe enlargement of the submandibular glands with homogeneous enhancement.

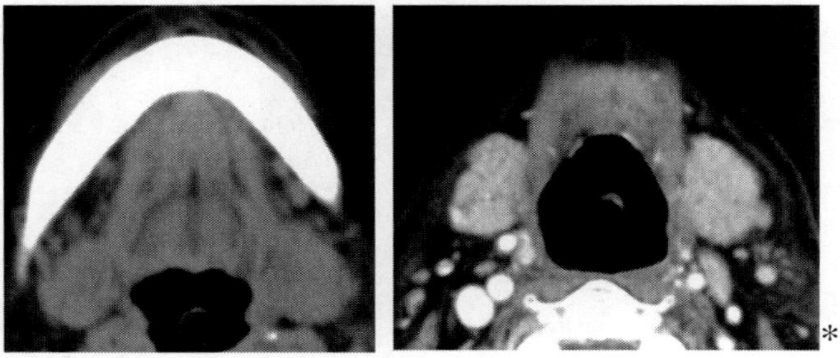

Figure 5. IgG4-related sialadenitis in a 76-year-old woman. Axial non-contrast and contrast enhanced CT images show moderate swelling of the submandibular glands with homogeneous enhancement.

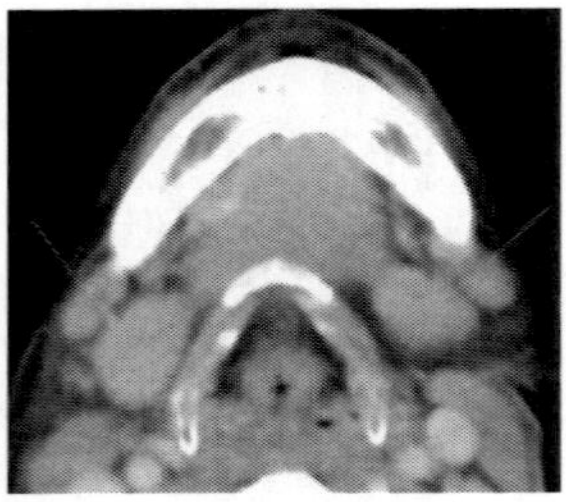

Figure 6. IgG4-related sialadenitis in a 72-year-old man. Axial contrast enhanced CT image shows mild enlargement of the submandibular glands with homogeneous enhancement.

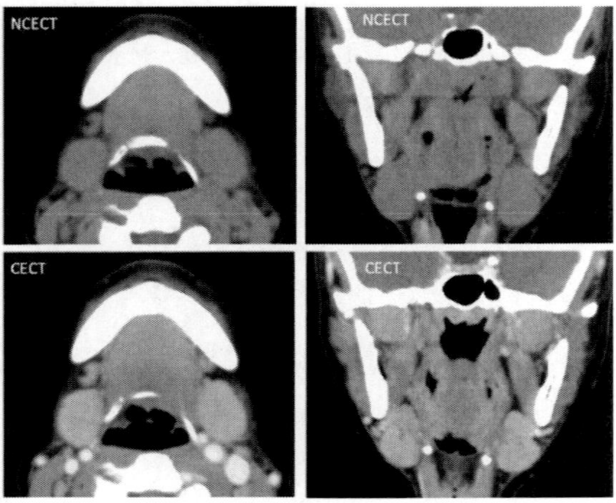

Figure 7. IgG4-related sialadenitis in a 43-year-old woman. Coronal and axial non-contrast enhanced and contrast enhanced CT images show mild enlargement of bilateral submandibular glands.

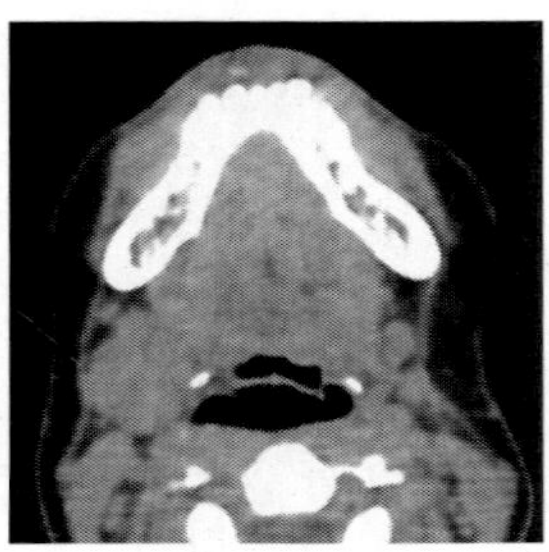

Figure 8. IgG4-related sialadenitis in a 44-year-old woman. Axial non-contrast enhanced (NCECT) CT image shows enlargement of the right submandibular gland pushed medially. Since excisional biopsy of the left submandibular gland was done, the location of the salivary gland is easier to identify.

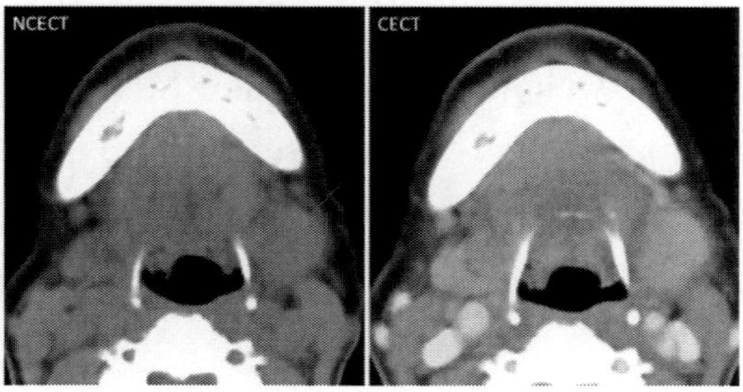

Figure 9. IgG4-related sialadenitis in a 50-year-old woman. Axial non-contrast enhanced and contrast enhanced CT images show enlargement of the unilateral left submandibular gland.

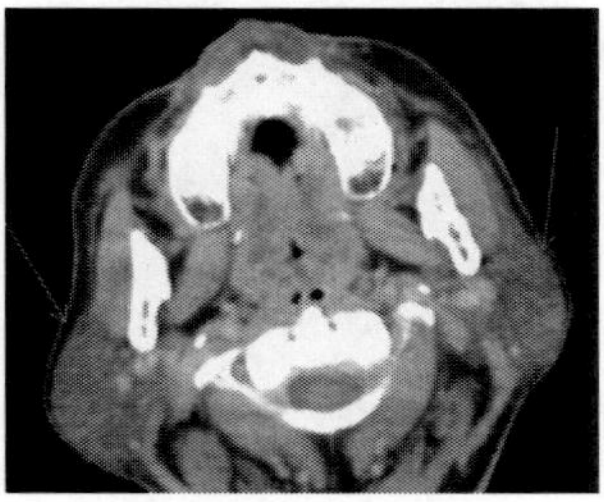

Figure 10. IgG4-related sialadenitis in a 72-year-old man. Axial contrast enhanced CT image shows enlargement of bilateral parotid glands.

MRI

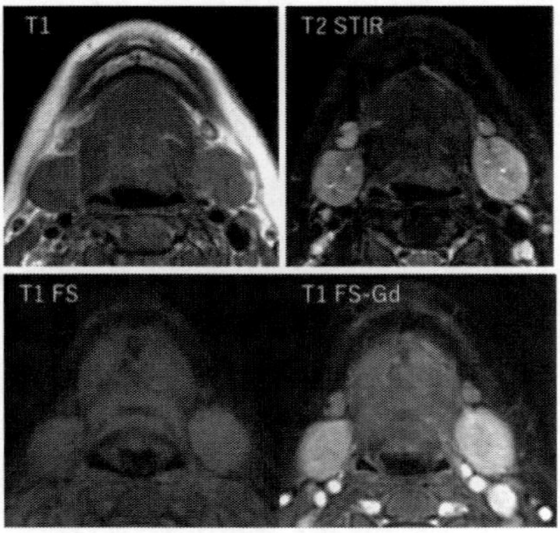

Figure 11. IgG4-related sialadenitis in a 43-year-old woman. Cervical MR images show bilateral submandibular gland swelling. Gadolinium-enhanced T1-weighted FS image shows enhancement of salivary glands. The contrast effect on the submandibular glands is stronger on the left than on the right.

In MR images, IgG4-associated sialadenitis has relatively low signal intensity on T2-weighted images due to fibrosis, and low signal intensity with homogenous enhancement on T1-weighted images (Fujita A 2012).

Gallium Scintigraphy

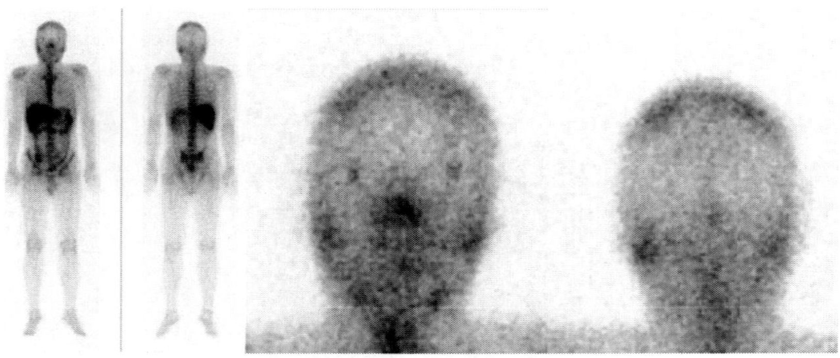

(A)

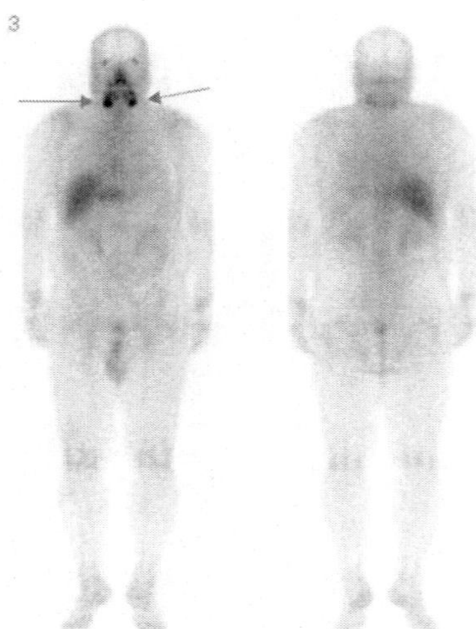

(B)

Figure 12. (A) IgG4-related sialadenitis in a 38-year-old man. Gallium scintigraphy shows abnormal uptake in the submandibular and parotid glands. (B) IgG4-related disease in a 66-year-old man. Gallium scintigraphy shows abnormal uptake of bilateral submandibular glands.

PET-CT

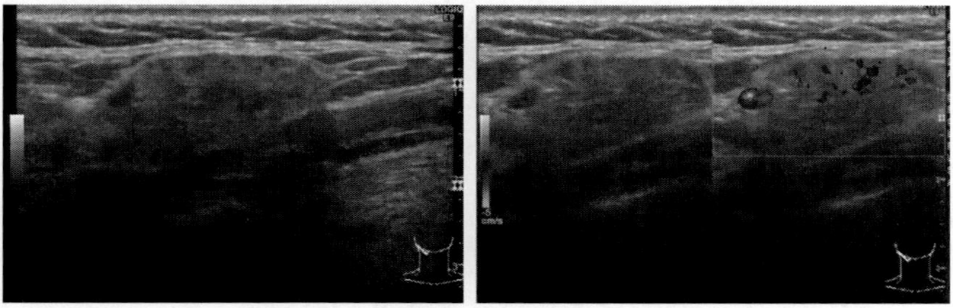

Figure 13. IgG4-related sialadenitis in a 75-year-old woman. B-mode and color Doppler US images show sialadenitis of the right submandibular gland. The gland is enlarged and slightly hypoechoic with increased blood flow. Color Doppler US image shows the inflamed right submandibular gland.

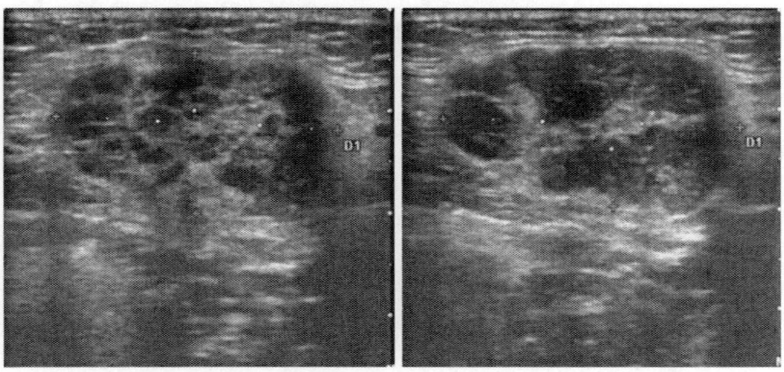

Figure 14. IgG4-related sialadenitis in a 35-year-old woman. Ultrasound images of the neck show that the left submandibular gland is hypoechoic and swollen.

Clinical Photography

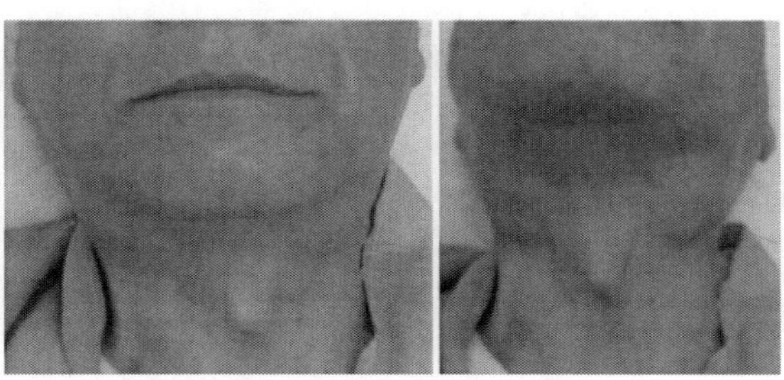

Figure 15. IgG4-related disease in a 66-year-old man. Clinical photographs show severe swelling of the submandibular glands on both sides of the neck (arrows).

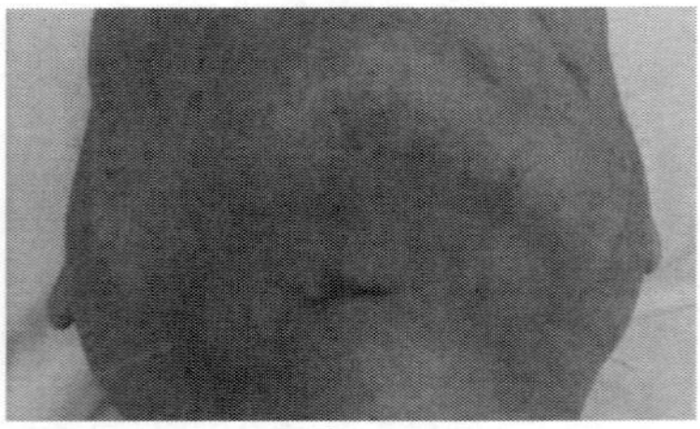

Figure 16. IgG4-related disease in a 72-year-old man. Clinical photograph shows moderate swelling of the submandibular glands on both sides of the neck (arrows).

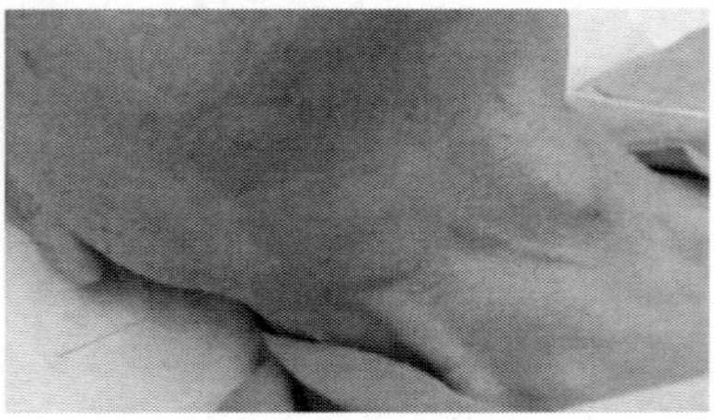

Figure 17. IgG4-related disease in a 66-year-old man. Clinical photograph shows the submandibular gland enlargement on the right side of the neck (arrow).

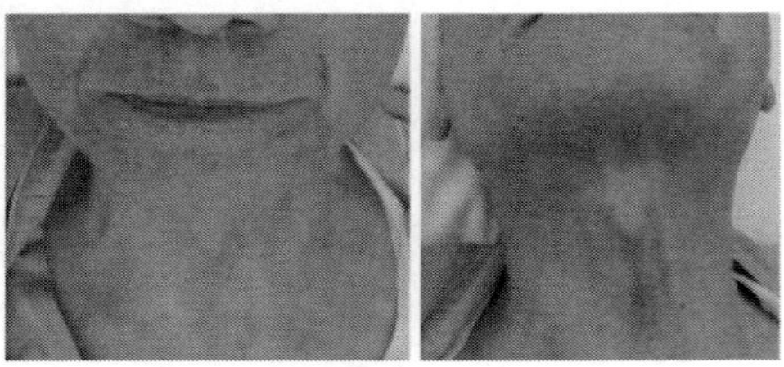

Figure 18. Clinical photographs of IgG4-related disease in a 66-year-old man (same patient as in previous figures). Enlarged submandibular glands were improved after glucocorticoid treatment.

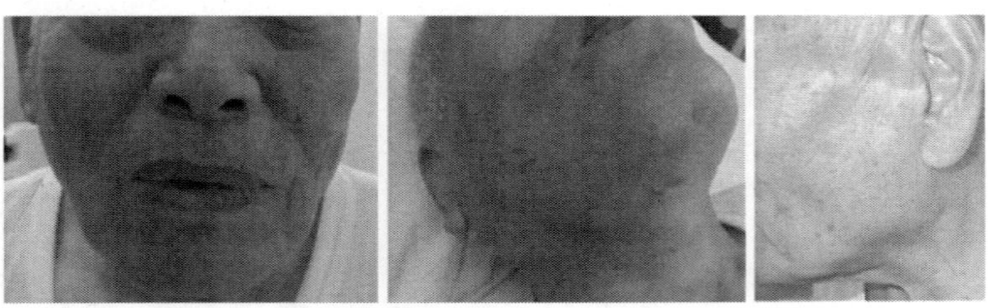

Figure 19. IgG4-related disease in a 72-year-old man. Clinical photographs show the parotid gland enlargement (arrows).

Histopathologic Features

Severe Fibrosis

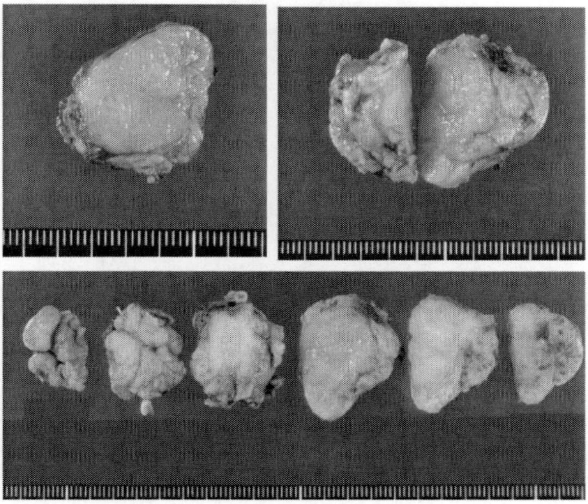

Figure 20. IgG4-related sialadenitis in a 49-year-old woman. Gloss pathology of resected submandibular gland saliva, with severe acinar atrophy and loss.

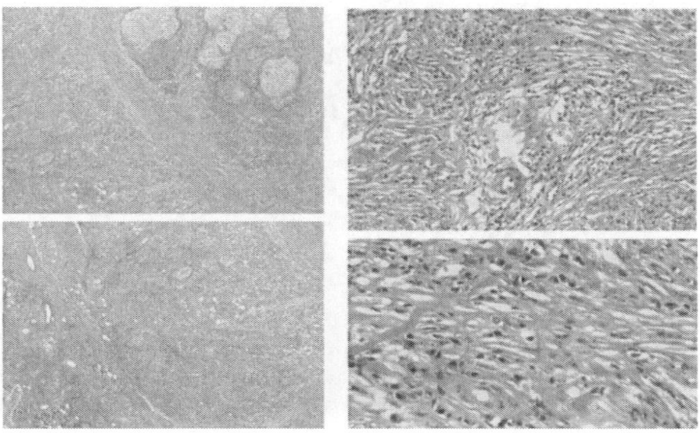

Figure 21. IgG4-related sialadenitis in a 49-year-old woman. Specimens from the submandibular gland are stained with hematoxylin and eosin. Histopathology shows severe atrophy and loss of acini, inflammatory cell infiltration of lymphocytes and plasma cells, fibrosis and sclerosis of the stroma. Lymph follicle formation is also prominent. The findings are consistent with the histology of chronic sclerosing sialadenitis.

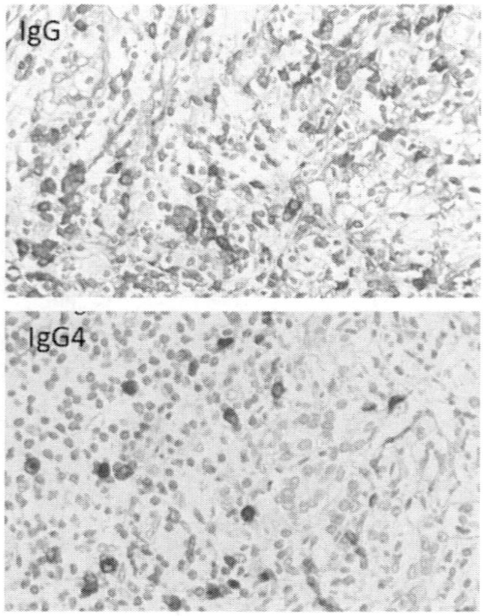

Figure 22. IgG4-related sialadenitis in a 49-year-old woman. Immunostaining of pathological specimens from the submandibular gland with IgG and IgG4. IgG4 is positive on most IgG-positive plasma cells. The tissue IgG4 (+) / IgG (+) cell ratio is over 50%.

Moderate Fibrosis

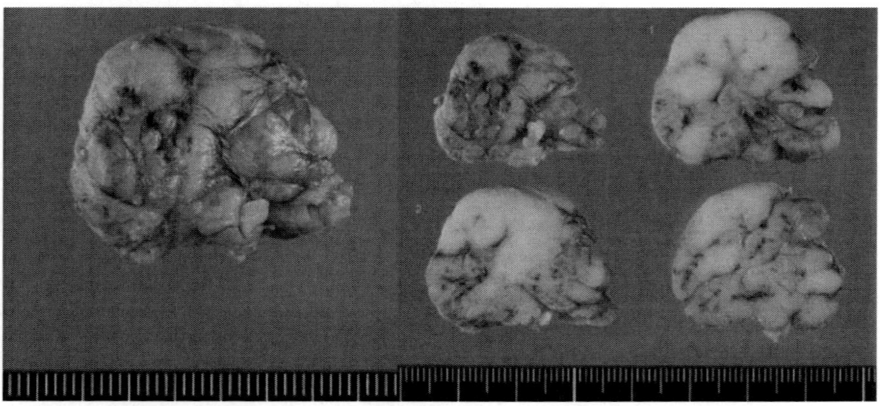

Figure 23. IgG4-related sialadenitis in a 43-year-old woman. Gloss pathology of resected submandibular gland saliva, with moderate acinar atrophy and loss.

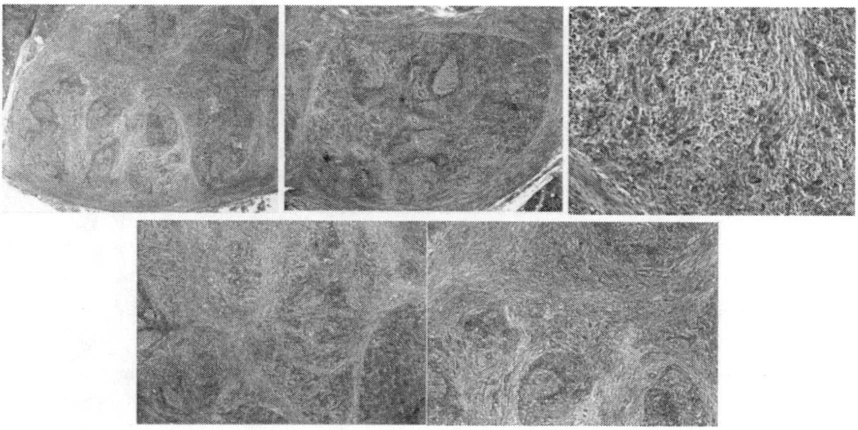

Figure 24. IgG4-related sialadenitis in a 43-year-old woman. Specimens from the submandibular gland are stained with hematoxylin and eosin. Histopathology shows atrophy and loss of acini, high levels of inflammatory cell infiltration of lymphocytes and plasma cells around the ducts in the lobules, fibrosis and sclerosis of the stroma. Lymph follicle formation with irregular germinal center enlargement is also prominent. These findings are consistent with the histology of chronic sclerosing sialadenitis.

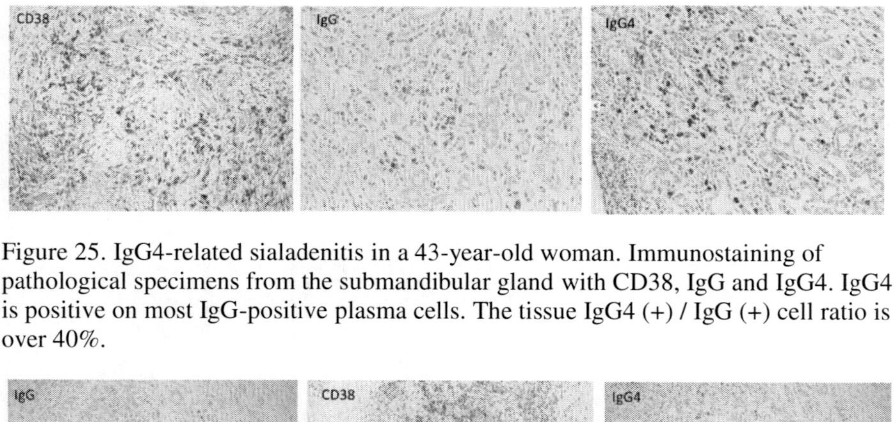

Figure 25. IgG4-related sialadenitis in a 43-year-old woman. Immunostaining of pathological specimens from the submandibular gland with CD38, IgG and IgG4. IgG4 is positive on most IgG-positive plasma cells. The tissue IgG4 (+) / IgG (+) cell ratio is over 40%.

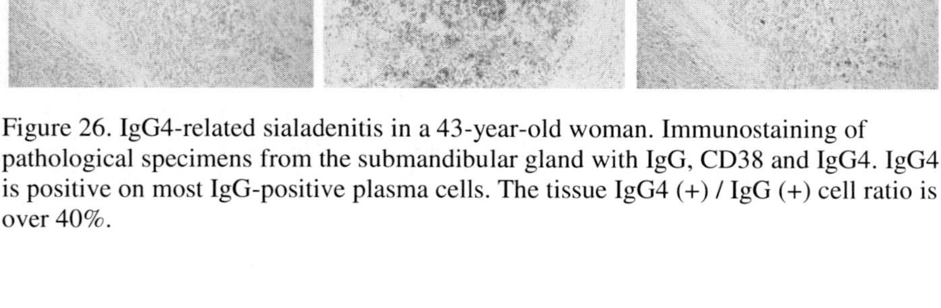

Figure 26. IgG4-related sialadenitis in a 43-year-old woman. Immunostaining of pathological specimens from the submandibular gland with IgG, CD38 and IgG4. IgG4 is positive on most IgG-positive plasma cells. The tissue IgG4 (+) / IgG (+) cell ratio is over 40%.

Mild Fibrosis

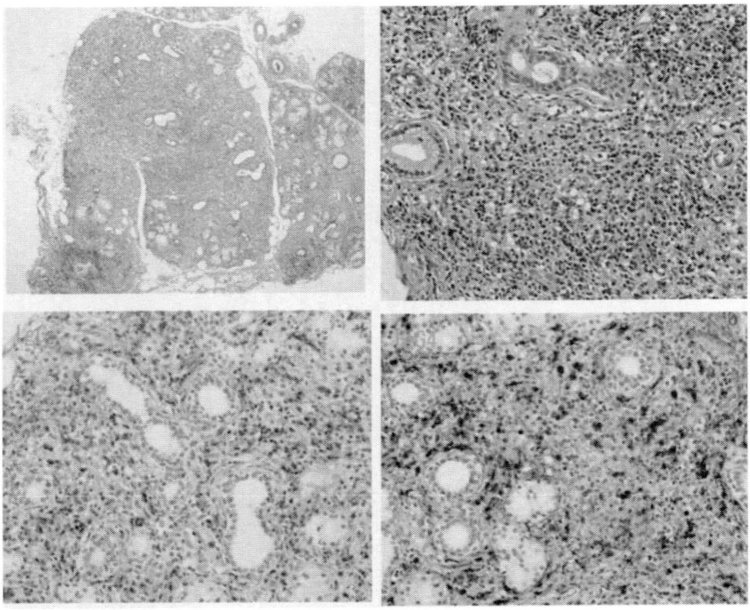

Figure 27. IgG4-related sialadenitis in a 64-year-old man. Specimens from the submandibular gland are stained with hematoxylin and eosin (the upper panels). Infiltration of plasma cells into the submandibular gland is observed. In the immunohistochemical staining (the lower panels), most of the IgG positive cells are IgG4 positive. The tissue IgG4 (+) / IgG (+) cell ratio is over 40%.

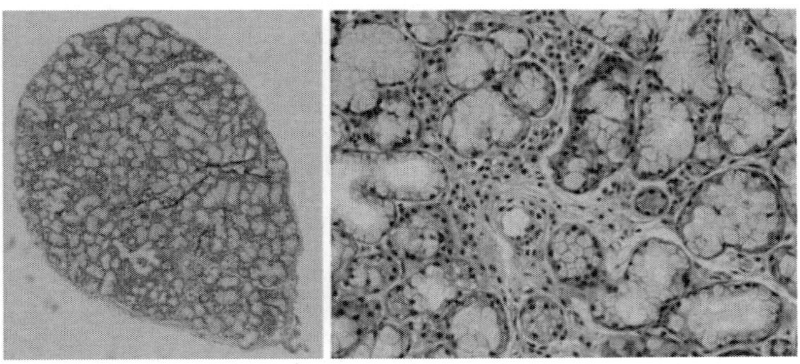

Figure 28. IgG4-related disease in a 68-year-old man. Histological images of the minor salivary gland of the lip show infiltration of lymphocytes and plasma cells by hematoxylin and eosin staining.

IgG4-Related Ophthalmic Disease, Lacrimal Gland Involvement

IgG4-related ophthalmic disease is a name proposed to integrate ocular adnexa lesions and IgG4-related lacrimal gland lesions (Sogabe Y 2014). Patients with IgG4-related ophthalmic disease, mainly in the lacrimal glands, have been reported (Sato Y 2008) (Cheuk W. 2007).

However, IgG4-related orbital disease can cause proptosis due to enlargement of the lacrimal glands, extraocular muscle enlargement, trigeminal nerve branch enlargement, diffuse orbital fat lesions, orbital mass lesions or pseudotumors, eyelid lesions, and nasolacrimal duct lesions, (Kawa S 2019).

Anatomy

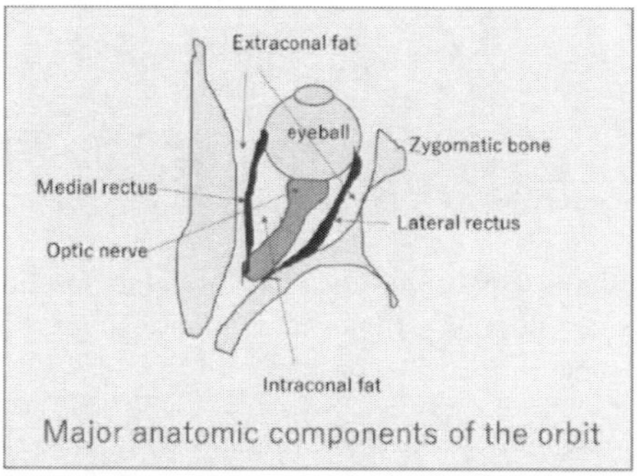

Figure 29. Major anatomic components of the orbit.

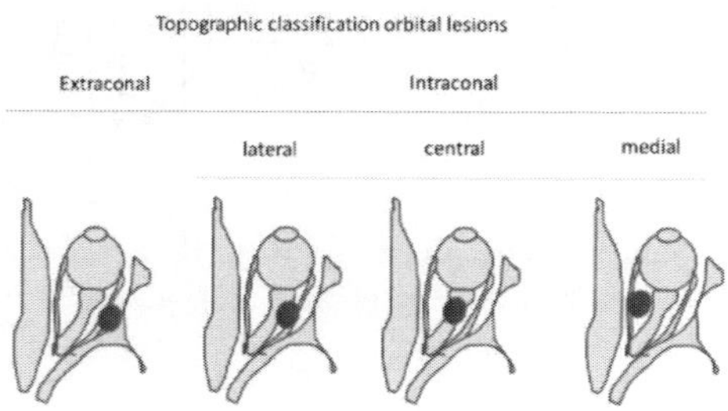

Figure 30. Topographic classification orbital lesions.

Dacryoadenitis

Patients with IgG4-related ophthalmic disease mainly has lacrimal gland lesions. Patients with IgG4-related dacryoadenitis exhibit enlargement of the lacrimal glands.

The lesions of lacrimal glands are usually bilateral, often with a concomitant of enlargement of salivary glands (Mikulicz's disease).

Some studies have reported that IgG4-related chronic sclerosing dacryoadenitis may predispose to lymphoma (Cheuk W.. 2008).

Imaging of IgG4-Relatedothalmic Disease with Dacryoadenitis

Clinical Photography

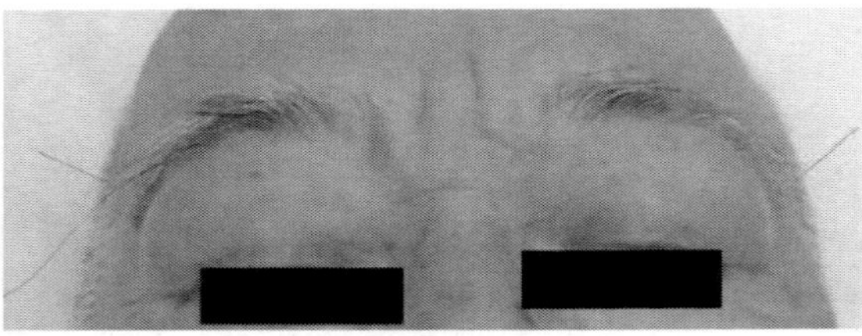

Figure 31. External ophthalmic photographs of IgG4-related ophthalmic disease with dacryoadenitis in a 66-year-old man. Bilateral eyelid swelling and palpable masses on the orbital rim were present.

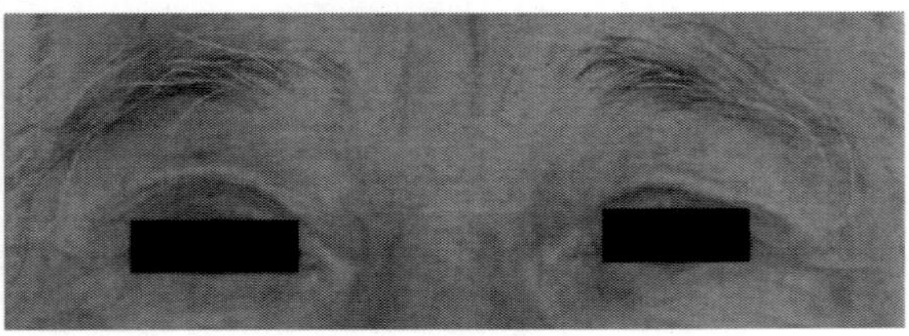

Figure 32. Photograph of IgG4-related ophthalmic disease with dacryoadenitis in a 66-year-old man (same patient as in previous figure). Bilateral eyelid swelling and palpable masses on the orbital rim were improved after glucocorticoid treatment.

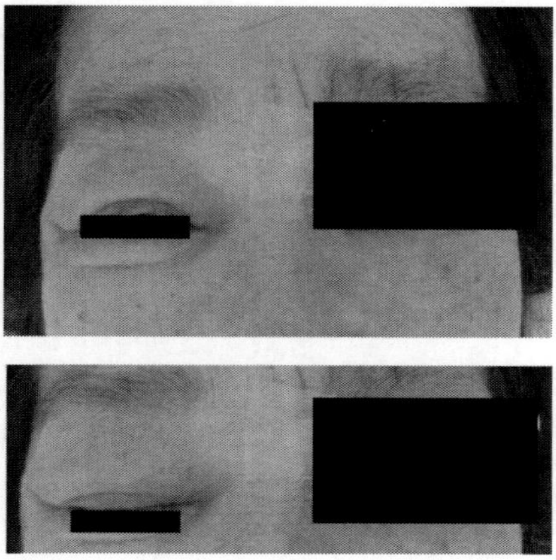

Figure 33. External ophthalmic photographs of IgG4-related ophthalmic disease with dacryoadenitis in a 73-year-old woman. Eyelid swelling and palpable masses on the orbital rim were present. Excisional biopsy of the left lacrimal gland was performed.

CT

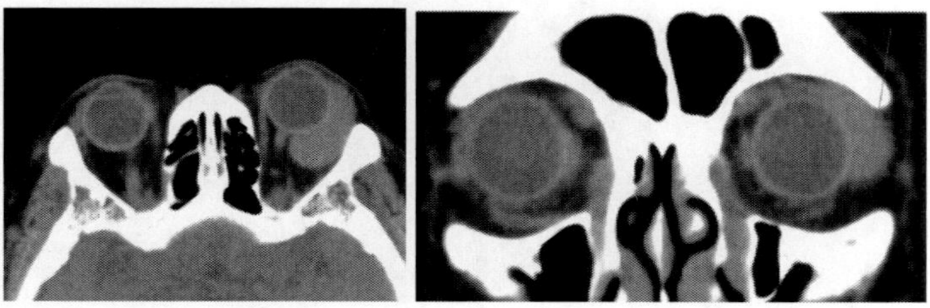

Figure 34. IgG4-related dacryoadenitis in an 80-year-old woman. Axial and coronal non-contrast enhanced CT (NCECT) images show enlargement of the left lacrimal gland.

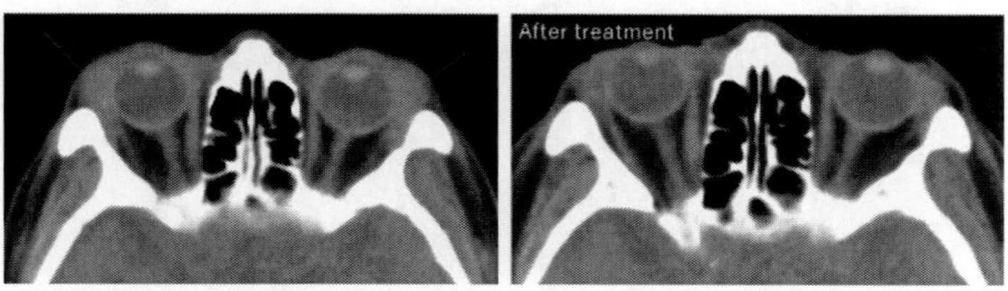

Figure 35. IgG4-related dacryoadenitis in a 76-year-old man. Axial non-contrast enhanced CT (NCECT) image (left panel) of the orbits shows symmetrical thickening of bilateral lacrimal glands before treatment. Follow-up axial CT image (right panel) obtained 6 months later after corticosteroid therapy shows resolution of the lesions.

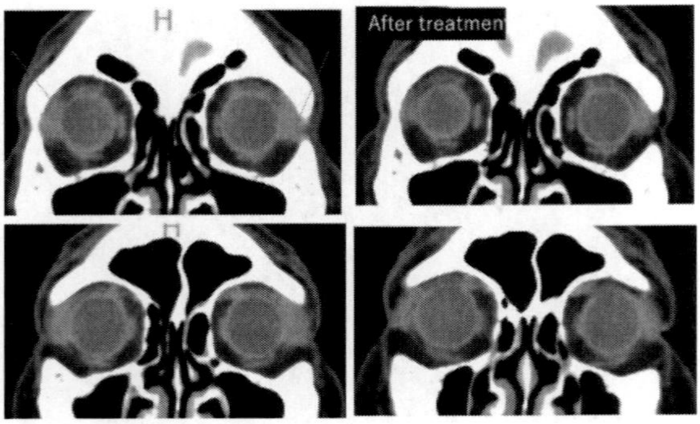

Figure 36. IgG4-related dacryoadenitis in a 76-year-old man. Coronal non-contrast enhanced CT (NCECT) images show enlarged bilateral lacrimal glands (arrows) before treatment. The enlargement of the lacrimal glands has been reduced by corticosteroid treatment on follow up coronal CT images.

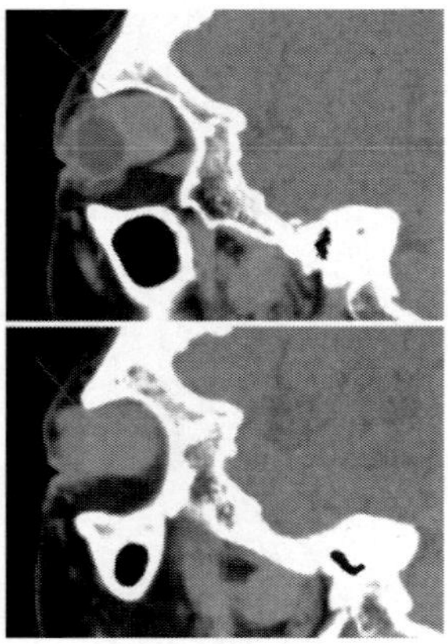

Figure 37. IgG4-related dacryoadenitis in an 80-year-old woman. Sagittal non-contrast enhanced CT (NCECT) images show enlargement of the left lacrimal gland.

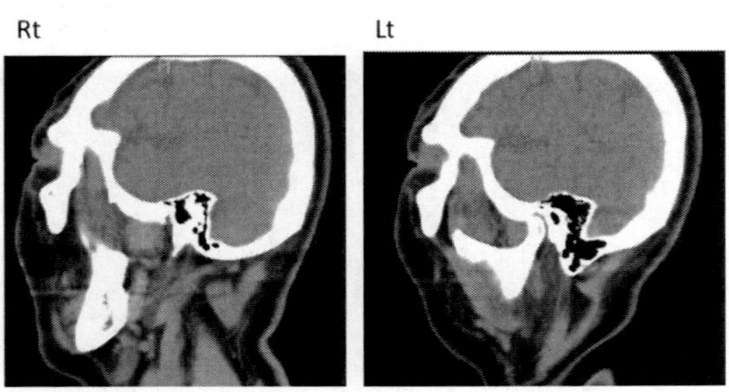

Figure 38. IgG4-related dacryoadenitis in a 76-year-old man. The sagittal non-contrast enhanced CT (NCECT) images show enlargement of bilateral lacrimal glands.

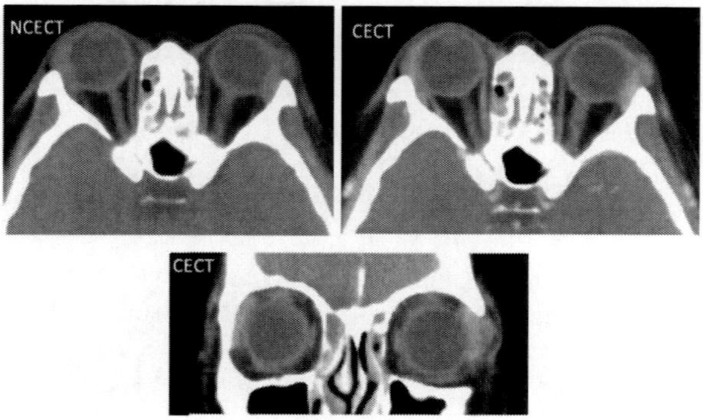

Figure 39. IgG4-related dacryoadenitis in a 43-year-old woman. Axial non-contrast enhanced CT (NCECT) image (left upper panel) of the orbits shows thickening of the left lacrimal gland and mild swelling of the right lacrimal gland. Axial and coronal contrast enhanced CT (CECT) images show homogenous enhancement of the lacrimal glands.

Orbital Pseudotumors

Idiopathic orbital inflammation, also called orbital pseudotumors, has been reported to be associated with IgG4-related disease (Wallace ZS. 2012).

IgG4-related orbital lesions can be unilateral or bilateral and may involve the entire orbit or certain components such as the extraocular muscles, lacrimal system, or optic nerves.

Imaging of Orbital Lesions

Clinical Photography

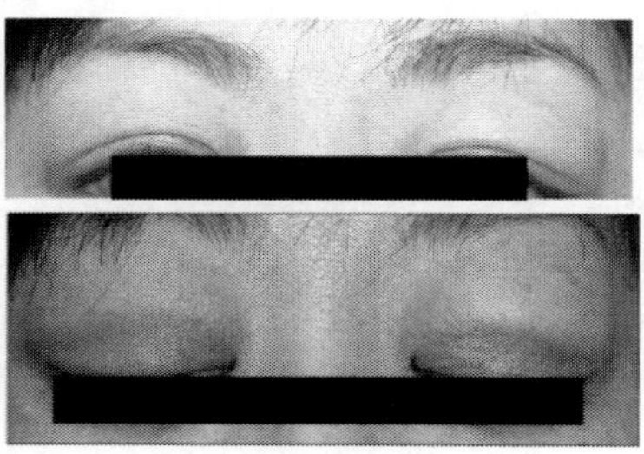

Figure 40. External ophthalmic photographs of IgG4-related ophthalmic disease with pseudotumor in a 43-year-old woman. Left eyelid swelling and palpable mass on the orbital rim were observed.

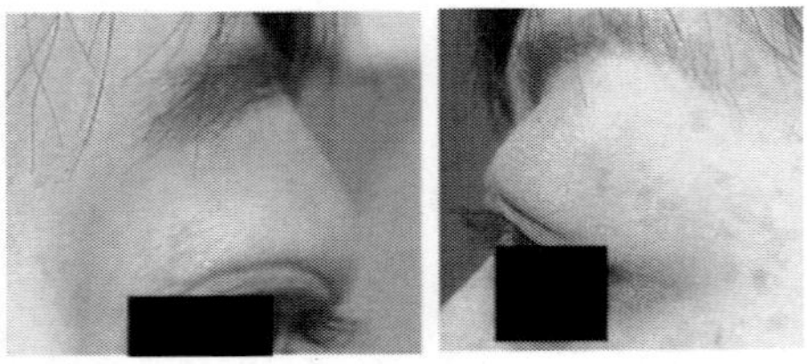

Figure 41. External ophthalmic photographs (eye side view) of IgG4-related ophthalmic disease with pseudotumor in a 43-year-old woman. Swelling of the eyelids was observed.

MRI

T1-Weighted MRI

Axial Images

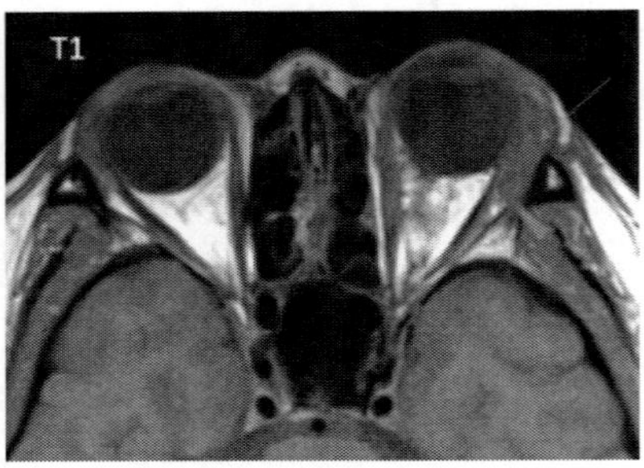

Figure 42. IgG4-related disease in a 43-year-old woman. Axial T1-weighted MR image shows swelling with relatively low signal intensity of the left eyelid (arrow) and left extraocular muscle (arrowhead) as an extraconal lesion.

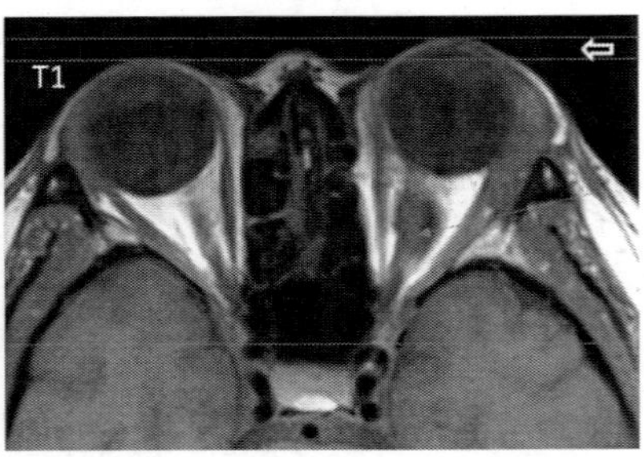

Figure 43. IgG4-related orbital pseudotumor in a 43-year-old woman. Axial T1-weighted magnetic resonance (MR) image shows a T1 hypointense interconal mass (arrow) in the left retrobulbar area and producing proptosis (open arrow).

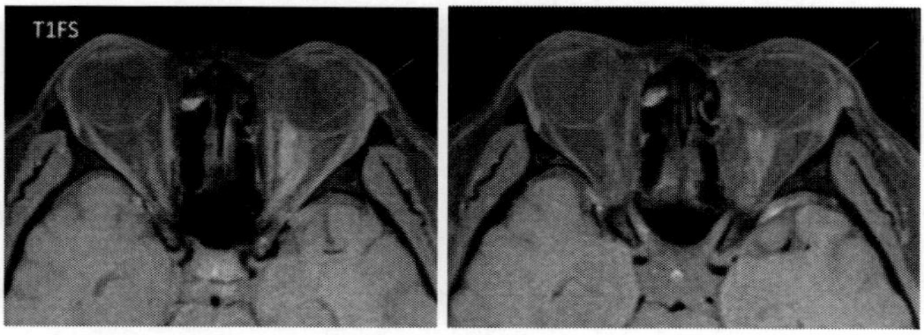

Figure 44. IgG4-related orbital pseudotumor in a 36-year-old woman. Axial T1-weighted fat-saturated (FS) MR images show an intraconal perineural spread lesion (arrows) near the left optic nerve.

Coronal Images

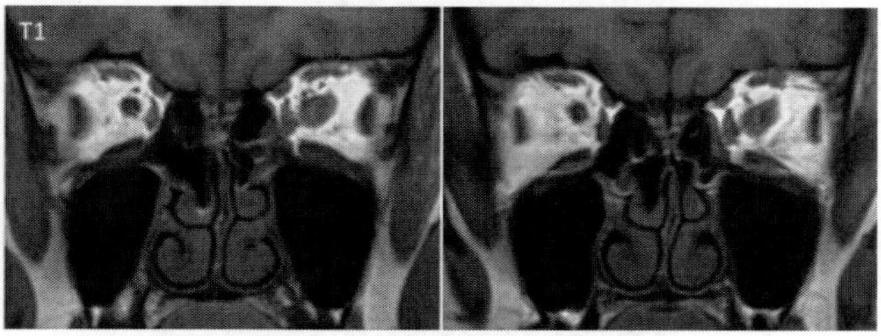

Figure 45. IgG4-related orbital pseudotumor in a 36-year-old woman. Coronal T1-weighted MR images show an intraconal perineural spread lesion (arrows) surrounding the left optic nerve.

Contrast Enhanced T1-Weighted MRI

Axial Images

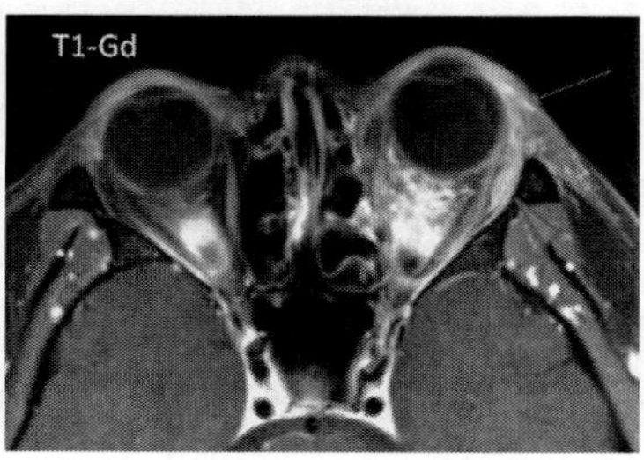

Figure 46. IgG4-related disease in a 43-year-old woman. Axial gadolinium-enhanced T1-weighted MR image of the orbits shows inflammatory process of the left eyelid (arrow) and left extraocular muscle (arrowhead).

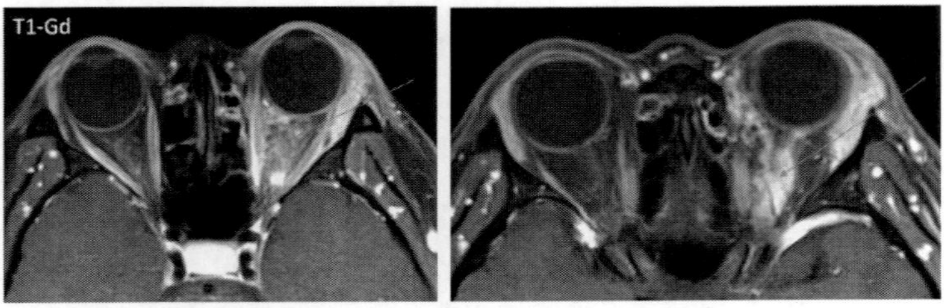

Figure 47. IgG4-related orbital disease in a 43-year-old woman. Axial gadolinium-enhanced T1-weighted MR image of the orbits shows a homogenous enhancement pattern in the left retrobulbar area (arrows).

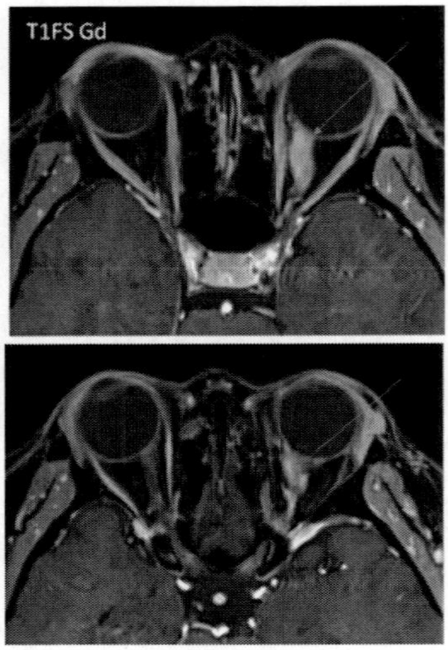

Figure 48. IgG4-related orbital pseudotumor in a 36-year-old woman.
Axial gadolinium-enhanced T1-weighted fat-saturated (FS) MR images show an intraconal perineural spread lesion (arrows) near the left optic nerve.

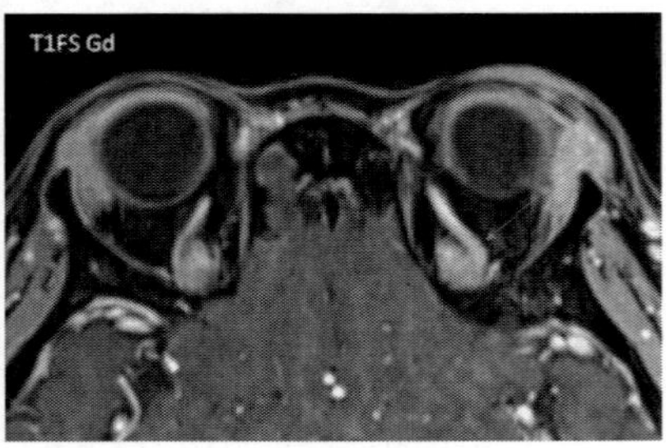

Figure 49. IgG4-related orbital disease in a 37-year-old woman. Axial gadolinium-enhanced T1-weighted fat-saturated (FS) MR image shows the dilatation of the posterior side of the left superior ophthalmic vein (arrow).

Coronal Images

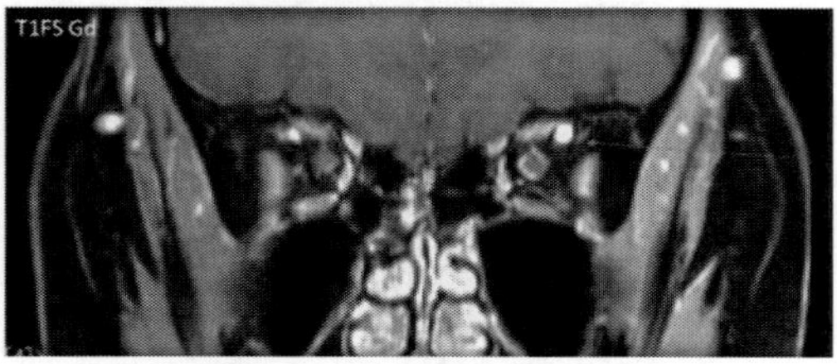

Figure 50. IgG4-related orbital disease in a 37-year-old woman. Coronal T2-weighted fat saturated (FS) MR image of the orbits shows the dilatation of the posterior side of the left superior ophthalmic vein as a hyperintense lesion (arrow).

T2-Weighted MRI

Axial Images

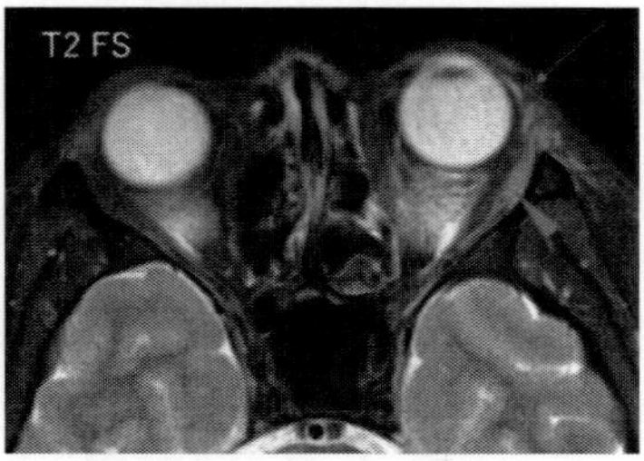

Figure 51. IgG4-related disease in a 43-year-old woman. Axial T2-weighted fat-saturated (FS) MR image of the orbits demonstrates swelling of the left eyelid (arrow) and left extraocular muscle (arrowhead) as an extraconal lesion.

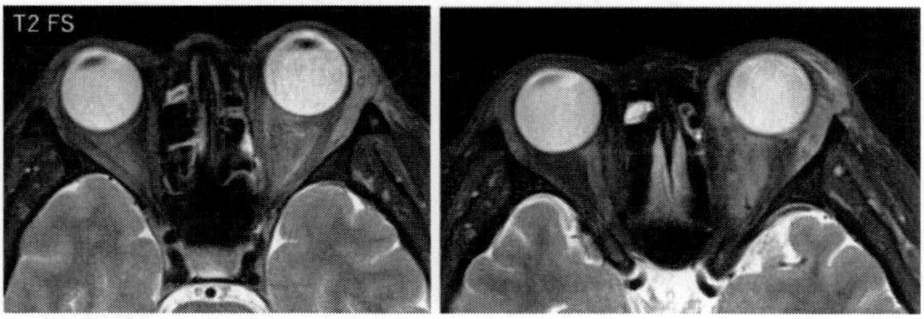

Figure 52. IgG4-related orbital disease in a 43-year-old woman. Axial T2-weighted fat saturated (FS) MR images of the orbits demonstrate a slightly hyperintense lesion in the left retrobulbar area (arrows) than the extraocular muscles or the optic nerve.

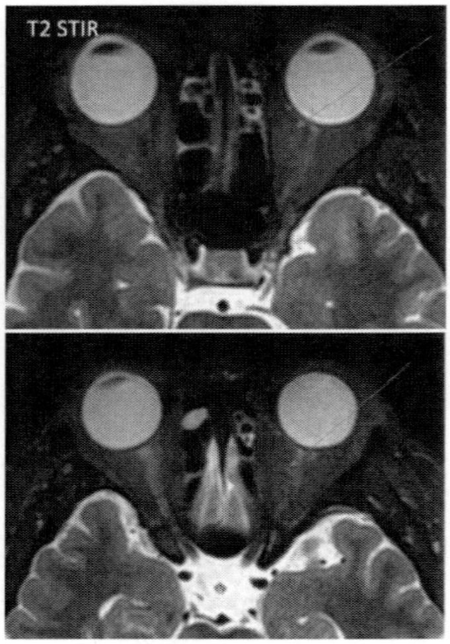

Figure 53. IgG4-related orbital pseudotumor in a 36-year-old woman. Axial T2-weighted short tau inversion recovery (T2-STIR) MR images show an intraconal perineural spread lesion (arrows) near the left optic nerve.

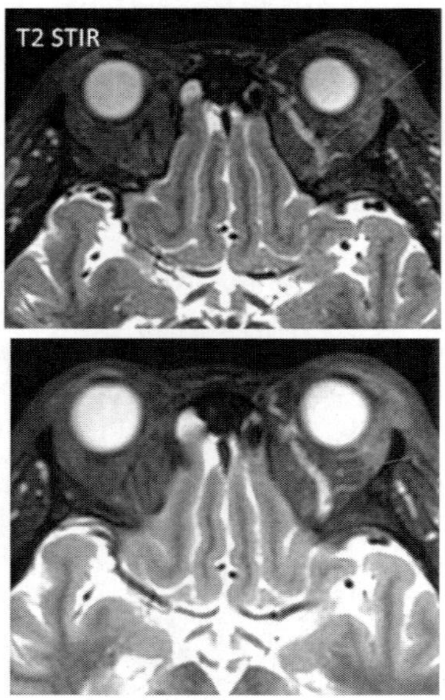

Figure 54. IgG4-related orbital disease in a 37-year-old woman. Axial T2-STIR MR images show the dilatation of the posterior side of the left superior ophthalmic vein as a hyperintense lesion (arrows). The dilatation is less noticeable on the front side of the vein. It may reflect venostasis due to the occupation effect of the IgG4-related orbital lesion.

Coronal Images

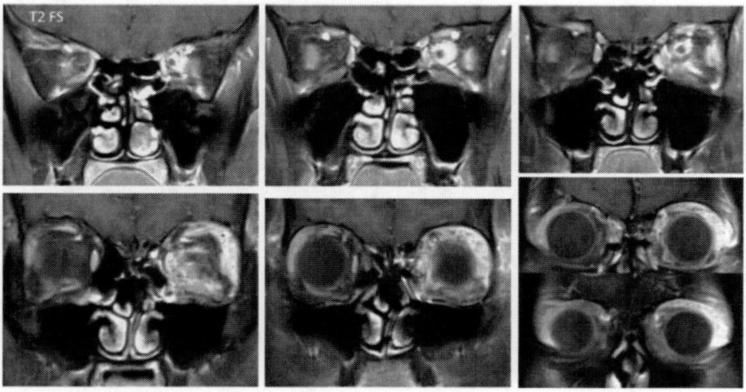

Figure 55. IgG4-related orbital pseudotumor in a 35-year-old woman. Coronal T2-weighted fat saturated (FS) MR images of the orbits demonstrates a slightly hyperintense lesions in the left retrobulbar area, eyelid, and extraocular muscle.

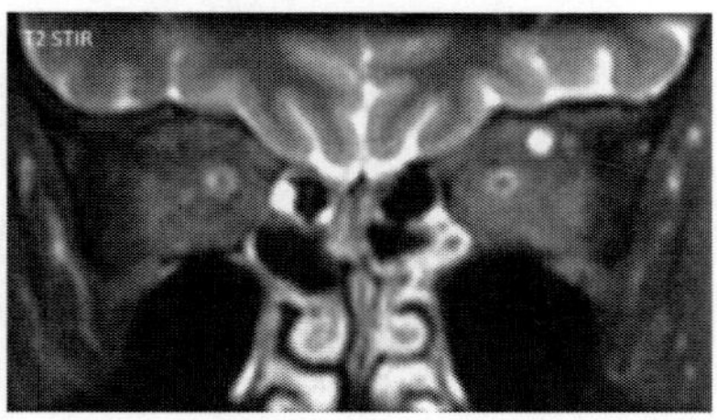

Figure 56. IgG4-related orbital disease in a 37-year-old woman. Coronal T2-weighted fat saturated (FS) MR image of the orbits shows the dilatation of the posterior side of the left superior ophthalmic vein as a hyperintense lesion (arrow).

Sagittal Images

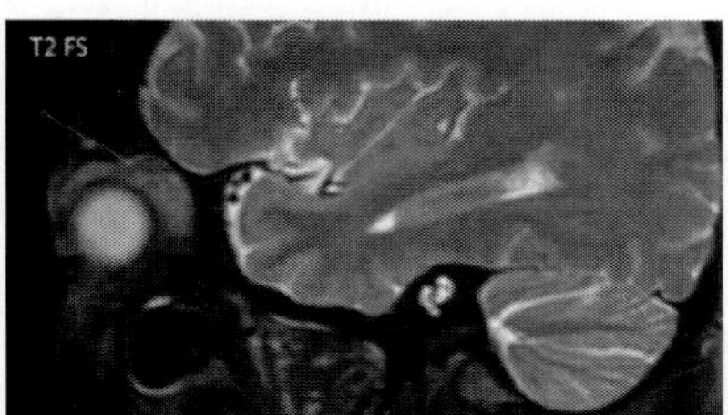

Figure 57. IgG4-related orbital pseudotumor in a 43-year-old woman. Sagittal T2-weighted fat-saturated (FS) MR image of the orbit demonstrates swelling of the left eyelid and left extraocular muscle (arrow).

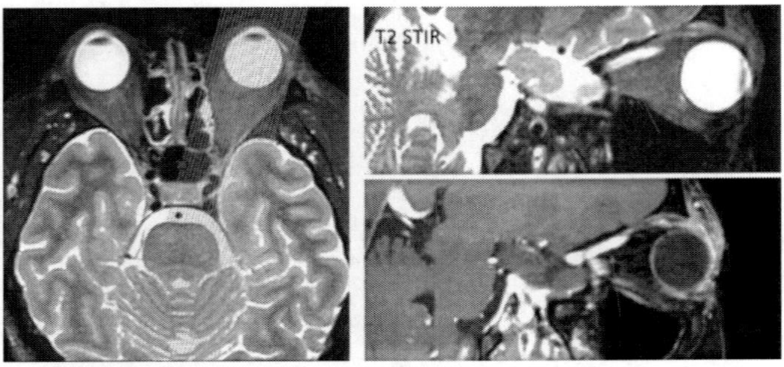

Figure 58. IgG4-related orbital disease in a 37-year-old woman. Sagittal T2-STIR MR images show the dilatation of the posterior side of the left superior ophthalmic vein as a hyperintense lesion (arrows). The dilatation is less noticeable on the front side of the vein. It may reflect venostasis due to the occupation effect of the IgG4-related orbital lesion.

Paranasal Sinusitis; IgG4-Related Chronic Rhinosinusitis

IgG4-related disease involves chronic rhinosinusitis (CRS) with nasal symptoms. The rhinosinusitis is a new clinical entity of nasal disease associated with elevated serum IgG4 levels (Moteki H 2011). Glucocorticoids are effective for IgG4-related chronic rhinosinusitis. The paranasal sinuses consist of four sets of air-filled spaces. The paranasal sinuses have several functions, reducing the weight of the head, air humidification and aiding in voice resonance. Sinuses are named after the facial bones where they are located, maxillary sinus, sphenoid sinus, ethmoid sinus and frontal sinus.

CT

CT is the most common method of evaluating sinusitis. CT allows for better anatomical delineation and assessment of extension, causes, and complications of inflammation.

The main findings of sinusitis are thickening of the peripheral mucosa, gas and fluid levels in the sinuses, gas bubbles within fluid, and obstruction of the ostiomeatal complexes (OMC).

Rhinitis is often characterized by thickening of the turbinates due to obstruction of the surrounding air channels.

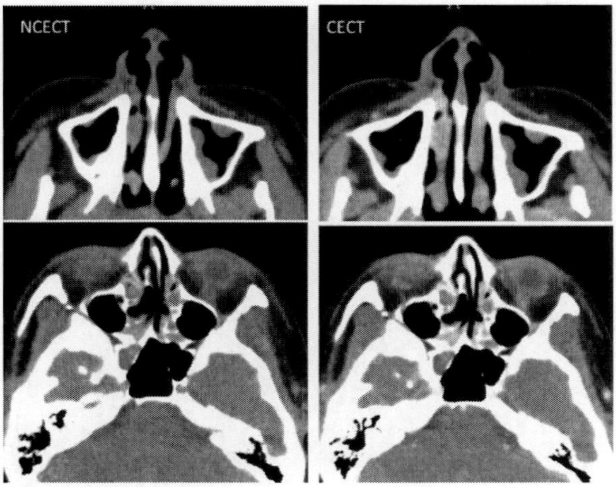

Figure 59. IgG4-related rhinosinusitis in a 43-year-old woman. Axial non-contrast enhanced CT (NCECT) and contrast enhanced CT (CECT) images show bilateral opaque areas located in the maxillary and ethmoid sinuses.

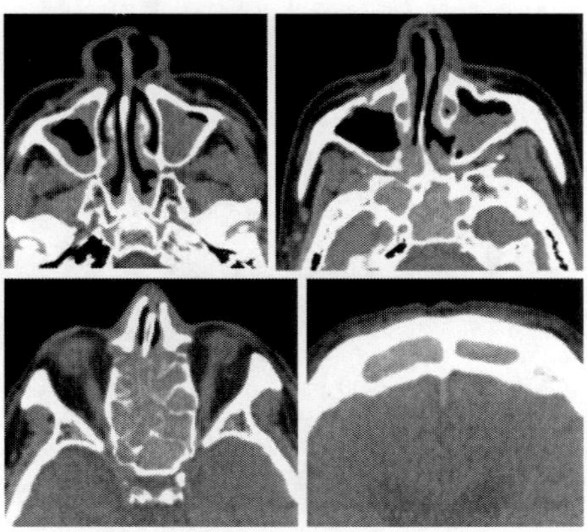

Figure 60. IgG4-related rhinosinusitis in a 67-year-old man. Axial non-contrast enhanced CT (NCECT) images show opaque areas located in every sinus.

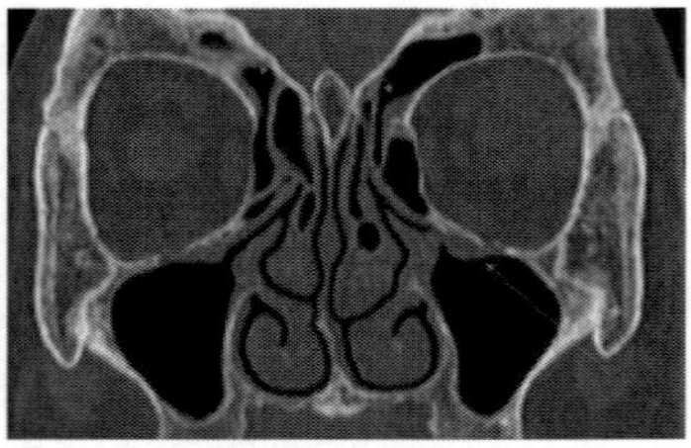

Figure 61. IgG4-related rhinosinusitis in an 80-year-old woman. Coronal non-contrast enhanced CT (NCECT) image shows mild mucosal thickening in the maxillary and ethmoid sinuses.

Maxillary Sinuses

Non-Contrast Enhanced Head CT

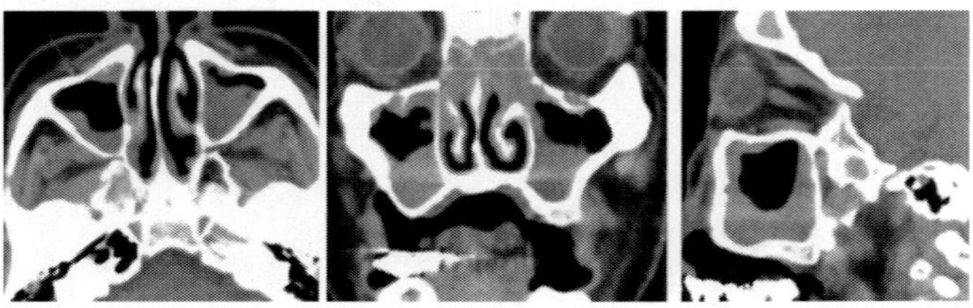

Figure 62. IgG4-related rhinosinusitis in a 66-year-old man. Axial, coronal and sagittal non-contrast enhanced head CT (NCECT) images show bilateral opaque areas located in the maxillary sinuses.

Contrast Enhanced Head CT

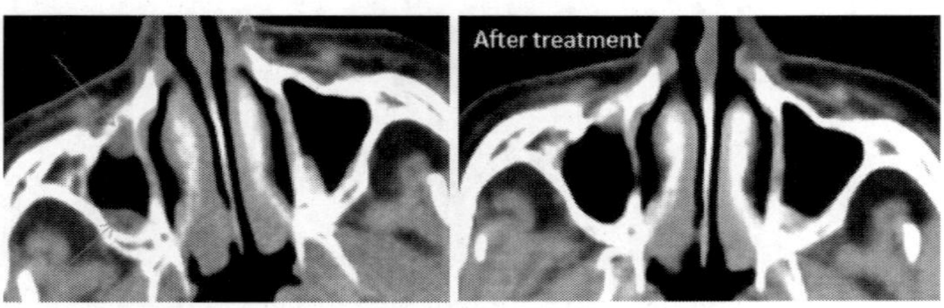

Figure 63. IgG4-related rhinosinusitis in a 72-year-old man. Axial contrast enhanced head CT (CECT) images show opaque areas located in the right maxillary sinus (arrows) and improvement of opacification after corticosteroid therapy.

Ethmoid Sinuses

Non-Contrast Enhanced Head CT

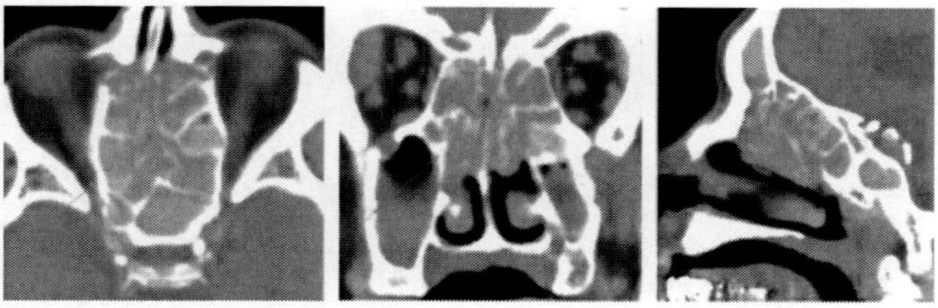

Figure 64. IgG4-related rhinosinusitis in a 66-year-old man. Axial, coronal and sagittal non-contrast enhanced head CT (NCECT) images show bilateral severe opaque areas located in the ethmoid sinuses.

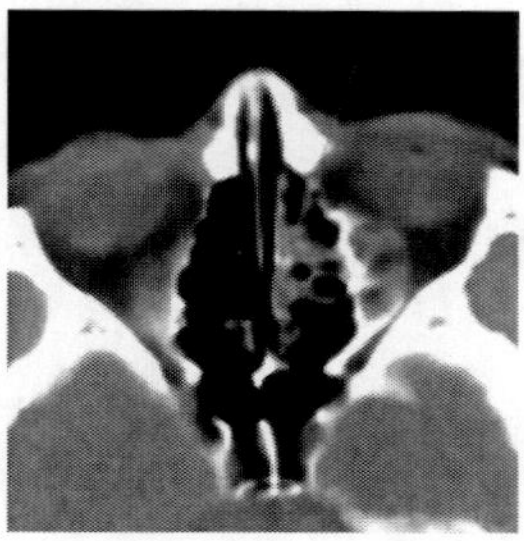

Figure 65. IgG4-related rhinosinusitis in a 49-year-old woman. Axial non-contrast enhanced head CT (NCECT) image shows mild opaque area located in the left ethmoid sinus (arrow).

Contrast Enhanced Head CT

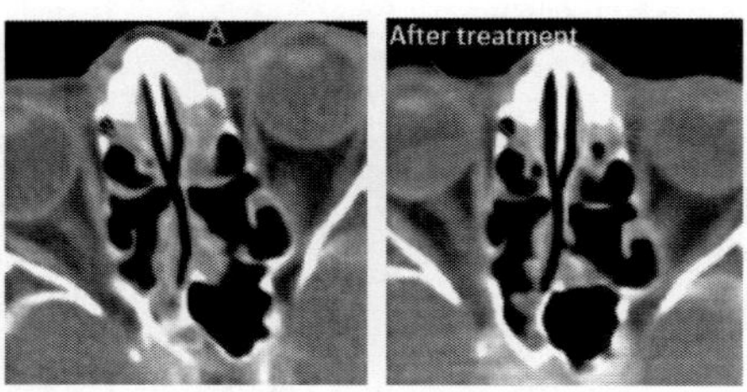

Figure 66. IgG4-related rhinosinusitis in a 72-year-old man. Axial contrast enhanced head CT (CECT) images show opaque areas located in the ethmoid sinuses (arrows) and slight improvement of opacification after corticosteroid therapy.

Sphenoid Sinus

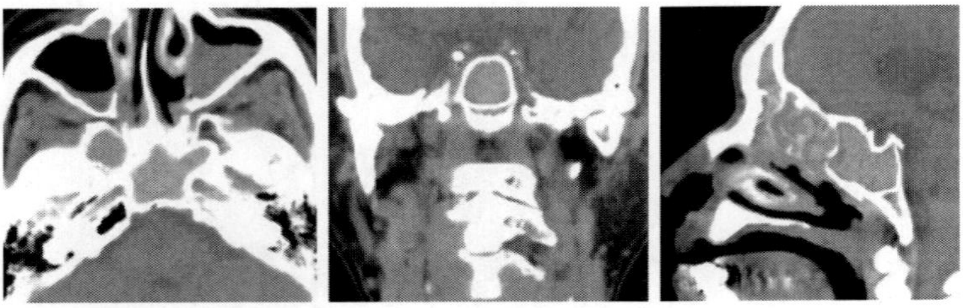

Figure 67. IgG4-related rhinosinusitis in a 66-year-old man. Axial, coronal and sagittal non-contrast enhanced head CT (NCECT) images show bilateral opaque areas located in the sphenoid sinus.

Frontal Sinuses

Non-Contrast Enhanced Head CT

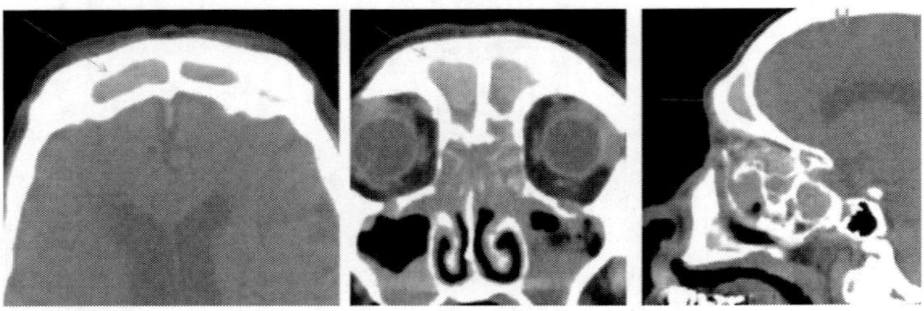

Figure 68. IgG4-related rhinosinusitis in a 66-year-old man. Axial, coronal and sagittal non-contrast enhanced head CT (NCECT) images show bilateral opaque areas located in the frontal sinuses.

Contrast Enhanced Head CT

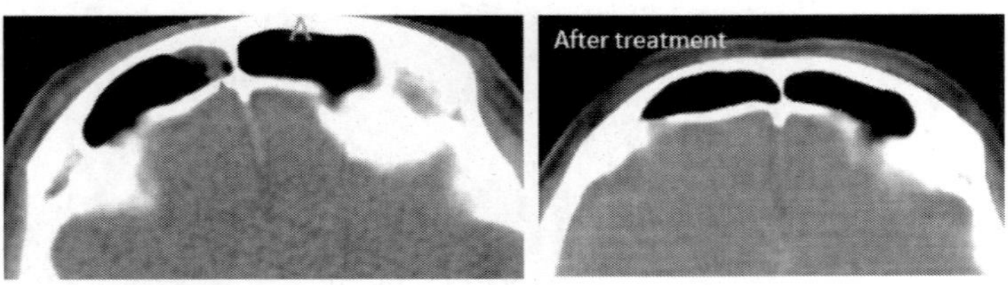

Figure 69. IgG4-related rhinosinusitis in a 72-year-old man. Axial contrast enhanced head CT (NCECT) images show mild opaque area located in the right frontal sinus.

MRI

CT has played a central role in diagnostic imaging of sinusitis. Among the modalities of diagnostic imaging, MRI has higher resolution and is increasingly being used to evaluate sinusitis. However, the indication of MRI is not yet clear in IgG4-related rhinosinusitis.

Signal characteristics of the lesions affected by sinusitis, in T1-weighted MR images, are mucosal thickening with isointense to soft tissue and are the fluid with hypointense. In T2-weighted MR images, both mucosal thickening and the fluid are of varying degrees but hyperintense. On the other hand, in gadolinium-enhanced MR imaging, signals of the inflamed mucous membranes increase in intensity, but those of the fluid remain unchanged.

T1-Weighted MRI

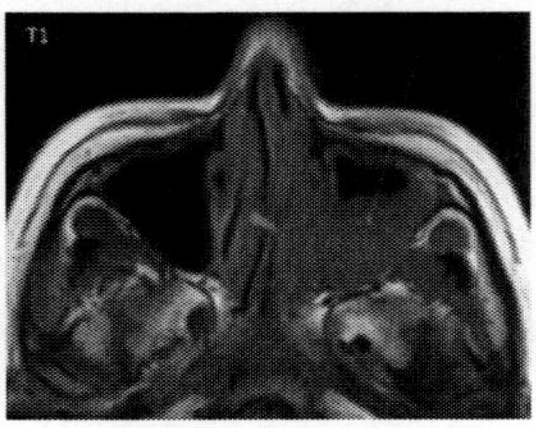

Figure 70. IgG4-related rhinosinusitis in a 41-year-old woman. The lesion of the maxillary sinus was asymmetrical. T1-weighted MR image demonstrates mucosal thickening (arrowhead) with isointensity to soft tissue, and the fluid with hypointensity (arrow).

Gadolinium-Enhanced T1-Weighted MRI

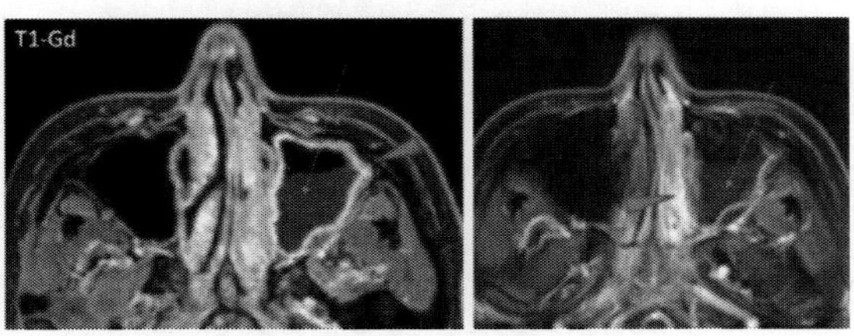

Figure 71. IgG4-related rhinosinusitis in a 41-year-old woman. Axial gadolinium-enhanced T1-weighted MR images demonstrate that signals of the inflamed mucosal membranes (arrowhead) of the left maxillary sinus increase in intensity, but those of the fluid (arrow) remains unchanged.

T2-Weighted MRI

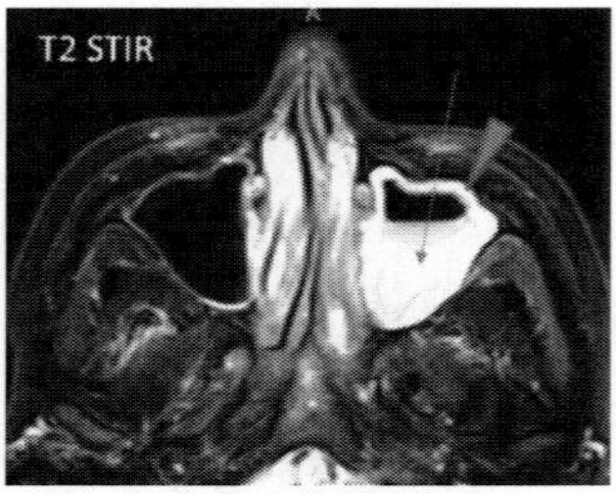

Figure 72. IgG4-related rhinosinusitis in a 41-year-old woman. Axial T2-weighted STIR MR image demonstrates both mucosal thickening (arrowhead) and the fluid (arrow) in the left maxillary sinus.

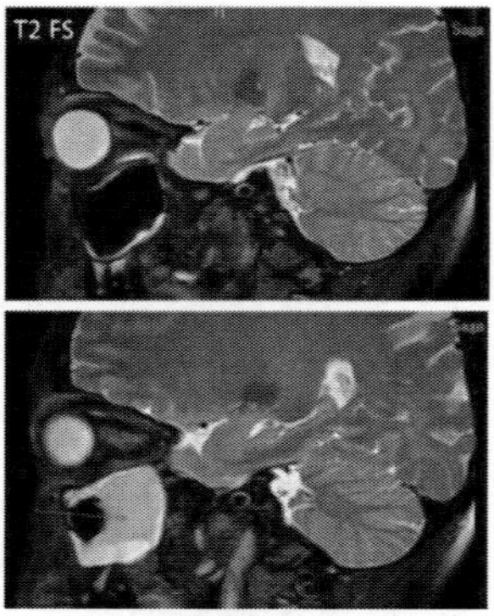

Figure 73. IgG4-related rhinosinusitis in a 41-year-old woman. Sagittal T2-weighted fat-saturated (FS) MR images show both mucosal thickening (arrowhead) and the fluid (arrow) in the left maxillary sinus. The lesion of the maxillary sinus is asymmetric.

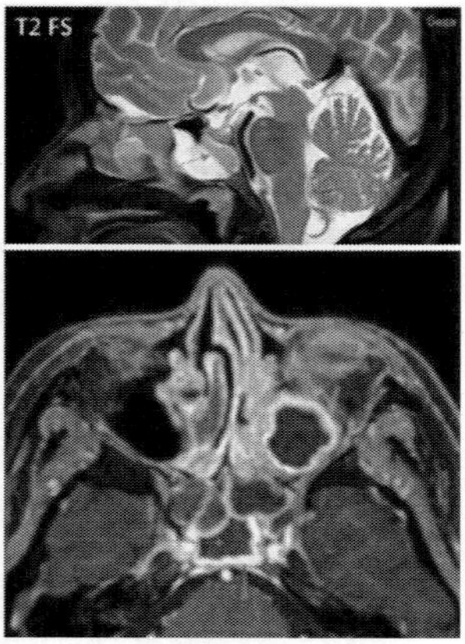

Figure 74. IgG4-related rhinosinusitis in a 41-year-old woman. Sagittal and axial T2-weighted fat saturated (FS) MR images show both mucosal thickening (arrowhead) and the fluid (arrow) in the sphenoid sinus.

IgG4-Related Mastoiditis

Several cases of IgG4-related disease in the mastoid sinuses represent a new anatomic location for the disease (Deshpande V 2016) (Schiffenbauer AI 2012).

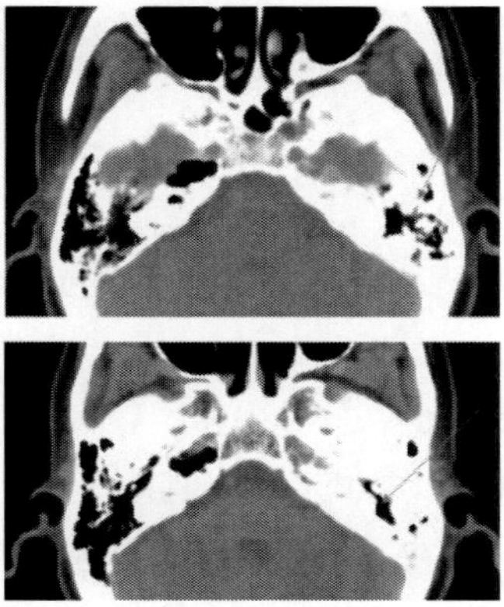

Figure 75. IgG4-related mastoiditis in a 76-year-old man. Axial head CT images show opacification of the left mastoid.

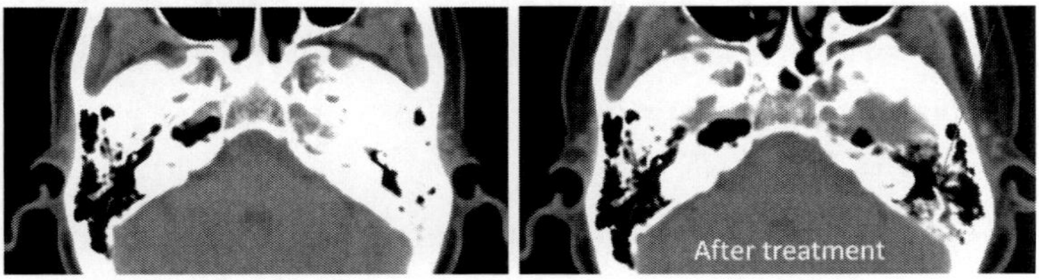

Figure 76. IgG4-related mastoiditis in a 76-year-old man. Axial non-contrast enhanced CT images show improved opacification of the left mastoid after corticosteroid therapy.

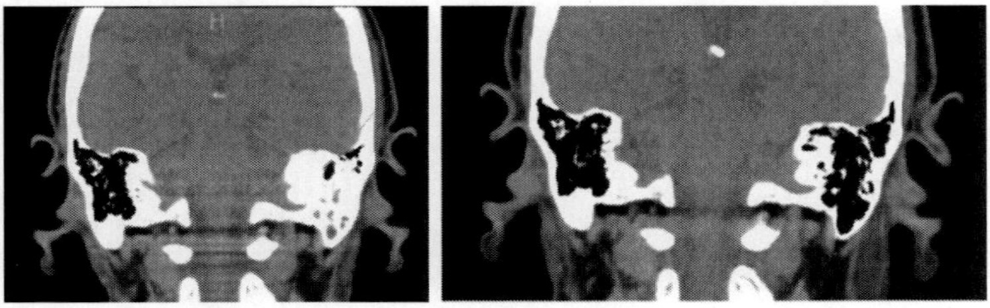

Figure 77. IgG4-related mastoiditis in a 76-year-old man. Coronal non-contrast enhanced CT images show improved opacification of the left mastoid after corticosteroid therapy.

THYROID DISEASE

Classification

In IgG4-related diseases, there are two types of thyroid lesions, Riedel's thyroiditis and the fibrous variant of Hashimoto thyroiditis.

Riedel Thyroiditis

Riedel's thyroiditis is a chronic, inflammatory condition with extensive fibrosis, a rock-hard, painless mass that involves the thyroid parenchyma and surrounding tissues. One third of patients with Riedel's thyroiditis have fibrosclerotic lesions in other organs (JV 2011) (Umehara H 2012).

IgG4-related disease is significantly associated with hypothyroidism, and this coexistence supports the existence of IgG4-associated thyroiditis (Watanabe T 2013). Hashimoto's thyroiditis is basically classified as IgG4-related thyroiditis or non-IgG4-related thyroiditis based on immunostaining profiles (Li Y 2012).

Imaging of Thyroid Lesions

Ultrasound Images

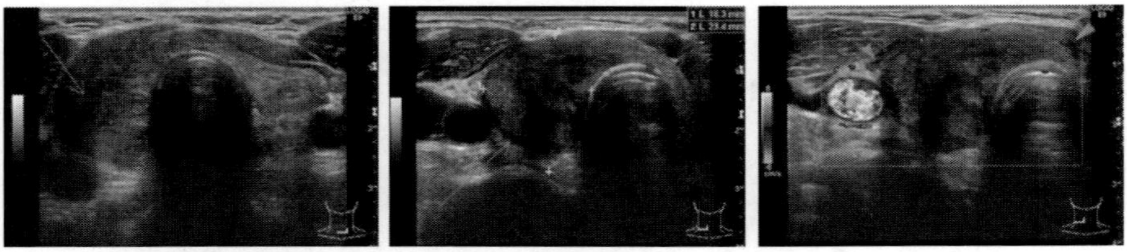

Figure 78. IgG4-related thyroiditis (Riedel thyroiditis) in a 58-year-old woman. Transverse ultrasound images show a large heterogeneous mass in the right lobe of the thyroid (arrows). Blood flow mainly around the periphery of the mass (arrowheads) is observed. There is no obvious calcification inside the mass.

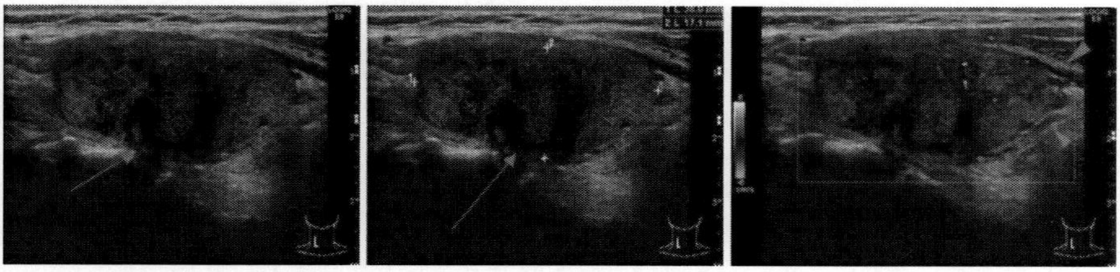

Figure 79. IgG4-related thyroiditis (Riedel thyroiditis) in the same patient as in previous figure. Longitudinal ultrasound images show a large heterogeneous mass in the right lobe of the thyroid (arrows).

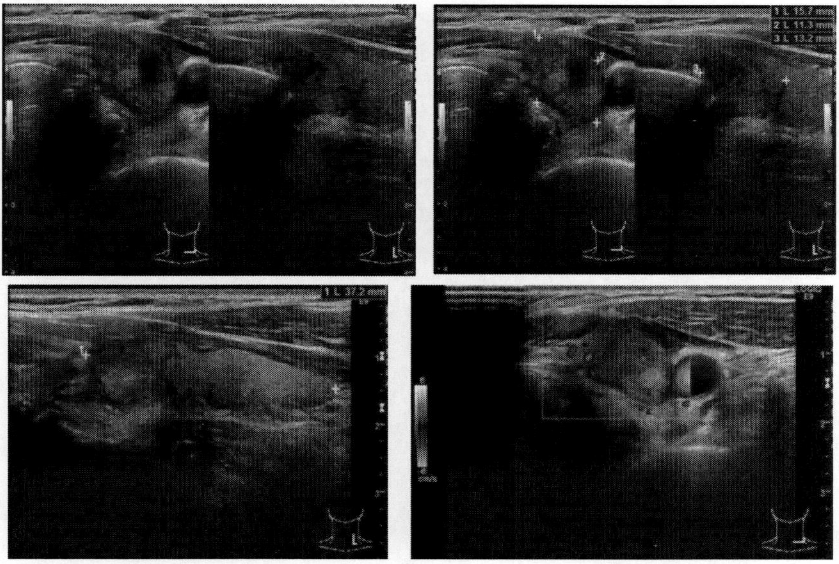

Figure 80. IgG4-related thyroiditis (Riedel thyroiditis) in a 58-year-old woman. Transverse and longitudinal ultrasound images show a heterogeneous mass in the left lobe of the thyroid.

CT

On CT, contrast enhancement is weaker than in normal thyroid tissue, resulting in localized or diffuse low absorption of the thyroid (Fujita A 2012).

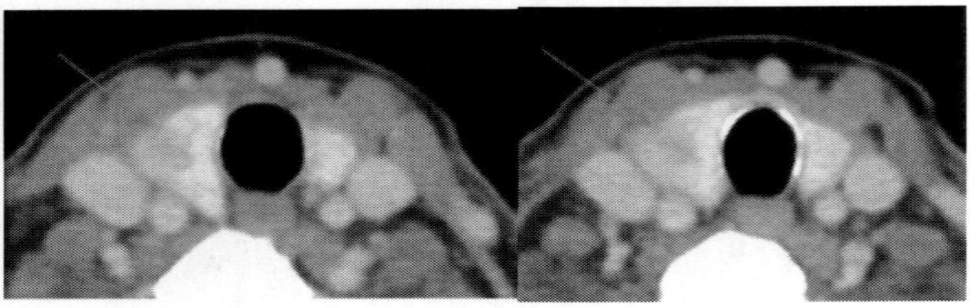

Figure 81. IgG4-related thyroiditis (Riedel thyroiditis) in a 58-year-old woman. Axial contrast-enhanced neck CT images show focal low attenuation area with minimal contrast enhancement relative to normal thyroid tissue.

Cervical Lymphadenopathy

IgG4-related lymphadenopathy often causes enlargement of lymph nodes close to the target organs (Choi YS 2017). When IgG4-related lymphadenopathy occurs to the head and neck lymph nodes, Mikulicz's disease and Riedel's thyroiditis are commonly associated (Kamisawa T. 2006). However, some patients with IgG4-associated lymphadenopathy have no underlying these lesions and can cause lymph node enlargement in the head and neck (Umehara H 2012). Differentiation of cervical lymphadenopathy should include IgG4-related disease.

CT

Non-Contrast Enhanced Neck CT

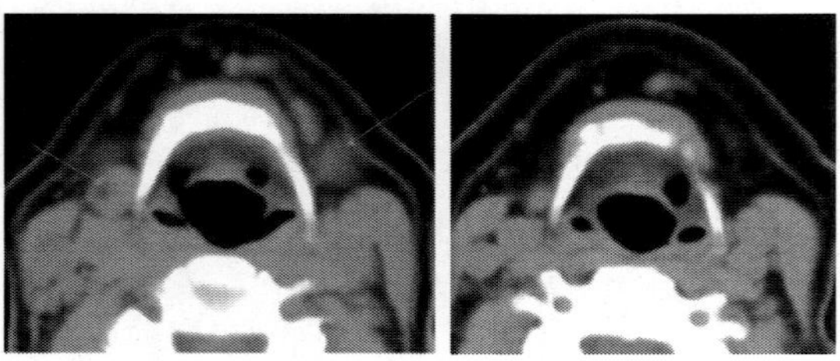

Figure 82. IgG4-related lymphadenopathy in a 76-year-old man. Axial non-contrast enhanced neck CT images show multiple cervical lymph node enlargement (left panel). Post-corticosteroid treatment image (right panel). The size of the cervical lymph nodes decreased after corticosteroid therapy.

Contrast Enhanced Neck CT

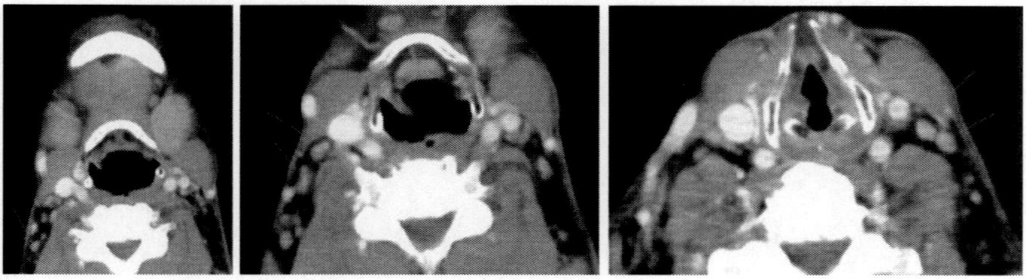

Figure 83. IgG4-related lymphadenopathy in a 67-year-old man. Contrast enhanced neck CT images show several small lymph nodes from both submandibular to the neck. The lymph nodes have a homogenous enhanced contrast effect.

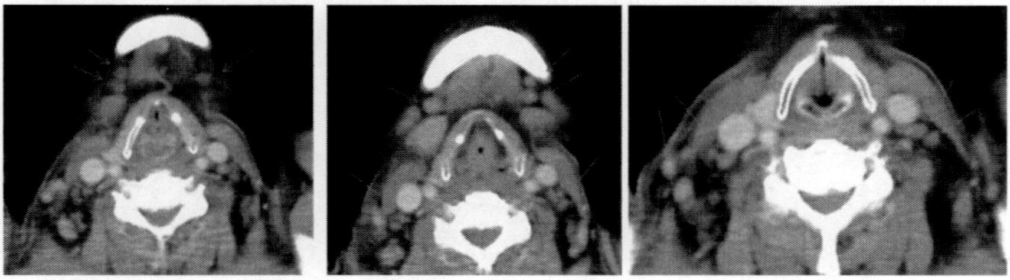

Figure 84. IgG4-related lymphadenopathy in a 73-year-old man. Contrast enhanced neck CT images show many small lymph nodes of the neck. The lymph nodes have a homogenous enhanced contrast effect.

Histopathology

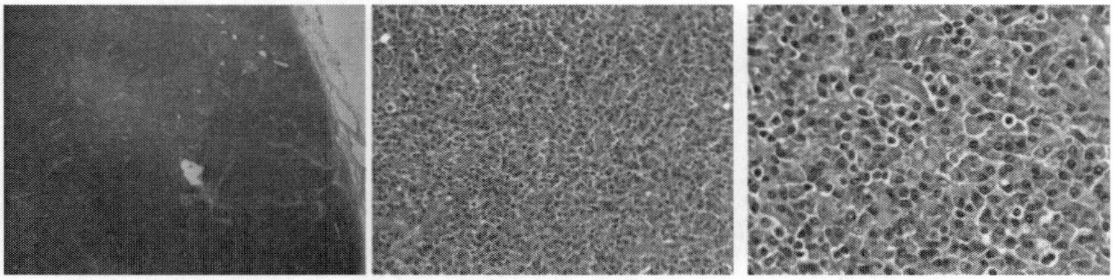

Figure 85. Histologically, cervical lymph node biopsy shows that most of the follicular structures have disappeared and plasmacytoid cells have grown densely. Medium to large lymphoid cells are mixed. Germinal center-like structures are observed.

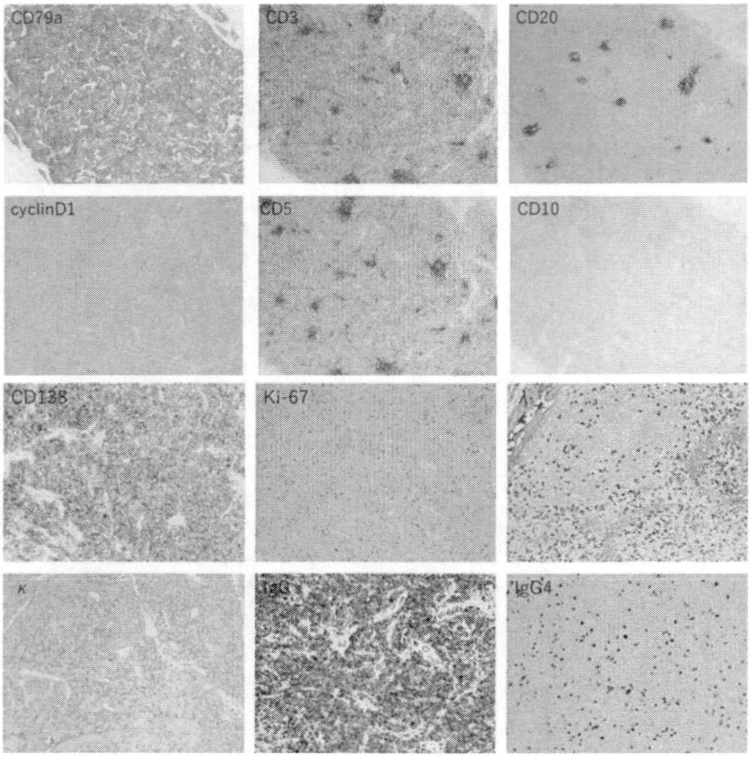

Figure 86. Proliferated cells are CD138 (+), CD79a (+), CD20 (-), CD3 (-), CD5 (-), CD10 (-), cyclinD1 (-), Kappa> Lambda, Ki-67 LI <3 %. The number of IgG4 positive cells exceeds 10 cells / HPF. Highly differentiated plasma cells are observed, and the Kappa chain and Lambda chain have no monoclonality.

Occipital Lymph Nodes

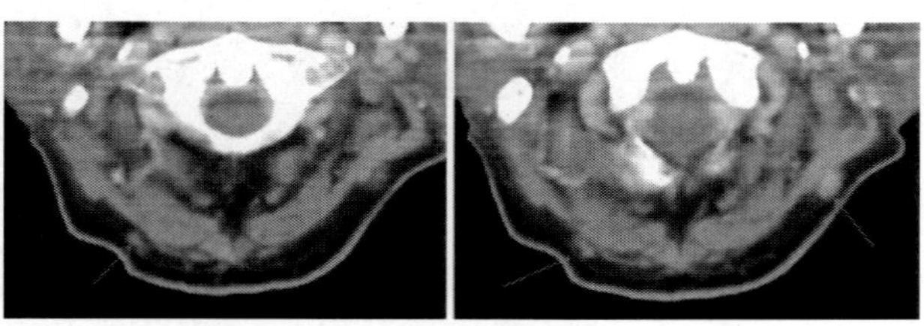

Figure 87. IgG4-related lymphadenopathy in a 71-year-old man. Contrast enhanced head CT images show swelling of the occipital lymph nodes. The lymph nodes have a homogenous enhanced contrast effect.

IgG4-Related Hypertrophic Pachymeningitis

Hypertrophic pachymeningitis is a member of IgG4-related disease and rare fibroinflammatory lesion that causes thickening of the dura of the skull and/or spinal canal, manifesting as radiculomyelopathy, headache, and cranial nerve palsy (Kawa S 2019) (Riku S 2009).

IgG4-Related Pituitary and Stalk Lesions

IgG4-related pituitary and pituitary stalk lesions present with symptoms of compressive optic neuropathy, panhypopituitarism, hypopituitarism, adrenocortical insufficiency, and syndromic inappropriate secretion of antidiuretic hormone (Kawa S 2019) (Shimatsu A 2009).

T1-Weighted MRI

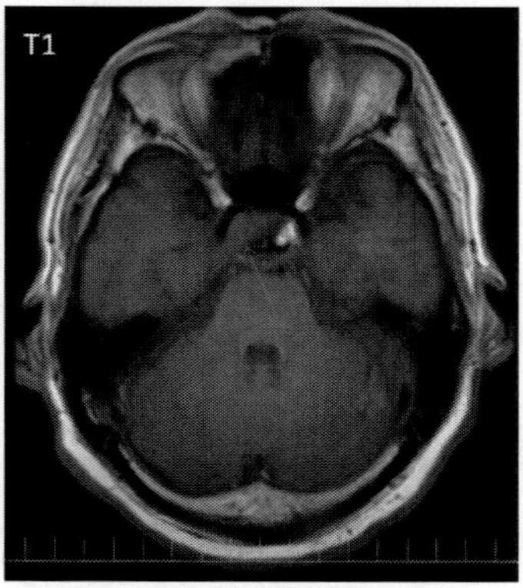

Figure 88. Axial T1-weighted magnetic resonance image shows a nodule of about 1cm in diameter of the pituitary gland (arrow), and a lesion of hypophysitis is suspected.

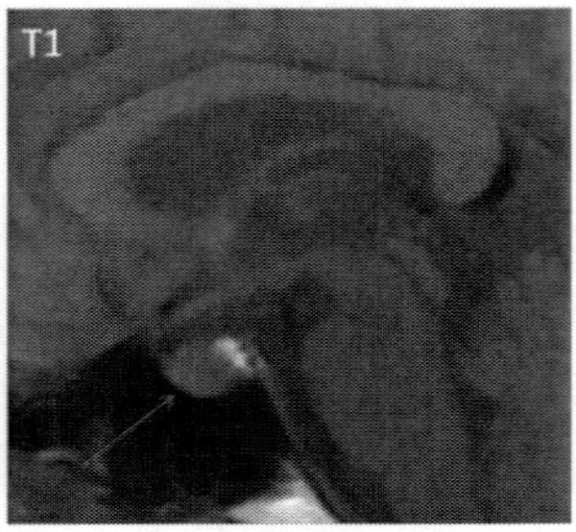

Figure 89. Sagittal T1-weighted magnetic resonance image shows a nodule of the pituitary gland (arrow).

Gadolinium-Enhanced MRI

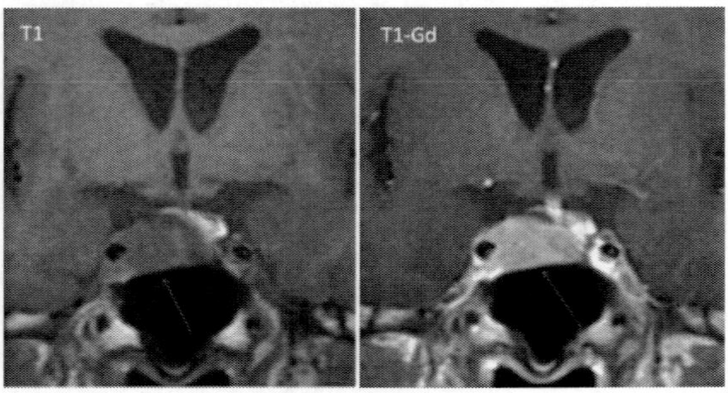

Figure 90. IgG4-related disease in a 63-year-old man. Coronal T1-weighted and gadolinium-enhanced T1-weighted MR images demonstrate that signals of an inflamed nodule (arrows) of the pituitary gland increase in intensity.

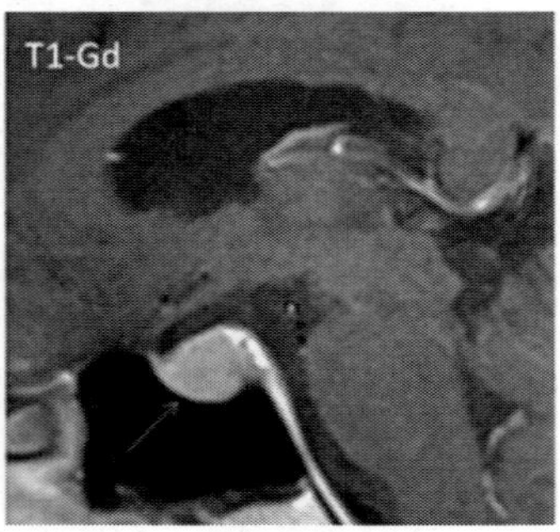

Figure 91. IgG4-related disease in a 63-year-old man. Sagittal gadolinium enhanced T1-weighted MR image demonstrates that signals of an inflamed nodule (arrows) of the pituitary gland increase in intensity.

T2-Weighted MRI

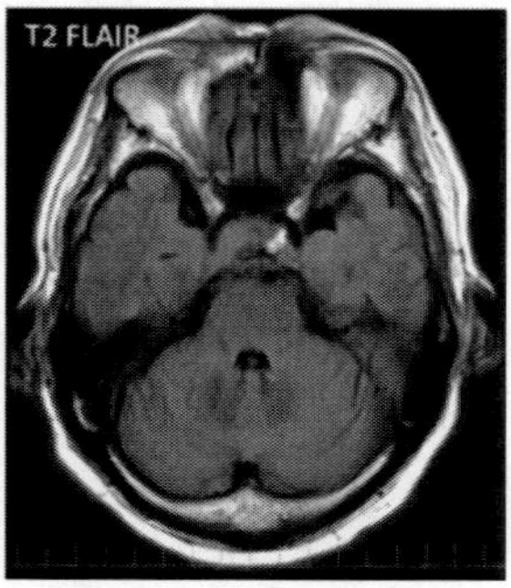

Figure 92. T2 Fluid-Attenuated Inversion Recovery (FLAIR) magnetic resonance image shows a nodule of about 1cm in diameter of the pituitary gland (arrow), and a lesion of hypophysitis is suspected.

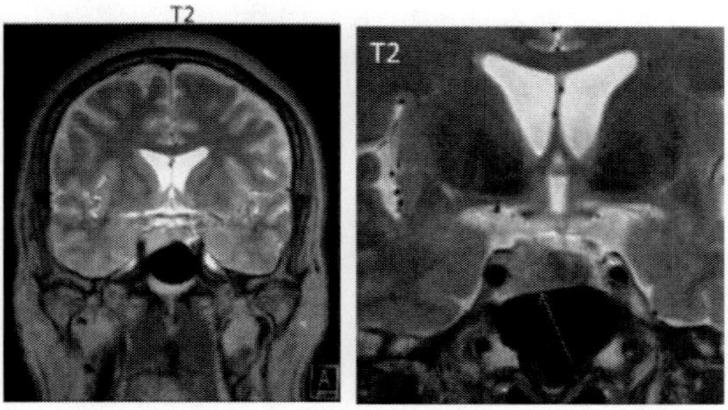

Figure 93. (a, b) Coronal T2-weighted magnetic resonance images show a nodule of the pituitary gland.

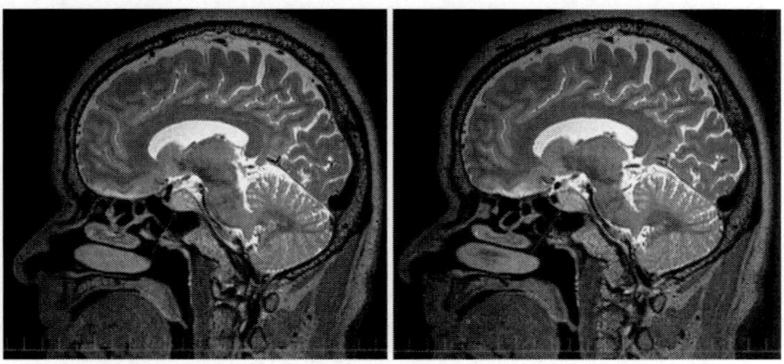

Figure 94. Sagittal T2-weighted magnetic resonance images show a nodule of about 1cm in diameter of the pituitary gland, and a lesion of hypophysitis is suspected.

Dynamic MRI

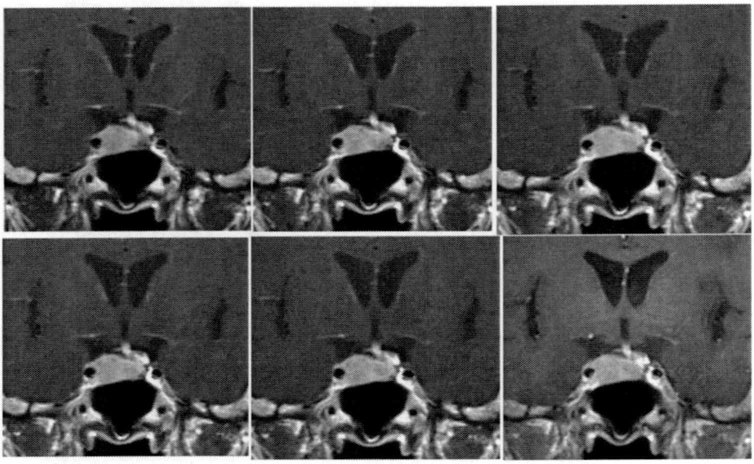

Figure 95. On dynamic MRI, a nodular lesion of the pituitary gland has increased intensity.

INFLAMMATORY PSEUDOTUMORS

Inflammatory pseudotumors in the central nervous system have also been reported. Various neurological symptoms may be present depending on where they occur. Although few cases have been reported, in which spontaneous remission has been achieved, corticosteroid administration may be useful in IgG4-related inflammatory pseudotumors of the nervous system (Zhang Z 2018).

REFERENCES

Cheuk W., Yuen HK, Chan JK. "Chronic sclerosing dacryoadenitis: part of the spectrum of IgG4-related Sclerosing disease?" *Am J Surg Pathol* 31 (2007): 643.

Cheuk W.., Yuen HK, Chan AC et al. "Ocular adnexal lymphoma associated with IgG4+ chronic sclerosing dacryoadenitis: a previously undescribed complication of IgG4-related sclerosing disease." *Am J Surg Pathol* 32 (2008): 1159-1167.

Choi YS, Kim SM, Sohn JS, Hwang JY, Chang TS, Cho DY. "IgG4-Related Disease with lymphadenopathy Presenting as a Cervical lymph node enlargement." *Kosin Med J* 32 (2017): 233-239.

Deshpande V, Zane NA, Kraft S, Stone JH, Faquin WC. "Recurrent Mastoiditis Mimics IgG4 Related Disease: A Potential Diagnostic Pitfall." *Head Neck Pathol* 10 (2016): 314-20.

Fujita A, Sakai O, Chapman MN, Sugimoto H. "IgG4-related disease of the head and neck: CT and MR imaging manifestations." *Radio Graphics* 32 (2012): 1945-1958.

Geyer JT, Ferry JA, Harris NL et al. "Chronic sclerosing sialadenitis (Küttner tumor) is an IgG4-associated disease." *Am J Surg Pathol* 34 (2010): 202-210.

Hamano H, Arakura N, Muraki T, Ozaki Y, Kiyosawa K, Kawa S. "Prevalence and distribution of extrapancreatic lesions complicating autoimmune pancreatitis." *J Gastroenterol* 41 (2006): 1197-1205.

Himi T, Takano K, Yamamoto M, Naishiro Y, Takahashi H. "A novel concept of Mikulicz's disease as IgG4-related disease." *Auris Nasus Larynx* 39 (2012): 9-17.

JV, Hennessey. "Riedel's thyroiditis: a clinical review." *J Clin Endocrinol Metab* 96 (2011): 3031–3041.

Kamisawa T., Nakajima H, Egawa N, Funata N, Tsuruta K, Okamoto A. "IgG4-related sclerosing disease incorporating sclerosing pancreatitis, cholangitis, sialadenitis and retroperitoneal fibrosis with lymphadenopathy." *Pancreatology* 6 (2006): 132-137.

Kawa S. "Immunoglobulin G4-related Disease: An Overview." *JMA J* 2 (2019): 11-27.

Li Y, Zhou G, Ozaki T, et al. "Distinct histopathological features of Hashimoto's thyroiditis with respect to IgG4-related disease." *Mod Pathol* 25 (2012): 1086-97.

Masaki Y, Sugai S, Umehara H. "IgG4-related diseases including Mikulicz's disease and sclerosing pancreatitis: diagnostic insights." *J Rheumatol* 37 (2010): 1380–1385.

Moteki H, Yasuo M, Hamano H, Uehara T, Usami S. "IgG4-related chronic rhinosinusitis: a new clinical entity of nasal disease." *Acta Otolaryngol* 131 (2011): 518-26.

Riku S, Hashizume Y, Yoshida M, et al. "[Is hypertrophic pachymeningitis a dural lesion of IgG4-related systemic disease?]." *Rinsho Shinkeigaku. 2009;49(9):594-6.* 49 (2009): 5946.

Sato Y, Ohshima K, Ichimura K, et al. "Ocular adnexal IgG4-related disease has uniform clinicopathology." *Pathol Int* 58 (2008): 465.

Schiffenbauer AI, Wahl C, Pittaluga S, et al. "IgG4-related disease presenting as recurrent mastoiditis." *The Laryngoscope* 122 (2012): 681-4.

Shimatsu A, Oki Y, Fujisawa I, et al. "Pituitary and stalk lesions (infundibulo-hypophysitis) associated with immunoglobulin G4-related systemic disease: an emerging clinical entity." *Endocr J* 56 (2009): 1033-41.

Sogabe Y, Ohshima K, Azumi A, et al. "Location and frequency of lesions in patients with IgG4-related ophthalmic diseases." *Graefes Arch Clin Exp Ophthalmol* 252 (2014): 531-8.

Umehara H, Okazaki K, Masaki Y, Kawano M, Yamamoto M, Saeki T, et al. "A novel clinical entity, IgG4-related disease (IgG4RD): general concept and details." *Mod Rheumatol* 22 (2012): 1-14.

Wallace ZS., Khosroshahi A, Jakobiec FA et al. "IgG4-related systemic disease as a cause of "idiopathic" orbital inflammation, including orbital myositis, and trigeminal nerve involvement." *Surv Ophthalmol* 57 (2012): 26-33.

Watanabe T, Maruyama M, Ito T, et al. "Clinical features of a new disease concept, IgG4-related thyroiditis." *Scand J Rheumatol* 42 (2013): 325-30.

Zhang Z, Fu W, Wang M, Niu L, Liu B, Jiao Y, Liu X. "IgG4-related inflammatory pseudotumor of the brain parenchyma: a case report and literature review." *Acta Neurol Belg* 118 (2018): 617-627.

In: IgG4 Related Disease
Editor: Syuichi Koarada
ISBN: 978-1-53618-050-3

Chapter 3

THORACIC MANIFESTATION OF IGG4-RELATED DISEASE

Syuichi Koarada*[*] and Yoshinobu Nakao
Division of Rheumatology, Faculty of Medicine,
Saga University, Nabeshima, Saga, Japan

ABSTRACT

Thorax lesions of IgG4-related disease are diverse. These lesions are like common and rare diseases, including malignancies, and can often be difficult to differentiate. Lung lesions present with interstitial pneumonia, nodules, masses, and consolidation. Airway lesions of IgG4-related disease include bronchial wall thickening. Pleural lesions include pleural thickening, pleural effusion, and pleurisy. Lymph node involvement can occur in the hilar and mediastinum in the lungs and the axillary lymph nodes outside the lungs. There may also be IgG4-related mastopathy outside the lungs.

---

[*] Corresponding Author's Email: koarada@cc.saga-u.ac.jp.

Introduction

IgG4-related disease is a multisystem fibrotic inflammatory disease with classical histopathological findings, often associated with elevated serum IgG4 levels. The thoracic symptoms of IgG4-related disease are so numerous that they can mimic the symptoms of other common and uncommon diseases (Corcoran J. P. 2017).

Physicians may encounter this disease, and knowledge and understanding of the diverse nature and status of thoracic IgG4-related disease are important.

IgG4-related lung disease is known to have several imaging patterns of lung involvement, including interstitium, hilar/mediastinal lymphadenopathy, bronchial wall and bronchovascular bundle thickening (airways), interlobular septal wall thickening nodular shadow, infiltrative shadow, and pleural thickening/effusion. In addition, they may appear as a combination of these lesions (Matsui S. 2016).

IgG4-related lung disease develops through the lymphatics of the lungs and exhibits various clinical features (Matsui S. 2016).

Lung and Pleural Disease

IgG4-related lung disease may appear with or without other organ involvement.

Interstitial pneumonia, asthma, inflammatory pulmonary pseudotumor, edema and thickening of bronchial mucosa, thickening of bronchial and bronchial perivascular bundles, pleural lesions, and the hilar and the mediastinal lymphadenopathy have been reported as respiratory lesions of IgG4-related disease.

Some inflammatory pseudotumors of the lung with lymphoplasmacytic infiltration, fibrosis, occlusive phlebitis, and IgG4-

positive plasma cell infiltration belong to the category of IgG4-related disease.

It has also been reported that IgG4-related lesions occur in visceral pleura or parietal pleural thickening, and in the subpleural lung parenchyma (Zen Y. 2009). IgG4-related lung and pleural disease need to be differentiated from idiopathic pulmonary fibrosis, sarcoidosis, and lung tumors (Zen Y. 2009).

IgG4-positive plasma cells infiltrate the lesion of the lung and patients with IgG4-related lung disease respond well to corticosteroid treatment.

Classification

Inoue D. et al., reported that there are four major forms of IgG4-related lung disease.

Table 1. IgG4-related intrathoracic disease

Lung parenchymal	Solid nodular type: solitary nodular lesion including mass Alveolar interstitial type: honeycombing, bronchiectasis or diffuse ground-glass opacity (GGOs) Round-shaped ground-glass opacity (GGO) type: multiple round-shaped GGOs Alveolar hemorrhage: rare.
Airways	Broncho-vascular type: thickening of bronchovascular bundles and/or interlobular septa.
Pleural	Pleural effusion Pleural nodules or thickening.
Mediastinal	Hilar and mediastinal lymphadenopathy Mediastinal mass Thoracic aortitis/periaortitis Pericardial effusion/pericardial thickening.

(a) a type characterized by nodular or massive solid lesions; (b) a type characterized by round ground-glass opacity; (c) alveolar interstitial disease (with honeycombing, bronchiectasis and diffuse ground-glass opacities); and (d) bronchovascular disease (with thickening of bronchovascular bundles and interlobular septa) (Inoue D. 2009) (Zen Y. 2009).

Also, Takao H. et al., described four subtypes of IgG4-related lung disease according to thoracic CT imaging: solid nodular type, round-shaped ground-glass opacity (GGO) type, alveolar interstitial type and bronchovascular type (Takato H. 2008).

Imaging of Thoracic Lesions

Lung Parenchymal

Interstitial Pneumonia

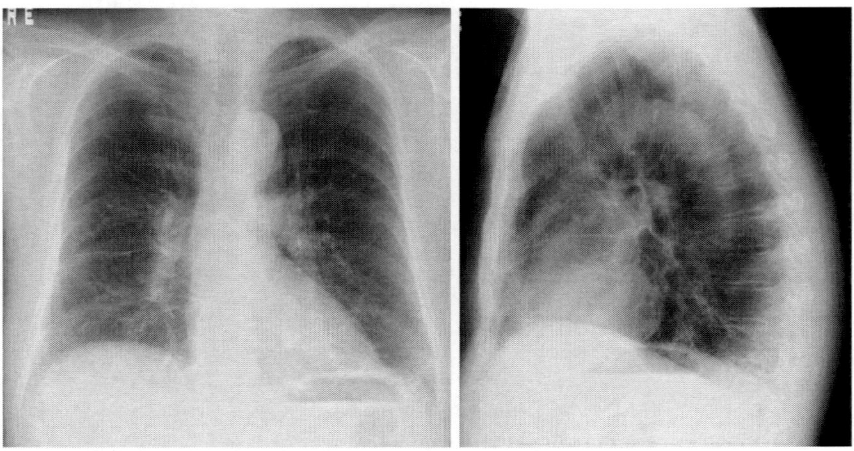

Figure 1. IgG4-related lung disease in a 73-year-old man. There are diffuse ground-glass opacities and reticular shadows in bilateral lower lung fields with volume loss.

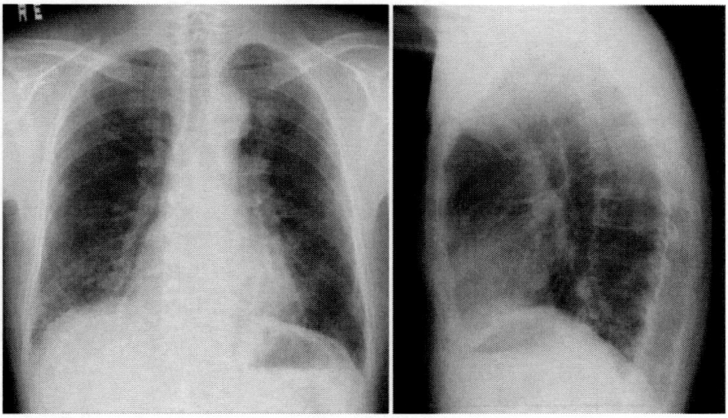

Figure 2. IgG4-related lung disease in a 60-year-old man. There are diffuse ground-glass opacities and reticular shadows in bilateral middle and lower lung fields with volume loss.

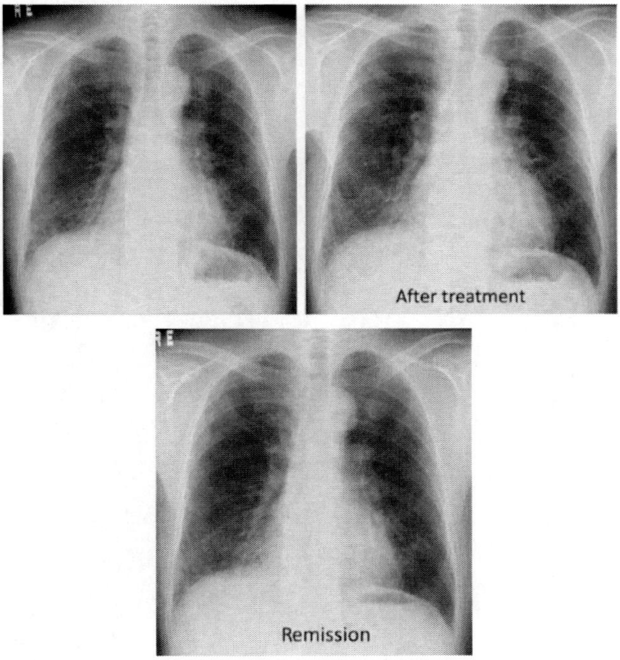

Figure 3. Chest radiograph on the day of admission. Ground-glass opacities and reticular shadows are visible in both middle and lower lung fields (left panel). Chest radiograph immediately after corticosteroid treatment on the 7th day of hospitalization. There is no improvement in interstitial pneumonia in the middle and lower lung fields (middle panel). Chest radiograph on day 30 of hospitalization shows an improvement in the interstitial shadows of both middle and lower lung fields (right panel).

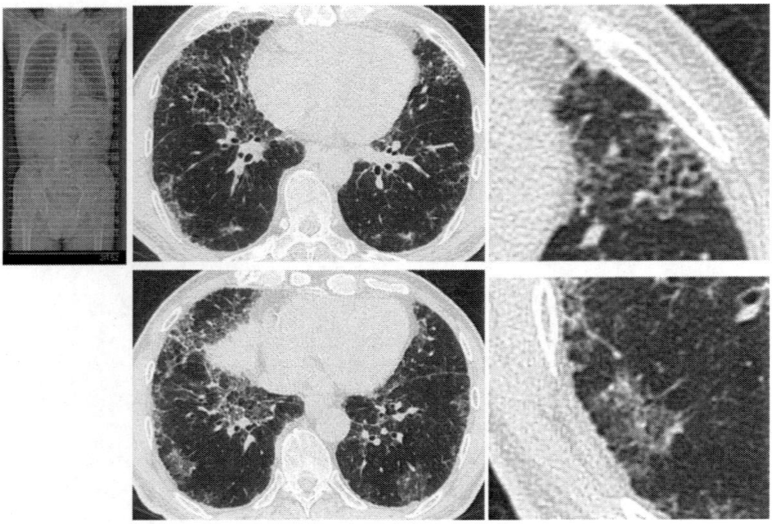

Figure 4. IgG4-related lung disease in a 60-year-old man. Axial non-contrast enhanced chest CT images show diffuse ground-glass opacities, linear reticular shadows, and small cystic changes with traction bronchiectasis in the areas of peripheral and lower lobes of both the lungs.

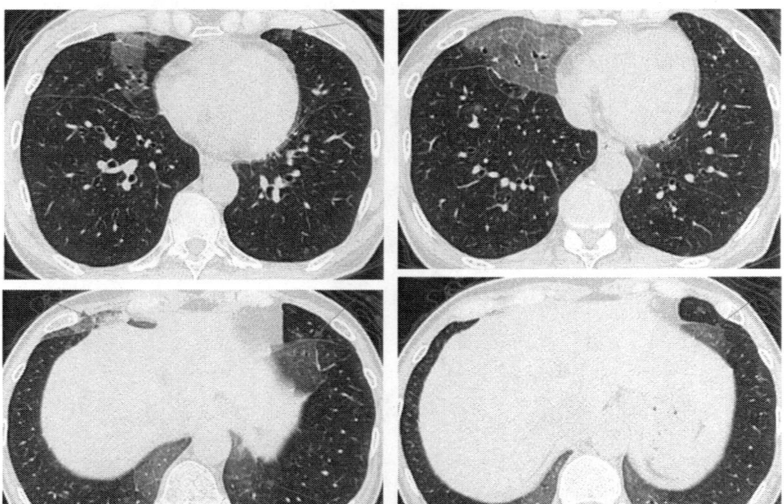

Figure 5. IgG4-related lung disease in a 60-year-old woman. Axial non-contrast enhanced chest CT images show focal ground glass opacities in the bilateral lower lobes and the right middle lobe.

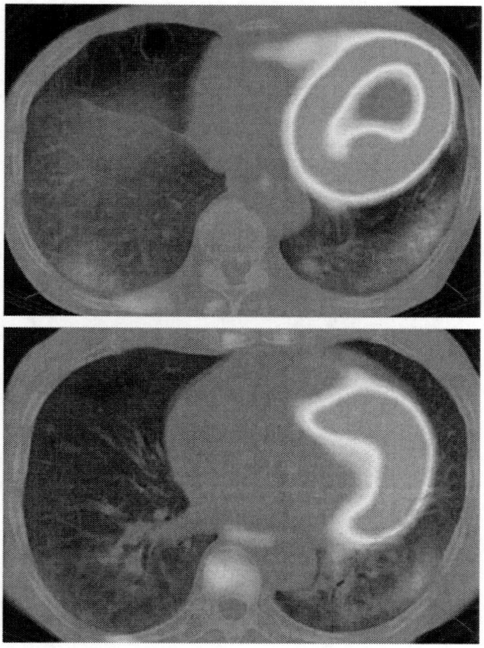

Figure 6. IgG4-related disease in a 66-year-old woman. FDG-PET/CT images show increased uptakes in the the bilateral lower lobes with interstitial pneumonia (arrows).

Mass Lesions

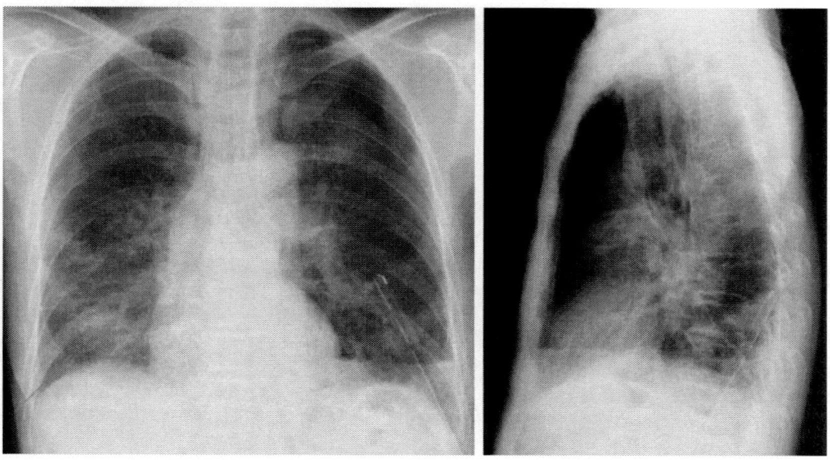

Figure 7. IgG4-related lung disease in a 55-year-old man. Plain radiograph images of the chest show a mass lesion in the right lung.

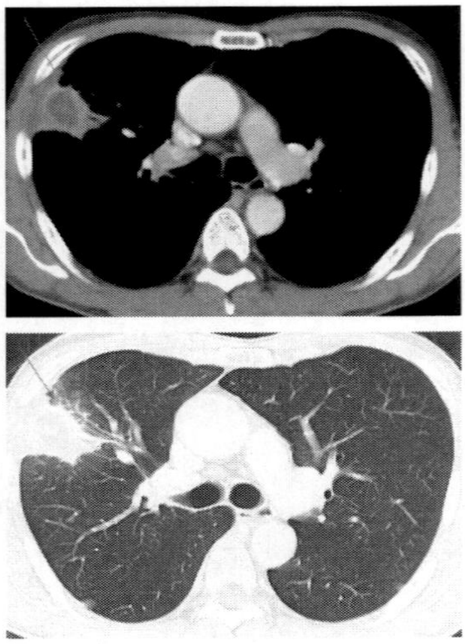

Figure 8. IgG4-related lung disease in a 55-year-old man. Chest CT images reveal a 4-cm right lung mass.

Nodular Lesions

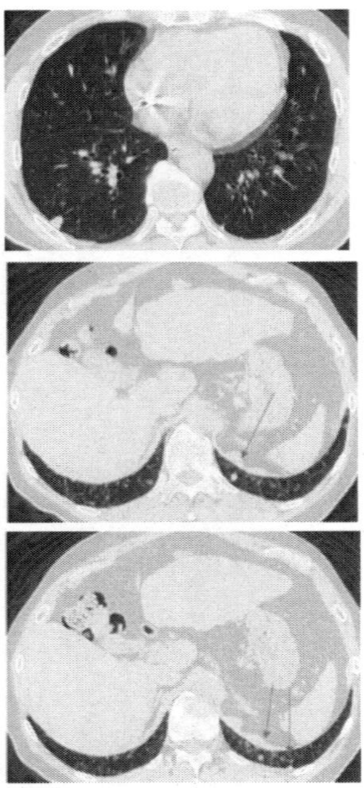

Figure 9. IgG4-related lung disease in a 66-year-old man. Axial non-contrast enhanced chest CT images show polygonal nodules (arrows) on the pleura side of the middle and lower lung fields in both the lungs.

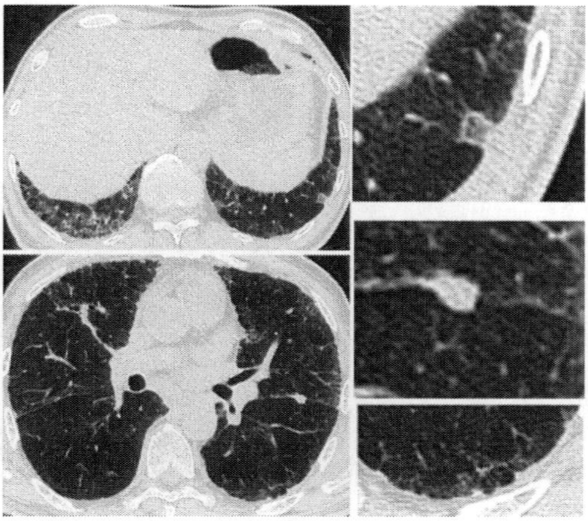

Figure 10. IgG4-related lung disease in a 60-year-old man. Flat nodules are scattered on both sides of the pleura and along the pulmonary veins.

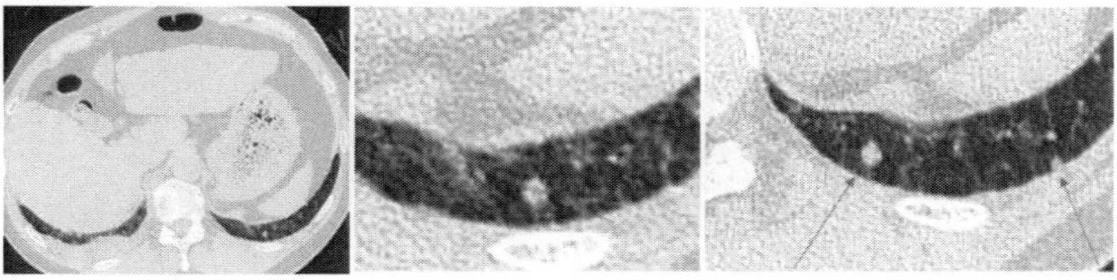

Figure 11. IgG4-related lung disease in a 66-year-old man. Axial non-contrast enhanced chest CT images show nodules (arrows) in the right lower lung field.

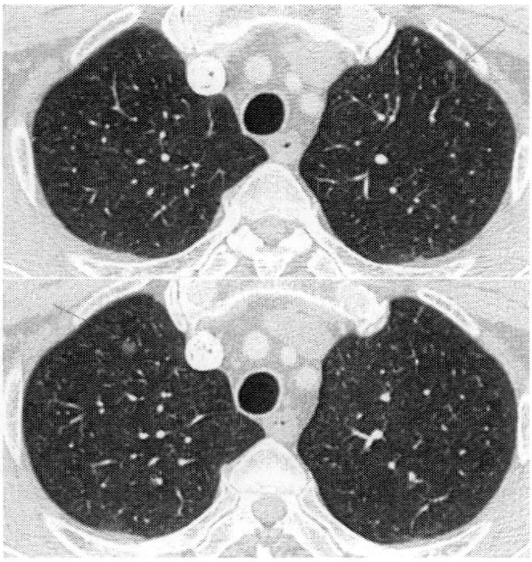

Figure 12. IgG4-related lung disease in a 63-year-old man. Axial non-contrast enhanced chest CT images show ground grass density nodules (arrows) in both upper lobes. They were resolved after corticosteroid therapy.

Consolidation

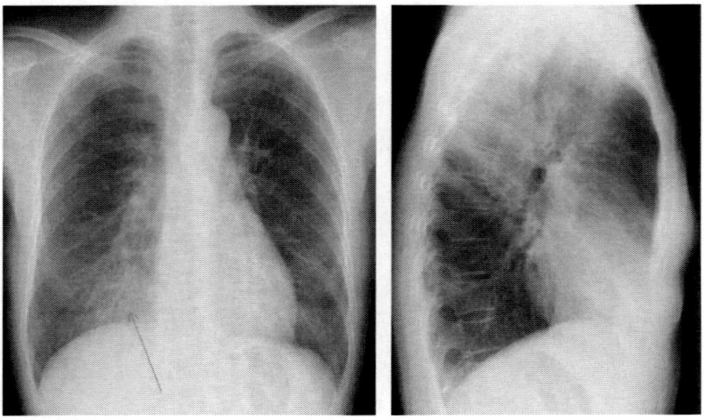

Figure 13. IgG4-related lung disease in a 66-year-old woman. Chest plain radiographs show consolidative infiltrate in the right lower lung field.

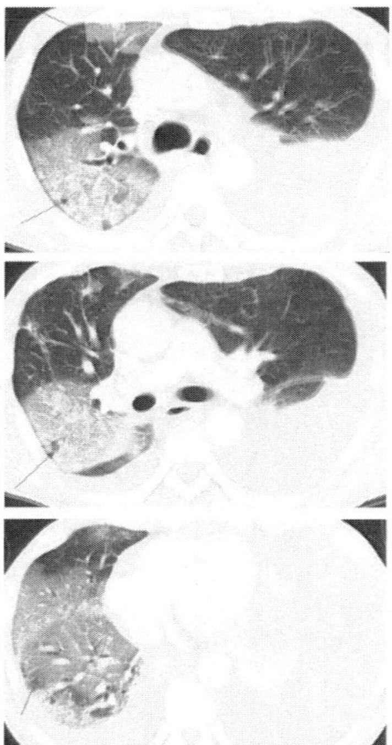

Figure 14. IgG4-related lung disease in a 55-year-old man. Axial contrast enhanced chest CT images demonstrates consolidative infiltrate and ground glass shadows in the right lung and massive pleural effusion in the left lung.

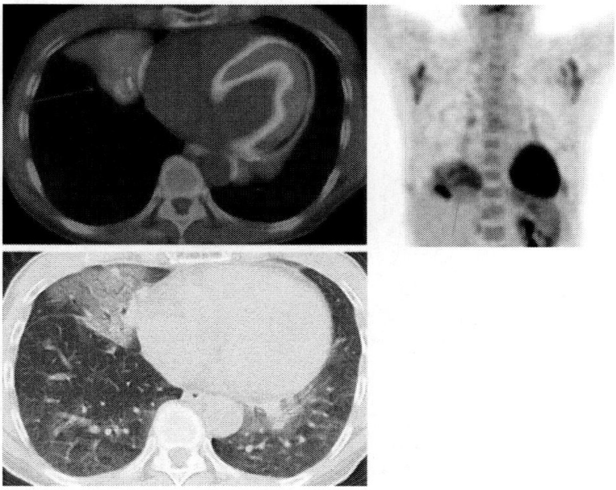

Figure 15. IgG4-related disease in a 61-year-old woman. FDG-PET/CT images show increased uptakes in the consolidation of the right lower lobe (arrows).

Alveolar Hemorrhage

Alveolar hemorrhage is rare in IgG4-related lung disease.

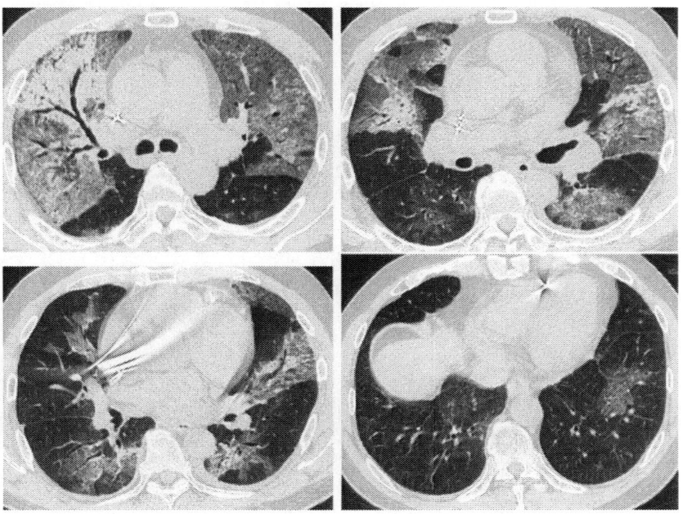

Figure 16. IgG4-related disease in a 66-year-old man. Axial non-contrast enhanced chest CT images show extensive ground-glass shadows and consolidation in both the lungs. The lesions are stronger in the upper lung fields and around the bronchial vascular bundles. The patient was diagnosed with alveolar hemorrhage by bronchoscopy and alveolar lavage fluid.

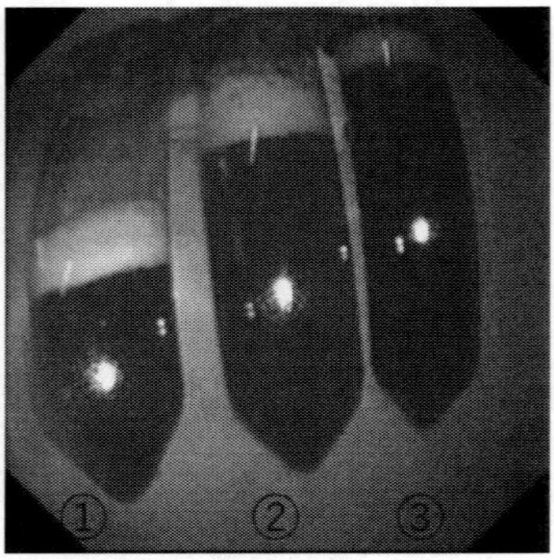

Figure 17. IgG4-related lung disease in a 66-year-old man. Bronchoalveolar lavage (BAL) was done in the right upper lobe. The progressive hemorrhagic BAL in the serial samples (left tube is the first BAL, middle tube is the second BAL, and right tube is the third BAL.). BAL fluid analysis shows a serial increase in the numbers of red blood cells.

Airways

Bronchovascular Type

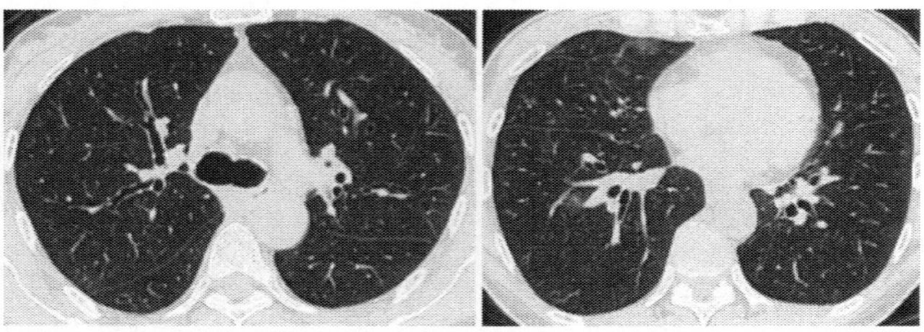

Figure 18. IgG4-related disease in a 60-year-old woman. Axial chest CT images show thickening of bronchovascular bundles in both the lungs.

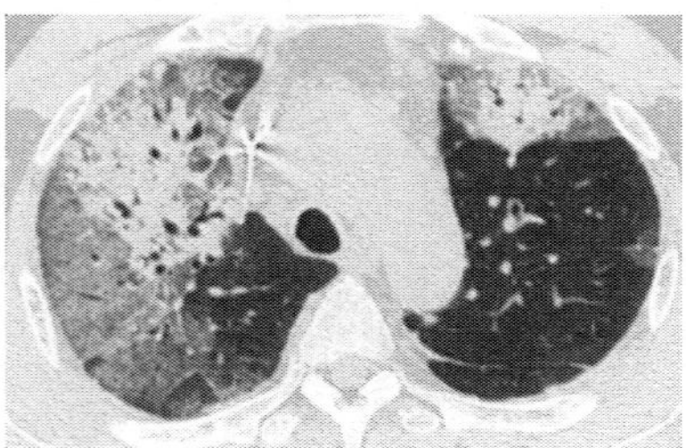

Figure 19. IgG4-related disease in a 66-year-old man. Axial non-contrast enhanced CT images of the chest show that the bronchi in the consolidation have an uneven expansion throughout.

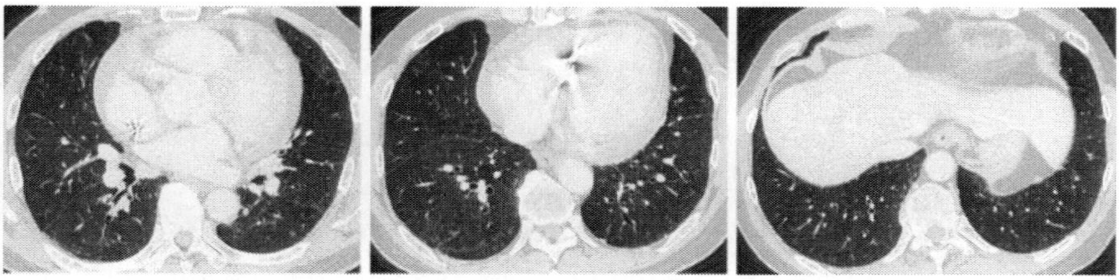

Figure 20. IgG4-related disease in a 67-year-old man. Axial contrast enhanced CT images of the chest show that the walls of bronchioles are thickened mainly in the lower lobes of both the lungs, and granular shadows appear.

Lymphadenopathy

See IgG4related lymphadenopathy in the thorax.

Pleural

Pleural Nodules or Thickening

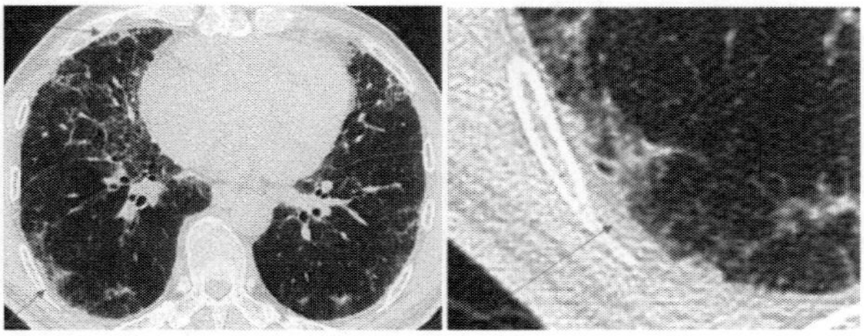

Figure 21. IgG4-related pleural disease in a 60-year-old man. Axial non-enhanced CT images show a pleural and subpleural lesion (arrows).

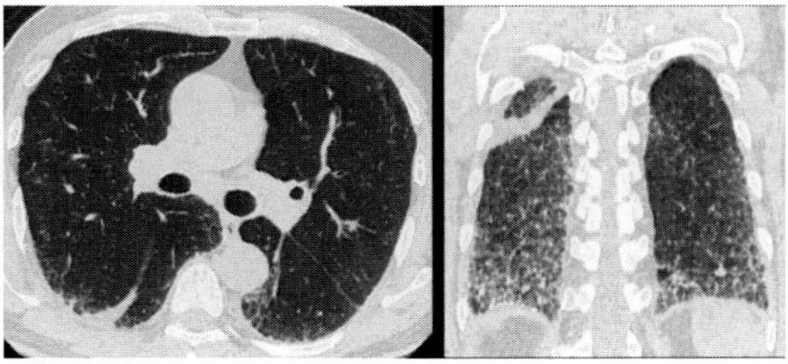

Figure 22. IgG4-related lung and pleural disease in a 76-year-old man. Axial chest CT scan (left panel) demonstrates thickening of the pleura of the right oblique fissure. Reconstructed coronal CT image (right panel) shows a thickened right pleura and mild emphysematous changes in both the upper lobes. Reticulo-nodular shadows and bronchiectasis predominate in the lower lung fields on the pleural side of both the lungs, suggesting interstitial pneumonia with a non-specific interstitial pneumonia (NSIP) pattern.

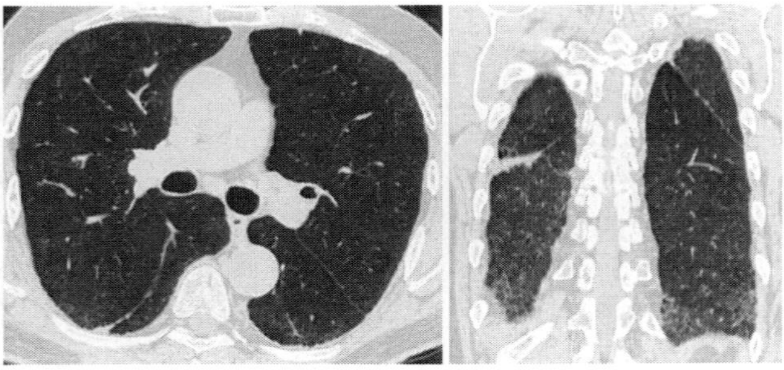

Figure 23. IgG4-related disease in a 76-year-old man. Axial CT scan after corticosteroid treatment shows an improvement in right pleural thickening. The interstitial pneumonia with reticular nodules of the NSIP pattern, which predominantly existed in the lower lung, also improved in the reconstructed coronal CT image.

Pleural Effusion

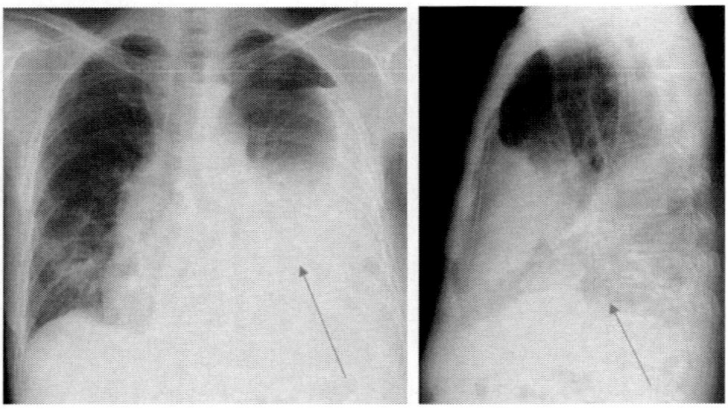

Figure 24. IgG4-related lung disease in a 55-year-old man. Plain radiographs show left massive pleural effusion.

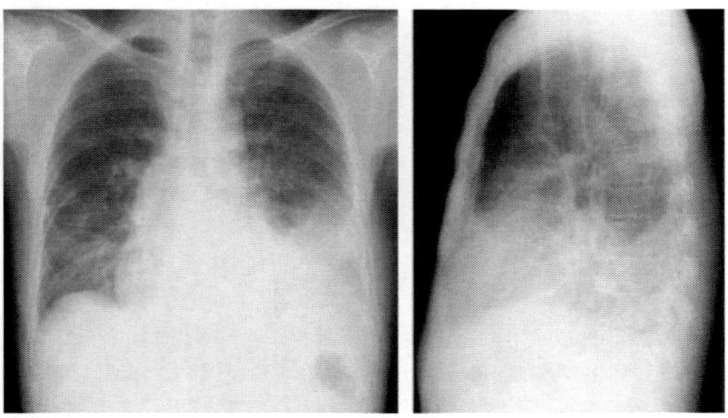

Figure 25. IgG4-related lung disease in a 54-year-old man. Plain radiograph shows moderate left pleural effusion.

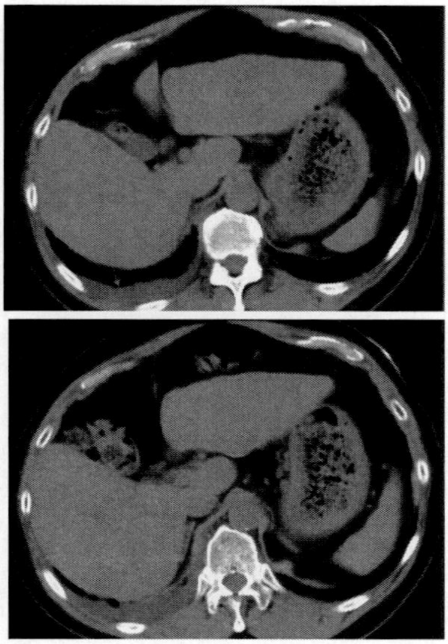

Figure 26. IgG4-related lung disease in a 66-year-old man. Axial non-contrast enhanced CT images of the chest show right pleural effusion (arrows).

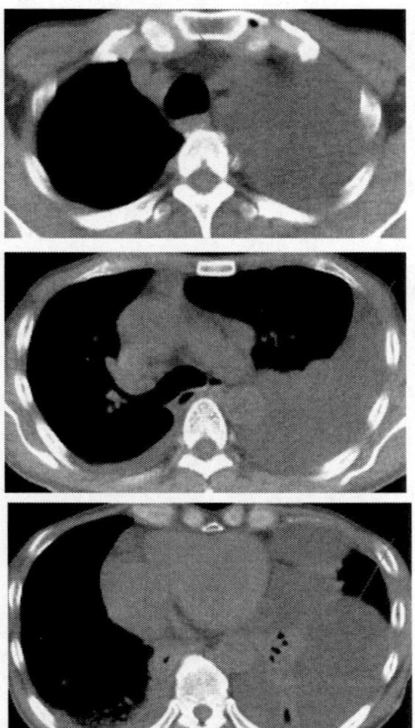

Figure 27. IgG4-related lung disease in a 55-year-old man. Axial non-contrast enhanced CT images of the chest show left massive pleural effusion (arrows).

Histopathology

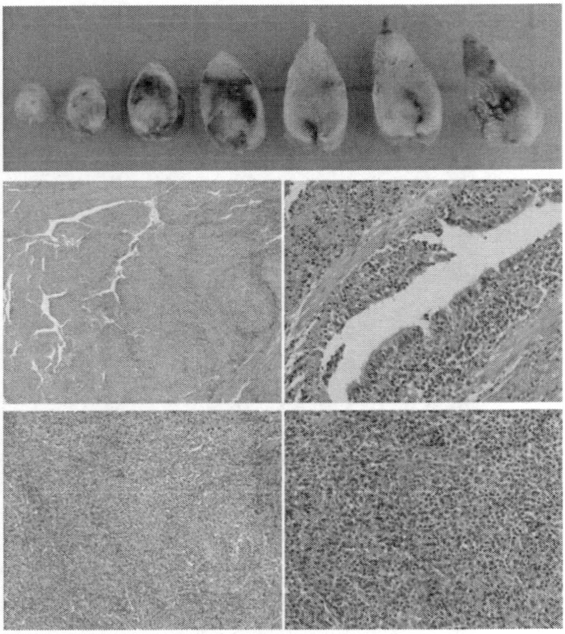

(a)

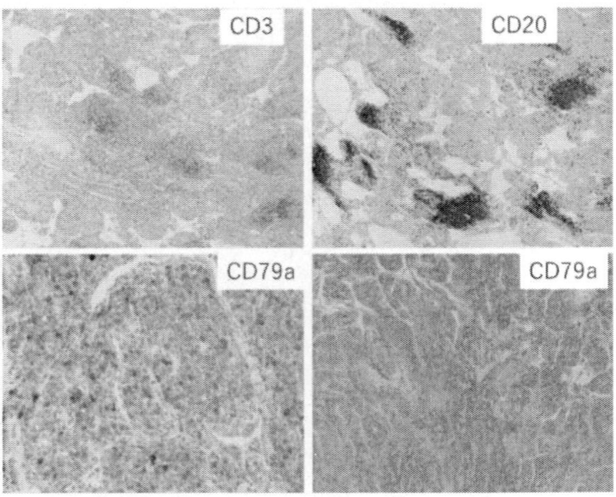

(b)

Figure 28. a, b. Pulmonary histopathology in IgG4-related sclerosing disease. Histologically, small to medium-sized lymphocytes (monocytoid cells and centrocyte-like cells) and plasma cells proliferate. B cells are predominant in immunohistology.

THORACIC LYMPHADENOPATHY

Enlargement of the hilar or mediastinal lymph nodes is also common in patients with IgG4 related lung disease (Patel M. 2011).

Hilar Lymphadenopathy

Plain Radiography

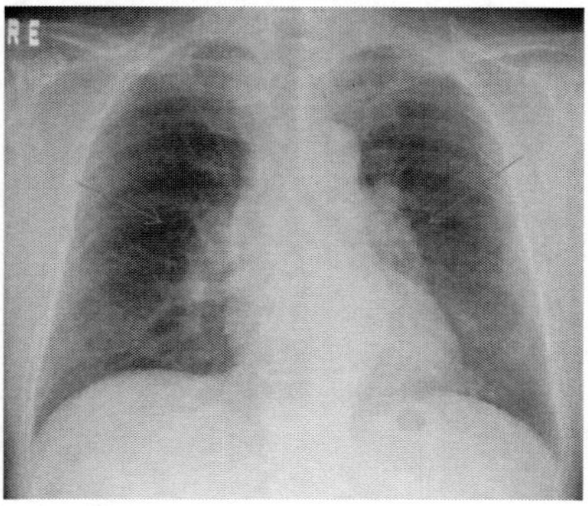

Figure 29. IgG4-related lung disease in a 72-year-old man. Chest radiograph shows bilateral hilum enlargement (arrows).

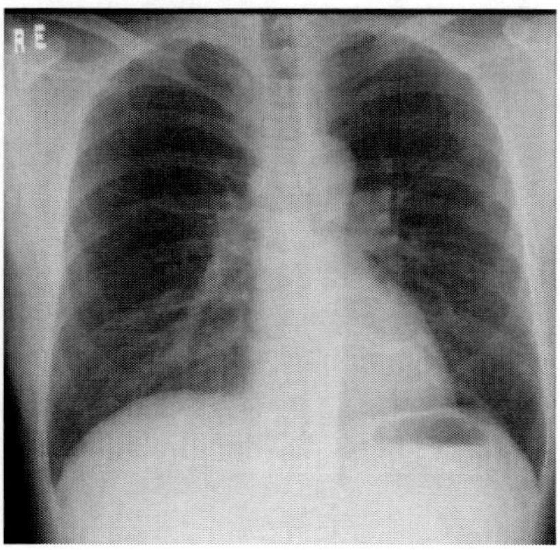

Figure 30. IgG4-related lung disease in a 38-year-old man. Chest radiograph shows mild bilateral hilum enlargement (arrows).

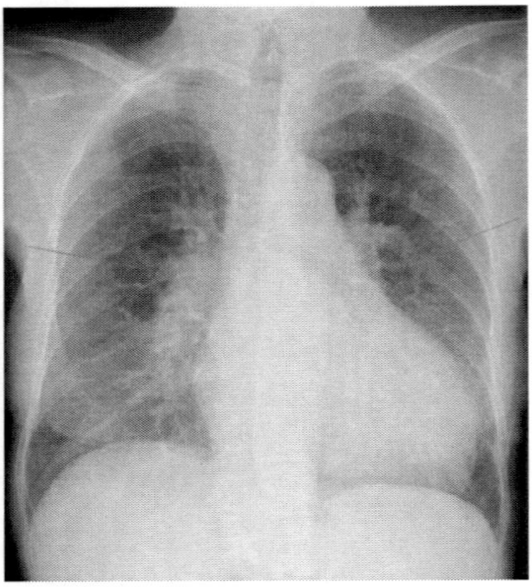

Figure 31. IgG4-related thoracic lymphadenopathy in a 66-year-old woman. Chest plain radiograph shows enlargement of the hilar lymph nodes.

Non-Contrast Enhanced Chest CT

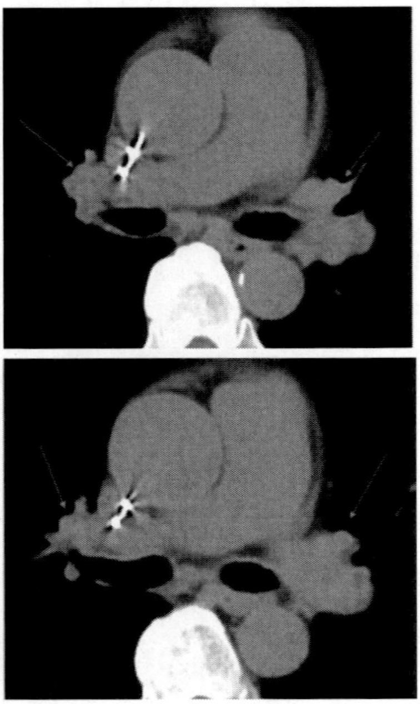

Figure 32. IgG4-related thoracic lymphadenopathy in a 66-year-old man. Axial non-contrast enhanced CT images of the chest demonstrate bilateral hilar lymphadenopathy (arrows).

Contrast Enhanced Chest CT

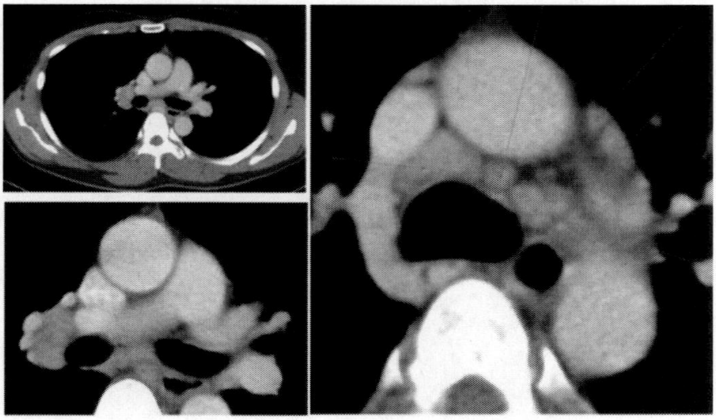

Figure 33. IgG4-related thoracic lymphadenopathy in a 38-year-old man. Axial contrast enhanced CT images of the chest demonstrate the mediastinal and bilateral hilar lymphadenopathy (arrows).

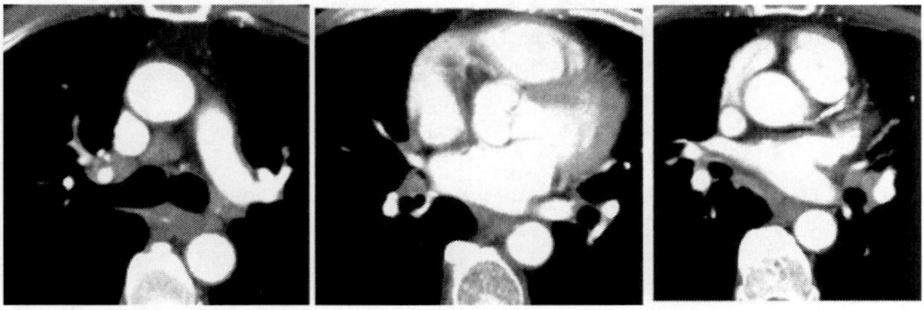

Figure 34. IgG4-related thoracic lymphadenopathy in a 60-year-old man. Axial contrast enhanced CT images show enlargement of the mediastinal and bilateral hilar lymph nodes.

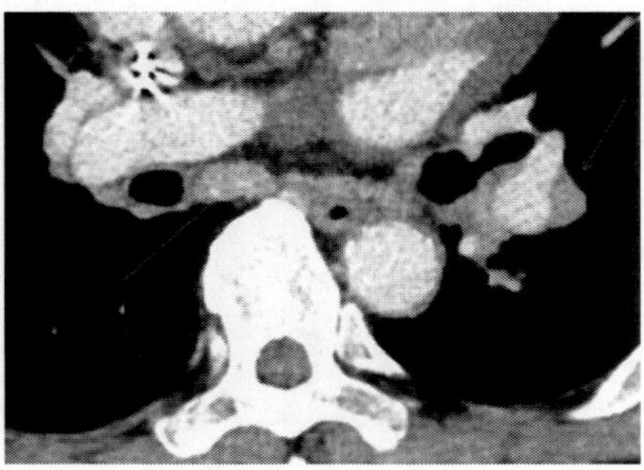

Figure 35. IgG4-related thoracic lymphadenopathy in a 67-year-old man. Axial contrast enhanced CT image shows enlargement of the hilar lymph nodes.

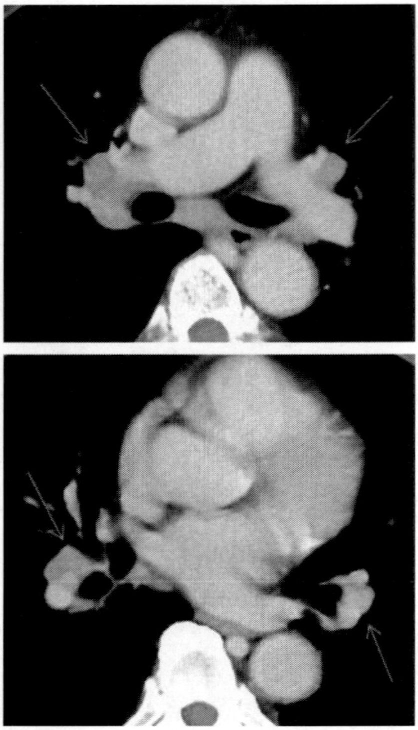

Figure 36. IgG4-related thoracic lymphadenopathy in a 72-year-old man. Axial contrast enhanced CT images show enlargement of the hilar lymph nodes.

PET/CT

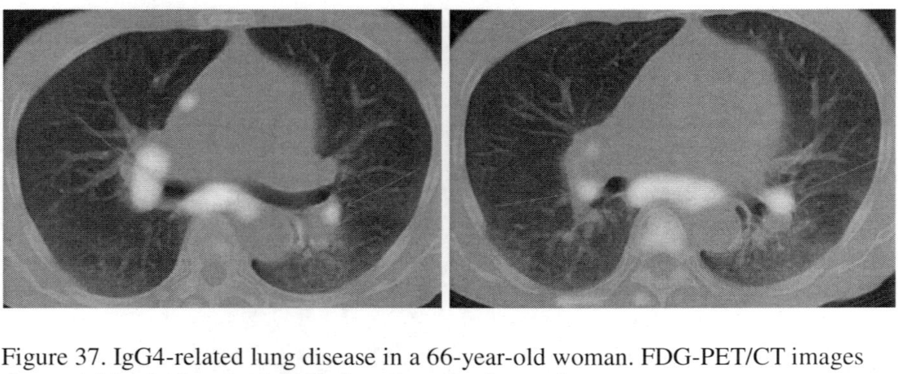

Figure 37. IgG4-related lung disease in a 66-year-old woman. FDG-PET/CT images show positive lesions in the hilar lymph nodes (arrows).

Mediastinal Lymphadenopathy

Non-Contrast Enhanced Chest CT

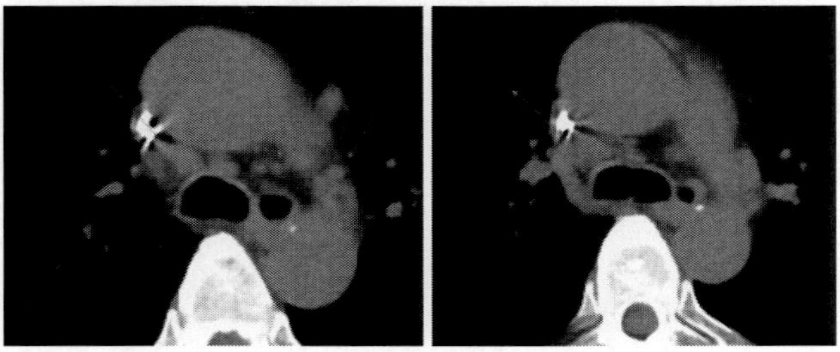

Figure 38. IgG4-related thoracic lymphadenopathy in a 66-year-old man. Axial non-contrast enhanced CT images show multiple enlarged mediastinal lymph nodes (arrows).

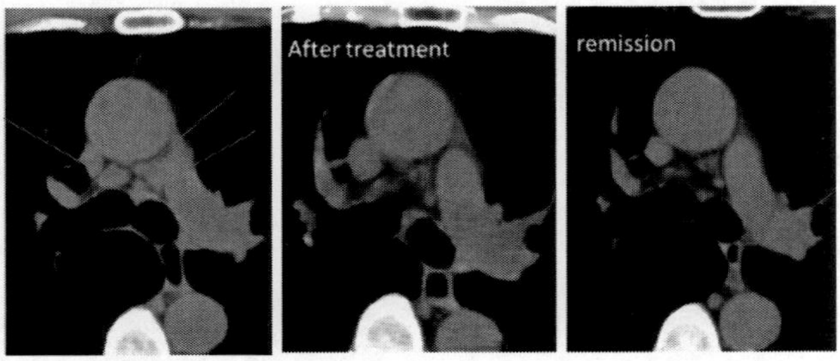

Figure 39. IgG4-related thoracic lymphadenopathy in a 76-year-old man. Axial non-contrast enhanced CT images show multiple enlarged mediastinal lymph nodes (arrows). The mediastinal involvement resolved completely after corticosteroid therapy and is in remission.

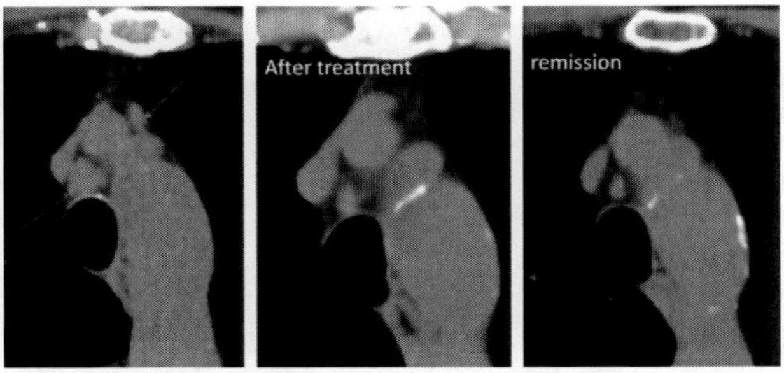

Figure 40. IgG4-related thoracic lymphadenopathy in a 76-year-old man. Axial non-contrast CT images show multiple enlarged mediastinal lymph nodes (arrows). The mediastinal lymphadenopathy resolved completely after corticosteroid therapy and is in remission.

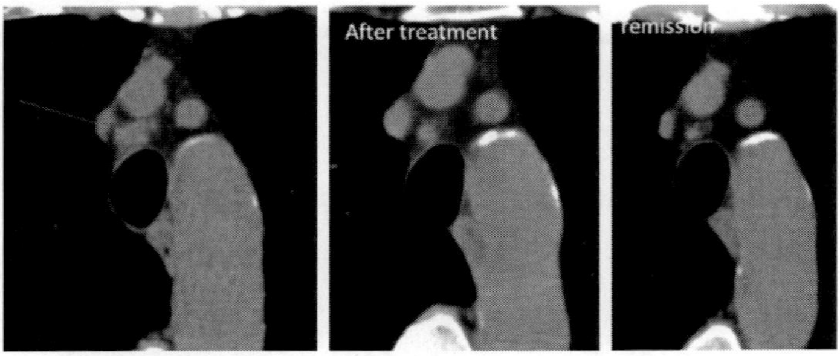

Figure 41. IgG4-related thoracic lymphadenopathy in a 76-year-old man. Axial non-contrast CT images show an enlarged mediastinal lymph node (arrow). The enlarged mediastinal lymph node diminished in size after corticosteroid therapy.

Contrast Enhanced Chest CT

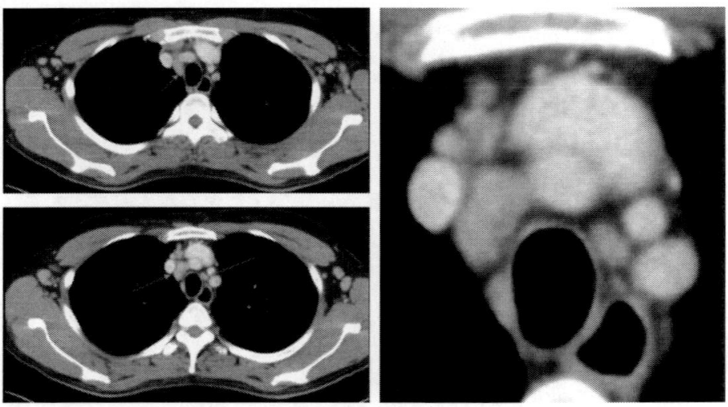

Figure 42. IgG4-related thoracic lymphadenopathy in a 38-year-old man. Axial contrast enhanced CT images show multiple enlarged mediastinal lymph nodes (arrows).

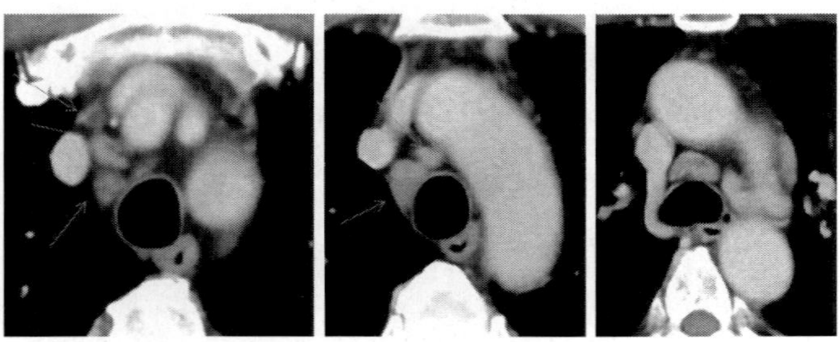

Figure 43. IgG4-related thoracic lymphadenopathy in a 72-year-old man. Axial contrast enhanced CT images show multiple enlarged mediastinal lymph nodes (arrows).

PET/CT

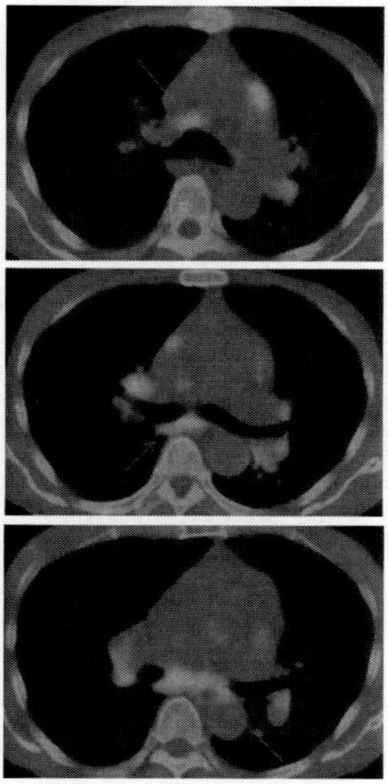

Figure 44. IgG4-related lung disease in a 66-year-old woman. FDG-PET/CT images show positive lesions in the mediastinal lymph nodes (arrows).

Axillary Lymphadenopathy

Right Axillary Lymph Nodes

CT

Contrast Enhanced Chest CT

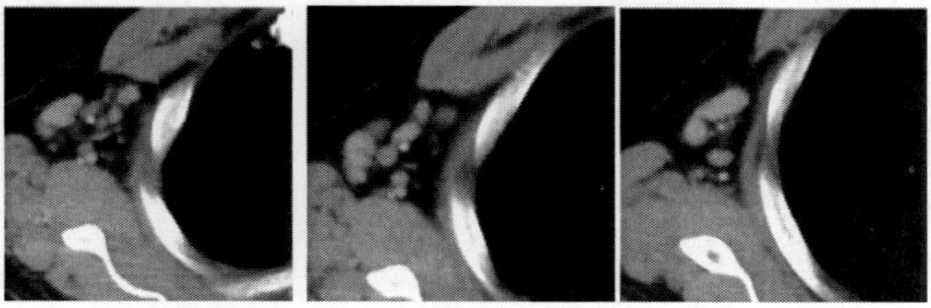

Figure 45. IgG4-related axillary lymphadenopathy in a 72-year-old man. Axial contrast enhanced CT images of the chest reveal multiple enlarged right axillary lymph nodes.

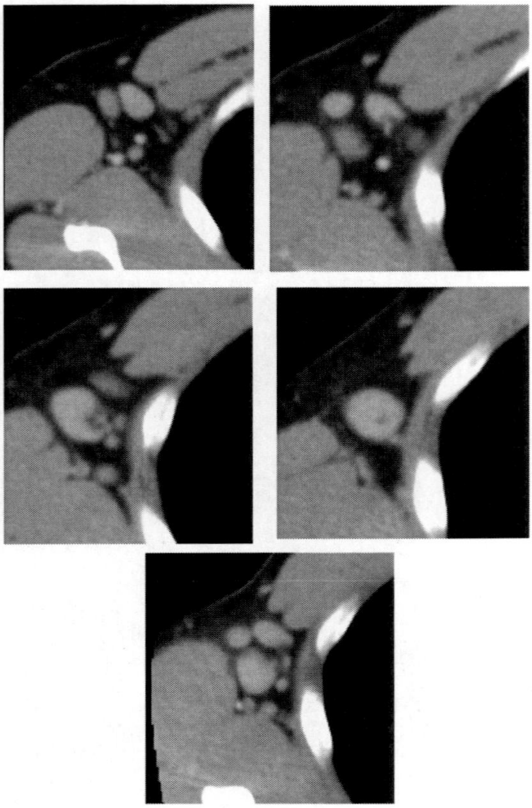

Figure 46. IgG4-related axillary lymphadenopathy in a 38-year-old man. Axial contrast enhanced CT images of the chest reveal multiple enlarged right axillary lymph nodes.

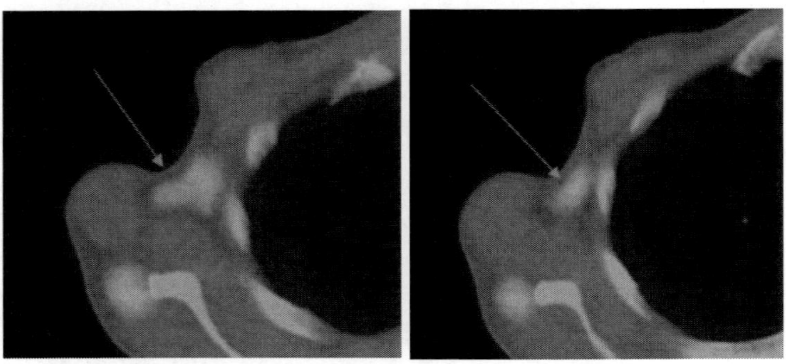

Figure 47. IgG4-related disease in a 66-year-old woman. FDG-PET/CT images show positive lesions in the right axillary lymph nodes (arrows).

Left Axillary Lymph Nodes

CT

Contrast Enhanced Chest CT

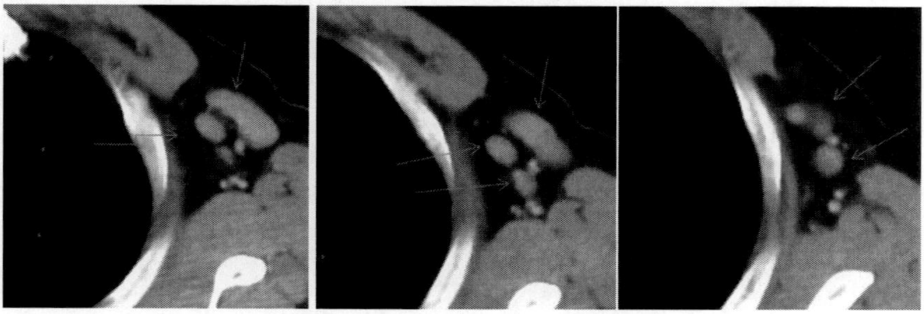

Figure 48. IgG4-related axillary lymphadenopathy in a 72-year-old man. Axial contrast enhanced CT images of the chest reveal multiple enlarged left axillary lymph nodes.

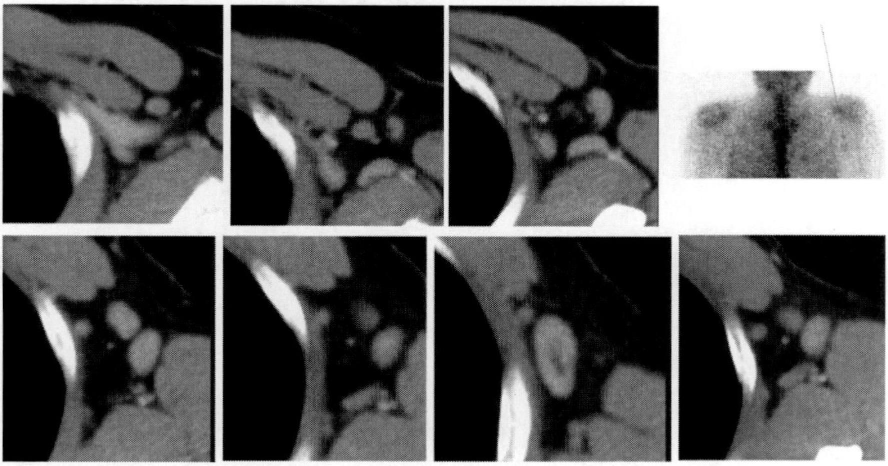

Figure 49. IgG4-related axillary lymphadenopathy in a 38-year-old man. Axial contrast enhanced CT images of the chest reveal multiple enlarged left axillary lymph nodes. Gallium scan shows abnormal uptake in left axillary lymph nodes (arrow).

PET/CT

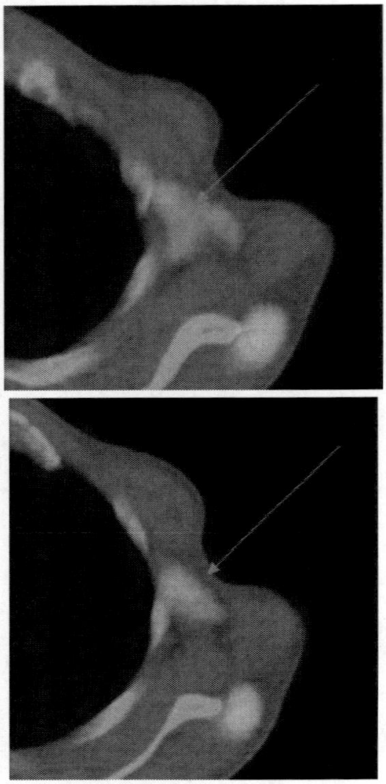

Figure 50. IgG4-related disease in a 66-year-old woman. FDG-PET/CT images show positive lesions in the left axillary lymph nodes (arrows).

IgG4-Related Mastopathy, Mastitis

IgG4-related mastopathy has been reported in case reports and small case series. IgG4-related mammary disorders include IgG4-related mastopathy (IgG4-RM), mastitis, sclerosing mastitis, and inflammatory pseudotumors of the breast (Cheuk W. 2009) (Zen Y. 2005) (Dite P. 2013) (Ogiya A. 2014) (Chougule A. 2015) (Moriya T. H. 2015) (Tan E. S. 2017) (Vitkovski T. 2017). Since no large IgG4-RM case series has been reported, IgG-related mastopathy is very rare (Yokoe T. 2018).

Mammography

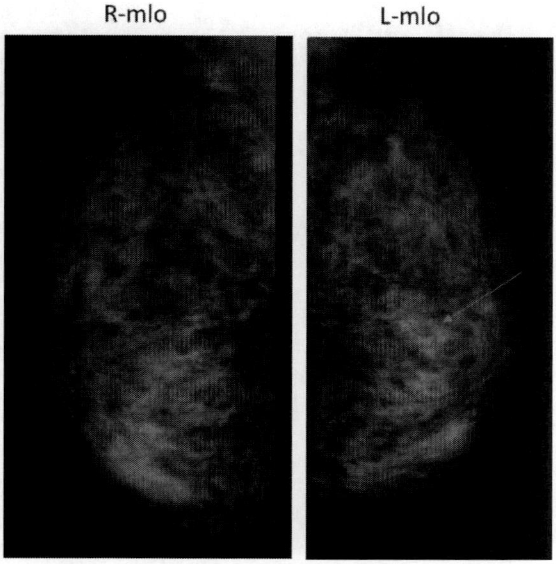

(a)

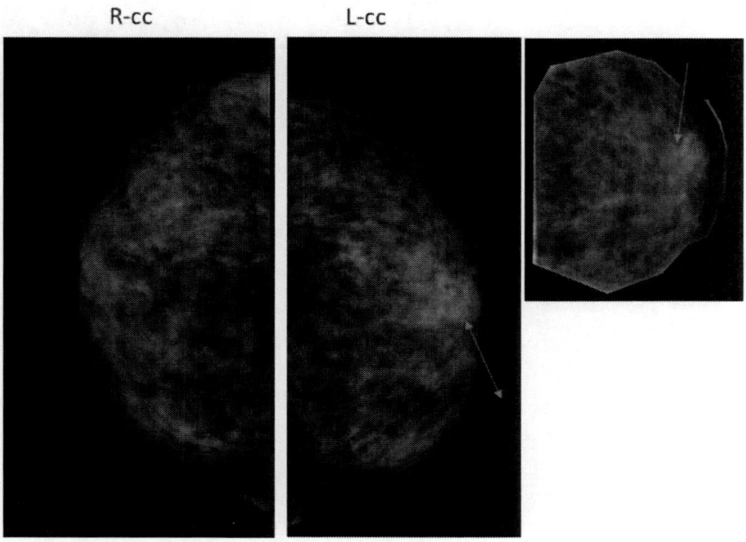

(b)

Figure 51 (a,b). IgG4-related mastopathy. Medio-lateral oblique (MLO) and cranio-caudal (CC) images show tumor-like shadow in the left mammary gland tissues.

CT

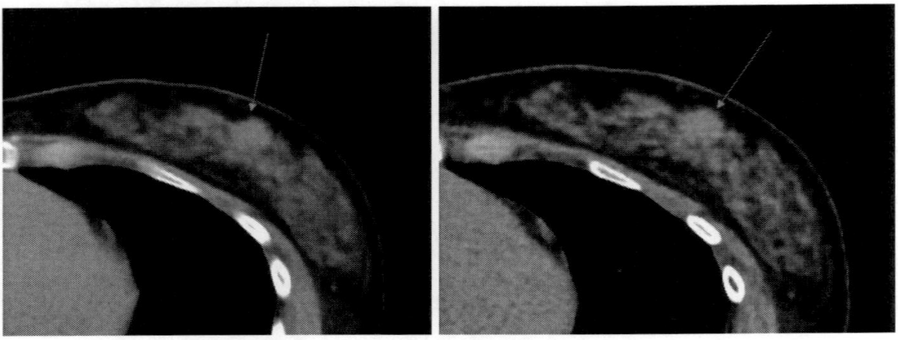

Figure 52. IgG4-related mastopathy in a 44-year-old woman. Non-contrast enhanced chest CT images show a hyperintensity flat nodule in the left mammary gland (arrows).

Ultrasound

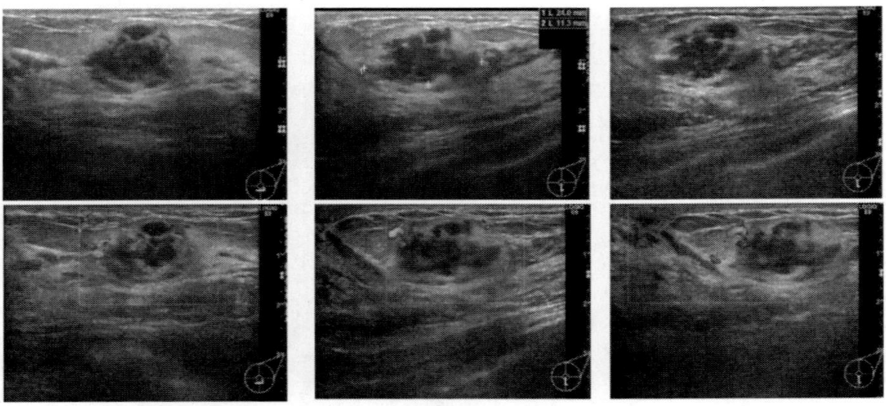

Figure 53. IgG4-related mastopathy in a 44-year-old woman. Breast ultrasound images show an irregular and lobulated hypoechoic nodule (arrows) measuring 19 × 10 × 21 mm large in the left mammary gland.

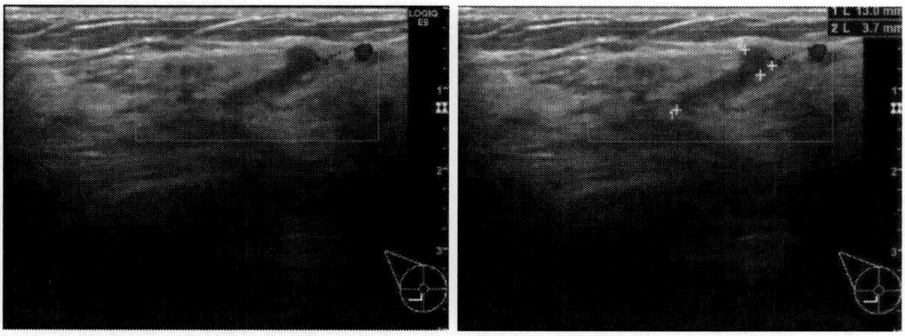

Figure 54. IgG4-related mastopathy in a 44-year-old woman. Breast ultrasound images show a hypoechoic area of about 13 × 4 mm, and a blood flow signal inside.

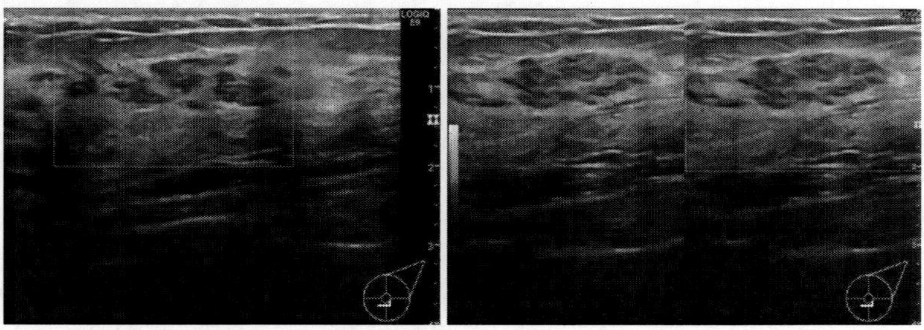

Figure 55. IgG4-related mastopathy in a 46-year-old woman. Breast ultrasound images show irregular and flat hypoechoic nodules in the left mammary gland.

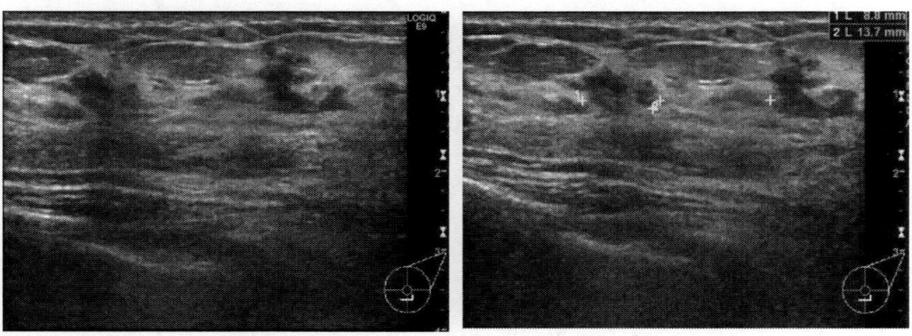

Figure 56. IgG4-related mastopathy in a 44-year-old woman. Breast ultrasound images show two irregular hypoechoic nodules (arrows) in the left mammary gland. There is a 13.7 mm distance between the two nodules.

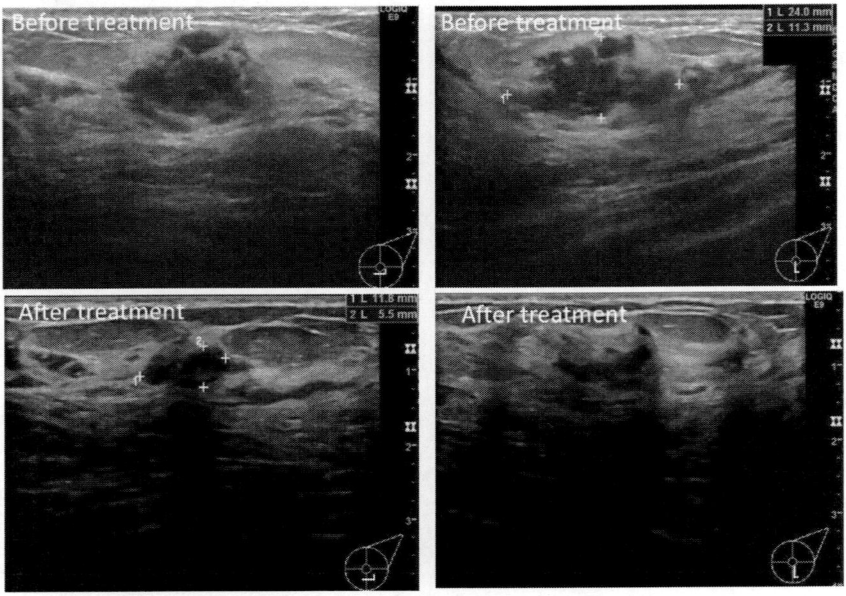

Figure 57. IgG4-related mastitis in a 45-year-old woman. Follow-up ultrasound images obtained before corticosteroid treatment (the upper panels) and 9 months after treatment (the lower panels) show shrinkage of the mass.

Elastography

Elastography may be useful in improving the specificity of US evaluation of breast lesions.

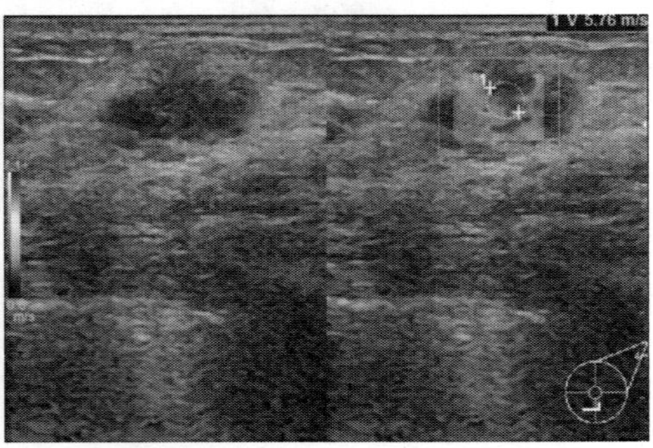

Figure 58. IgG4-related mastopathy in a 44-year-old woman. Elastogram of the left breast demonstrates a stiff mass indicated by the red and yellow color overlay.

Histopathology

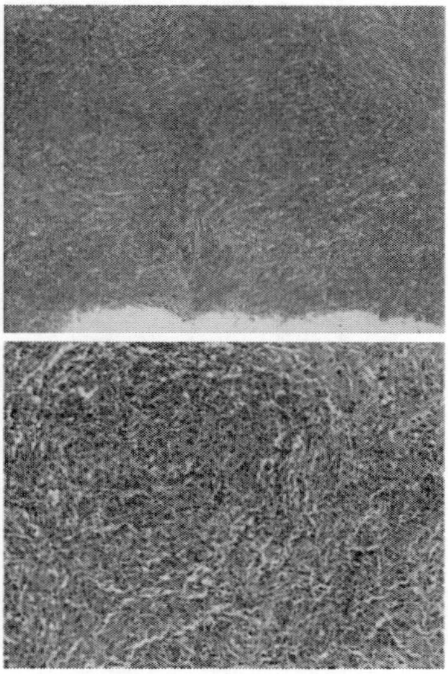

Figure 59. IgG4-related mastitis in a 44-year-old woman. Pathological specimens from the left breast mass by vacuum assisted biopsy. Micrographs of low magnification (left panel) and high magnification (right panel). Specimens are stained with hematoxylin and eosin. Although no epithelial neoplasm is identified, significant lymphoplasmacytic infiltration and fibrosis are observed.

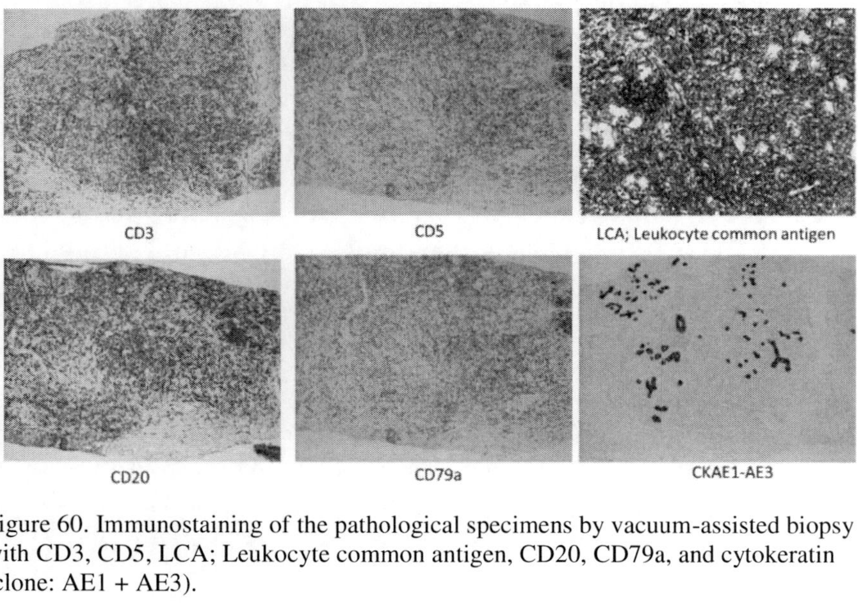

Figure 60. Immunostaining of the pathological specimens by vacuum-assisted biopsy with CD3, CD5, LCA; Leukocyte common antigen, CD20, CD79a, and cytokeratin (clone: AE1 + AE3).

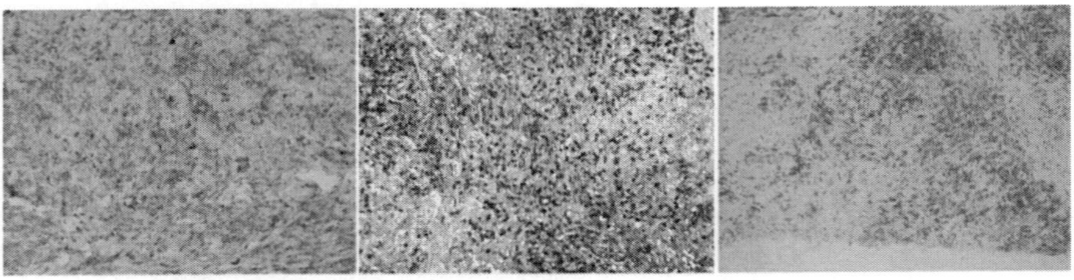

Figure 61. Immunostaining of pathological specimens by vacuum assisted biopsy with IgG, IgG4 and CD138. Infiltration of numerous plasma cells (CD138 positive) is observed. IgG4 is positive on most IgG-positive plasma cells. The tissue IgG4 (+) / IgG (+) cell ratio is over 40%.

REFERENCES

Cheuk W., Chan A. C., Lam W. L., et al., "IgG4-related sclerosing mastitis: s: description of a new member of the IgG4-related sclerosing diseases." *Am J Surg Pathol* 33 (2009): 1058-64.

Chougule A., Bal A., Das A., Singh G. "IgG4 related sclerosing mastitis: expanding the morphological spectrum of IgG4 related diseases." *Pathology.* 2015;47:27-33. 47 (2015): 27-33.

Corcoran J. P., Culver E. L., Anstey R. M., Talwar A., Manganis C. D., Cargill T. N., Hallifax R. J., Psallidas I., Rahman N. M., Barnes E. "Thoracic involvement in IgG4-related disease in a UK-based patient cohort." *Respir Med* 132 (2017): 117-121.

Dite P., Trna J., Kinkor Z., et al., "Unusual multiorgan immunoglobulin G4 (IgG4) inflammation: autoimmune pancreatitis, mikulicz syndrome, and IgG4 mastitis." *Gut Liv* 7 (2013): 621-4.

Inoue D., Zen Y., Abo H. et al., "Immunoglobulin G4-related lung disease: CT findings with pathologic correlations." *Radiology* 251 (2009): 260-270.

Matsui S., Yamamoto H., Minamoto S., et al., "Proposed diagnostic criteria for IgG4-related respiratory disease." *Respir Investig* 54 (2016): 130-2.

Moriya T. H., Nagashima H., Yasuda M., Kimijima I. "IgG4-related disease of the breast: a systemic disease whose mammary manifestations mimic breast cancer." *Int Cancer Conf J* 4 (2015): 67-72.

Ogiya A., Tanaka K., Tadokoro Y., et al., "IgG4-related sclerosing disease of the breast successfully treated by steroid therapy." *Breast cance* 21 (2014): 231-5.

Patel M., Kumar B., Diep M. L., Nandurkar D. "IgG4 Related Lung Disease." *Canadian Respiratory Journal* 2016 (2011): 1-3.

Takato H. M., Ichikawa Y., et al., Yasui. "Nonspecific interstitial pneumonia with abundant IgG4-positive cells infiltration, which was thought as pulmonary involvement of IgG4-related autoimmune disease." *Intern Med* 47 [2008]: 291-294.

Takato H., Yasui M., Ichikawa Y., et al., "Nonspecific interstitial pneumonia with abundant IgG4-positive cells infiltration, which was thought as pulmonary involvement of IgG4-related autoimmune disease." *Intern Med* 47 (2008): 291-294.

Tan E. S., Friesen B., Loh S. F., Fox J. "Immunoglobulin-G4 related mastitis: a case report." *Int J Surg Case Rep* 37 (2017): 169-72.

Tan E. S., Friesen B., Loh S. F., Fox J. "Immunoglobulin-G4 related mastitis: a case report." *Int J Surg Case Rep* 37 (2017): 169-72.

Vitkovski T. G. S, Filardi D. A., Gupta E., Breuer F. Marder. "IgG4-related sclerosing disease of the breast in a male patient." *Int J Surg Pathol* 25 [2017]: 711-5.

Vitkovski T., Marder G. S., Filardi D. A., Gupta E., Breuer F. "IgG4-related sclerosing disease of the breast in a male patient." *Int J Surg Pathol* 25 (2017): 711-5.

Yokoe T. T., Kikuchi M., et al., "IgG4-related mastopathy: A case report and literature review." *Clin Case Rep* 6 [2018]: 1549-1553.

Yokoe T., Hayashida T., Kikuchi M., et al., "IgG4-related mastopathy: A case report and literature review." *Clin Case Rep* 6 (2018): 1549-1553.

Zen Y., Inoue D., Kitao A. et al., “IgG4-related lung and pleural disease: a clinicopathologic study of 21 cases.” *Am J Surg Pathol* 33 (2009): 1886-1893.

Zen Y., Kasahara Y., Horita K., et al., “Inflammatory pseudotumor of the breast in a patient with a high serum IgG4 level: histologic similarity to sclerosing pancreatitis.” *Am J Surg Pathol* 29 (2005): 275-8.

In: IgG4 Related Disease
Editor: Syuichi Koarada

ISBN: 978-1-53618-050-3

Chapter 4

IgG4-Related Disease in Urinary Tract, IgG4-Related Retroperitoneal Fibrosis and Related Disorders

Syuichi Koarada[1,]* and Yukiko Takeyama[1]
[1]Division of Rheumatology, Faculty of Medicine,
Saga University, Nabeshima, Saga, Japan

Abstract

Urinary tract lesions of IgG4-related disease are variable. Often it takes the form of retroperitoneal fibrosis. Urinary tract lesions can include hydronephrosis and renal failure due to ureteral thickening and obstruction. It can also involve the prostate. Renal lesions are also variable, with diffuse lesions, patchy/wedge-shaped lesions, perirenal rim lesions, nodular lesions of the renal sinus, and wall thickening of the renal pelvis.

---

* Corresponding Author's Email: koarada@cc.saga-u.ac.jp.

In retroperitoneal fibrosis, urinary tract and vascular lesions, and spinal/sacral soft tissue lesions can coexist, but they also exist as single lesion. Urinary tract lesions are easier to understand if they are separated from vascular and musculoskeletal lesions.

There are rare cases of glomerular lesions and membranous nephropathy.

INTRODUCTION

Retroperitoneal fibrosis is one of the most common subsets of IgG4-related disease.

IgG4-related retroperitoneal fibrosis is detected by CT, MRI, and other imaging as lesions in around the ureter, around the aorta, near the vertebral body, in the pelvic cavity, and around the superior mesenteric artery.

In IgG4-related disease, blood vessels (aorta and other blood vessels) and ureters are involved in the retroperitoneal legions by the growth of soft tissue with infiltration of inflammatory cells and fibrosis. Clinically, patients present with pain, inflammatory abdominal aortic aneurysm, hydronephrosis, and postrenal failure (Kawano M 2016) (Hamano H. 2002).

Serum IgG4 levels are elevated in many patients with IgG4-related retroperitoneal fibrosis.

RETROPERITONEAL FIBROSIS

In IgG4-related retroperitoneal fibrosis, CT and MRI findings show thickening or mass of soft tissue surrounding the aorta and the ureter.

Retrograde Pyelography of the Left Ureter:

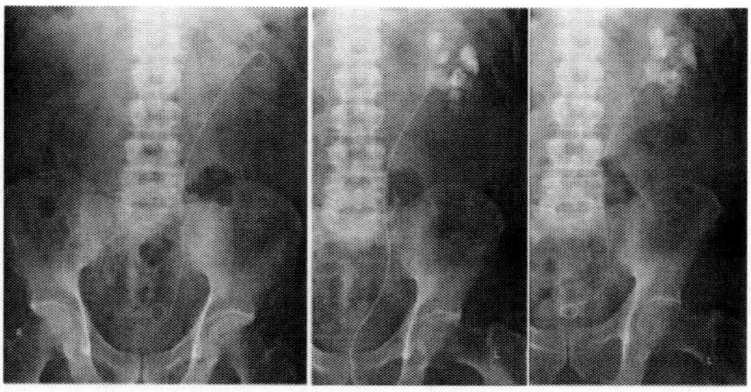

Figure 1. IgG4-related retroperitoneal fibrosis in a 67-year-old man. Retrograde pyelography of the left ureter shows hydronephrosis of the left kidney.

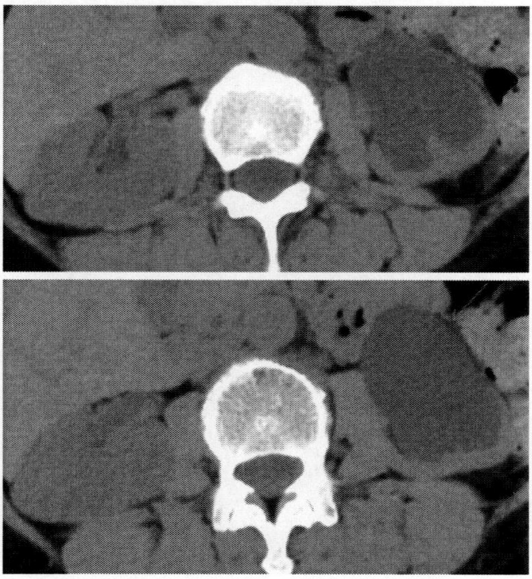

Figure 2. IgG4-related retroperitoneal fibrosis in a 49-year-old woman. Axial non-contrast enhanced abdominal CT images show severe left hydroureteronephrosis (arrows).

CT

Non-Contras Enhanced Abdominal CT (NCECT)

In cross-section imaging of CT, IgG4-related retroperitoneal fibrosis appears as soft tissue masses covering the abdominal aorta and its branches, and/or surrounding the ureters, causing hydronephrosis and hydroureter.

Axial Images

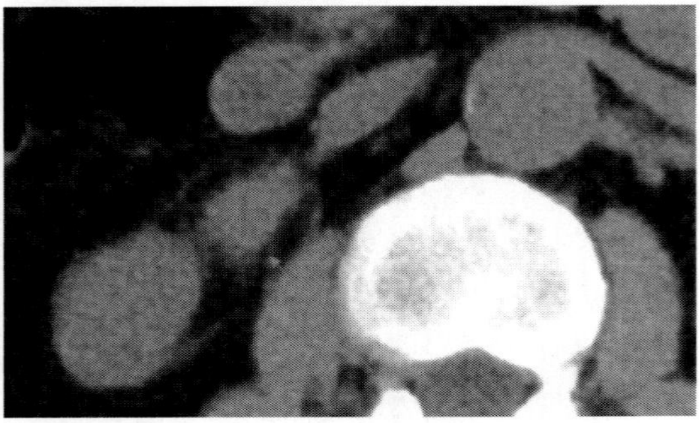

Figure 3. IgG4-related retroperitoneal fibrosis in a 67-year-old man. Axial non-contrast enhanced abdominal CT image shows a soft tissue mass suggesting thickening of the proximal right ureter wall at the ureteropelvic junction (UPJ) (arrow).

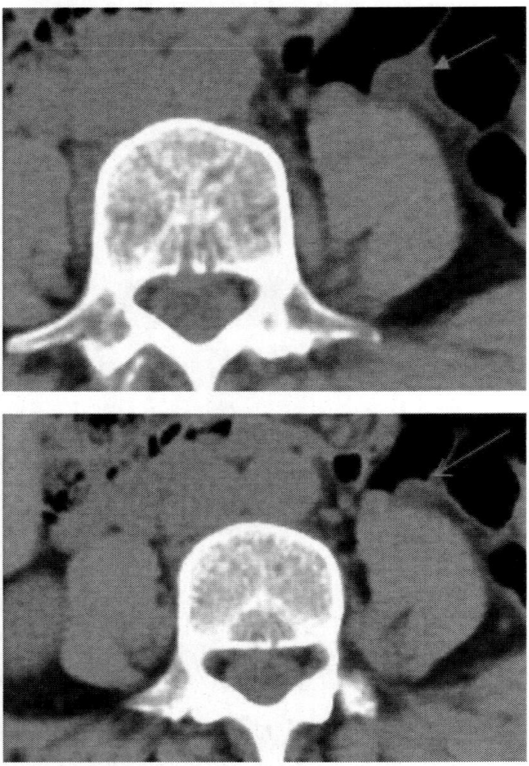

Figure 4. IgG4-related retroperitoneal fibrosis in a 59-year-old woman. Axial non-contrast enhanced abdominal CT images show the left hydroureter (arrow).

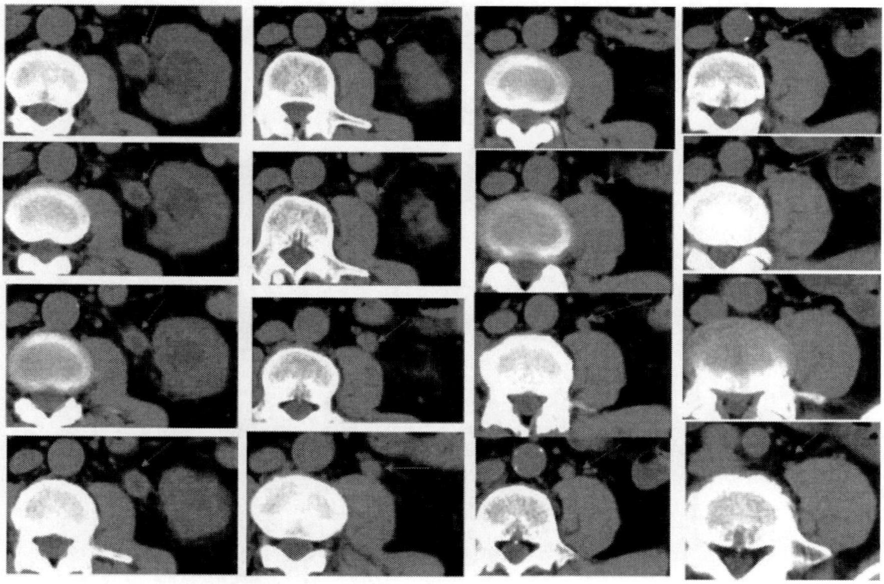

Figure 5. IgG4-related retroperitoneal fibrosis in a 67-year-old man. The non-contrast enhanced abdominal CT images show thickening of the wall from the left renal pelvis and the proximal ureter to middle part of the ureter (arrows).

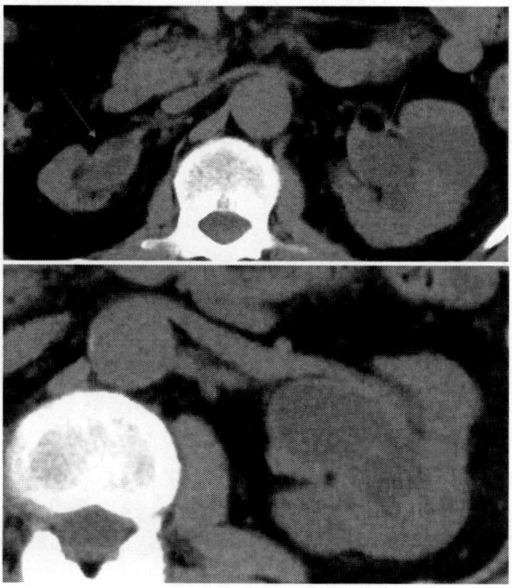

Figure 6. IgG4-related retroperitoneal fibrosis in a 67-year-old man. Non-contrast enhanced abdominal CT images show tissue swelling with hydronephrosis (arrows) and atrophy of the right kidney.

Contrast Enhanced Abdominal CT

Axial Images

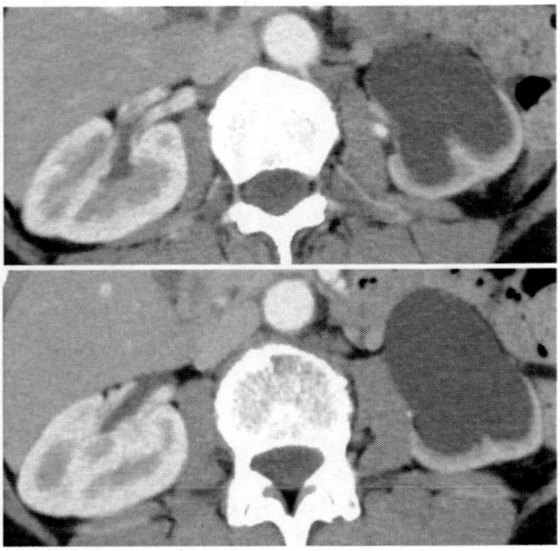

Figure 7. IgG4-related retroperitoneal fibrosis in a 49-year-old woman. Axial contrast enhanced abdominal CT images show severe left hydroureteronephrosis.

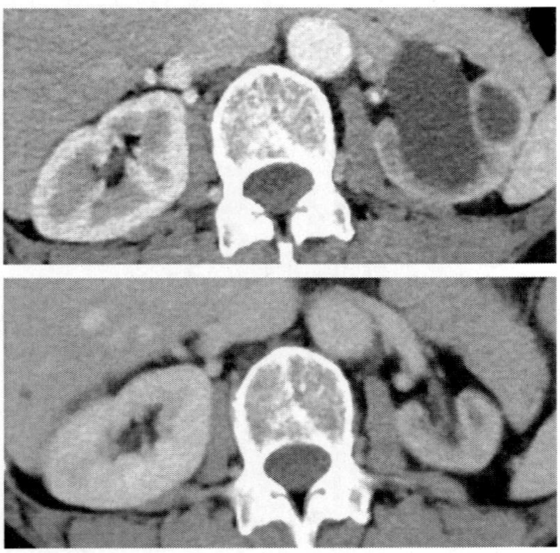

Figure 8. IgG4-related retroperitoneal fibrosis in a 55-year-old woman. Axial contrast enhanced abdominal CT images obtained before corticosteroid treatment (the upper panel) and after the therapy (the lower panel) show resolution of hydronephrosis and remarked atrophy of the left kidney.

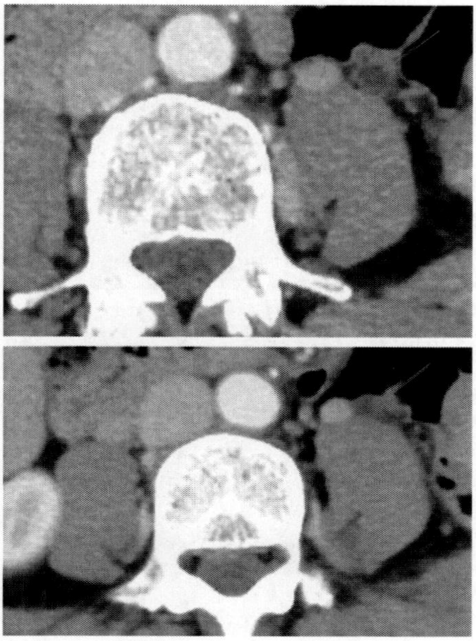

Figure 9. IgG4-related retroperitoneal fibrosis in a 59-year-old woman. Axial contrast enhanced abdominal CT images show the left hydroureter (arrows).

MRI

T1-Weighted MR Images

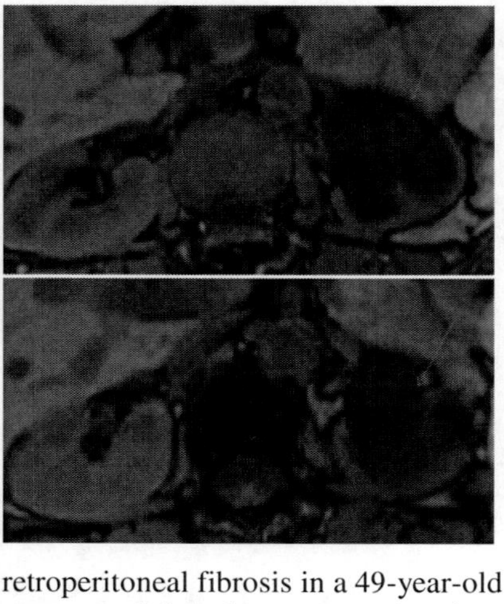

Figure 10. IgG4-related retroperitoneal fibrosis in a 49-year-old woman. Axial T1-weighted MR images show severe left hydroureteronephrosis (arrows).

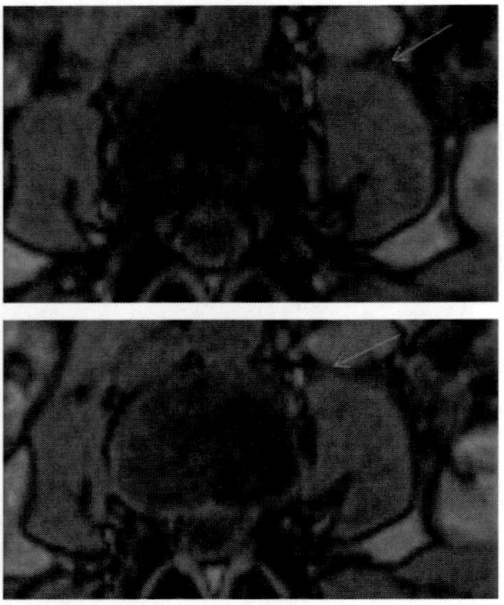

Figure 11. IgG4-related retroperitoneal fibrosis in a 49-year-old woman. Axial T1-weighted MR images show left hydroureter (arrows). However, the lesion has low signal intensity and is difficult to distinguish from surrounding tissues.

T2-Weighted MR Images

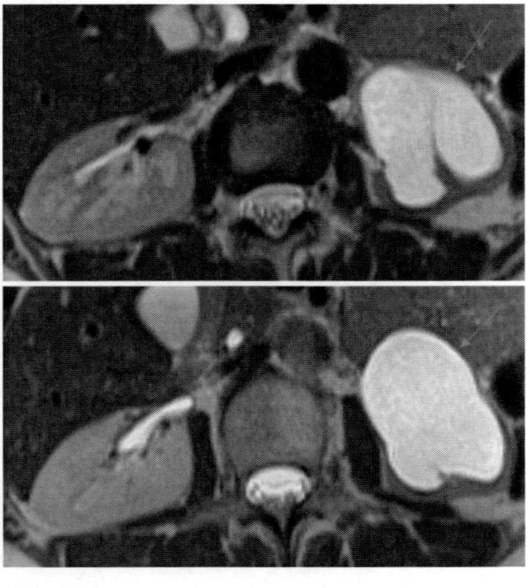

Figure 12. IgG4-related retroperitoneal fibrosis in a 49-year-old woman. Axial T2-weighted MR images show severe left hydronephrosis (arrows).

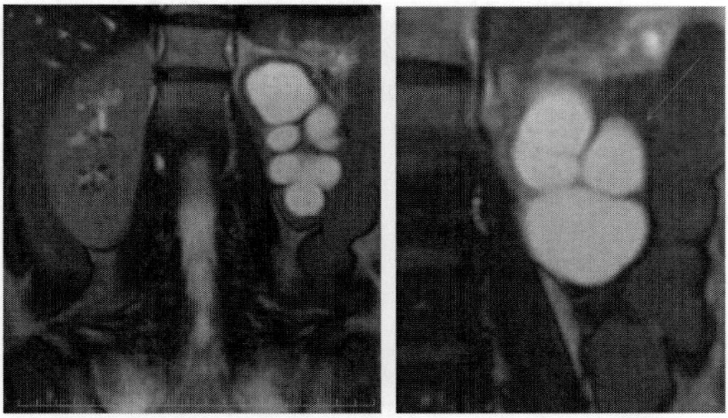

Figure 13. IgG4-related retroperitoneal fibrosis in a 49-year-old woman. Coronal T2-weighted MR images show severe left hydronephrosis (arrows).

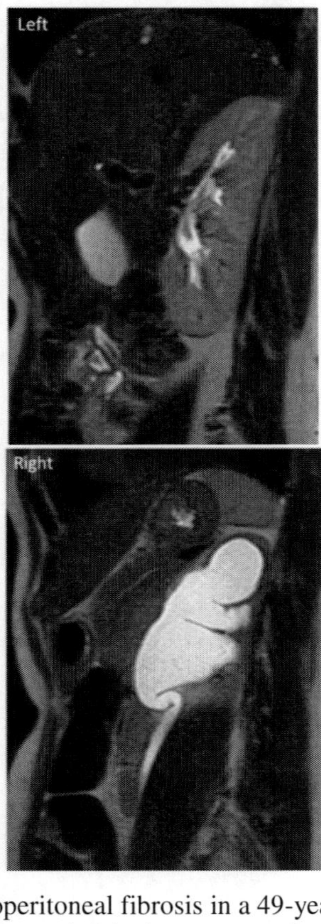

Figure 14. IgG4-related retroperitoneal fibrosis in a 49-year-old woman. Sagittal T2-weighted MR images show severe left hydroureteronephrosis. The right kidney is normal.

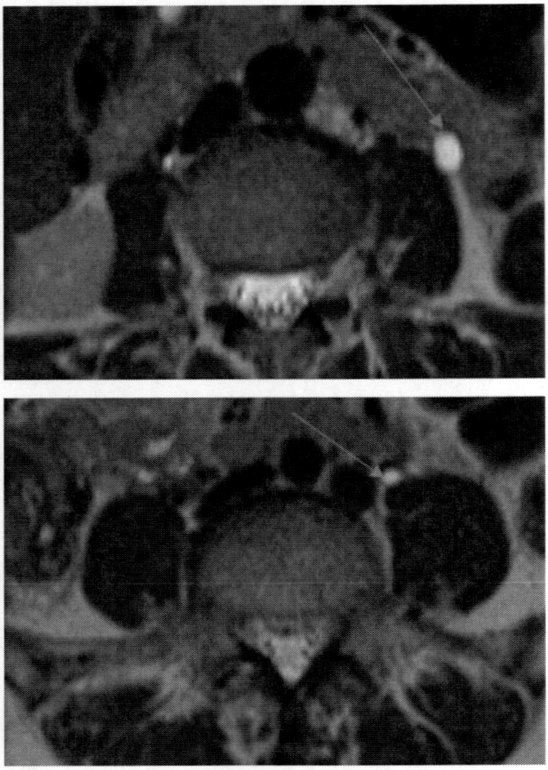

Figure 15. IgG4-related retroperitoneal fibrosis in a 49-year-old woman. Axial T2-weighted MR images show left hydroureter (arrows).

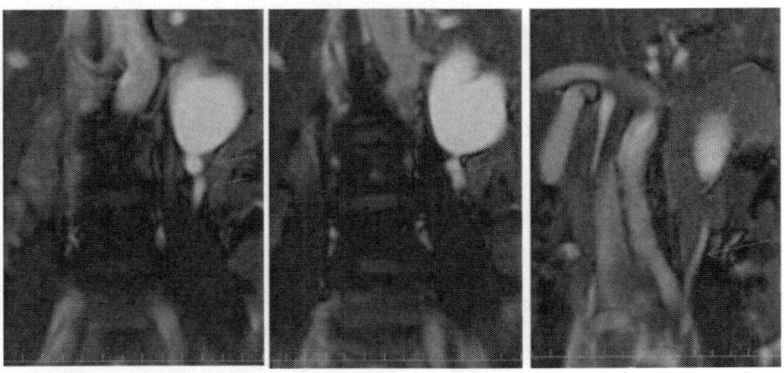

Figure 16. IgG4-related retroperitoneal fibrosis in a 49-year-old woman. Coronal T2-weighted MR images show left hydroureter (arrows).

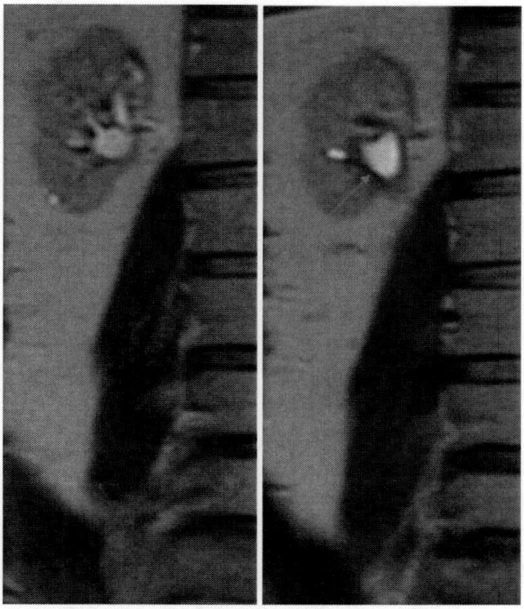

Figure 17. IgG4-related retroperitoneal fibrosis in a 67-year-old man. Coronal T2-weighted MR images through the right renal pelvis show mild hydronephrosis (arrow) and atrophy of the right kidney.

Diffusion-Weighted MR Images

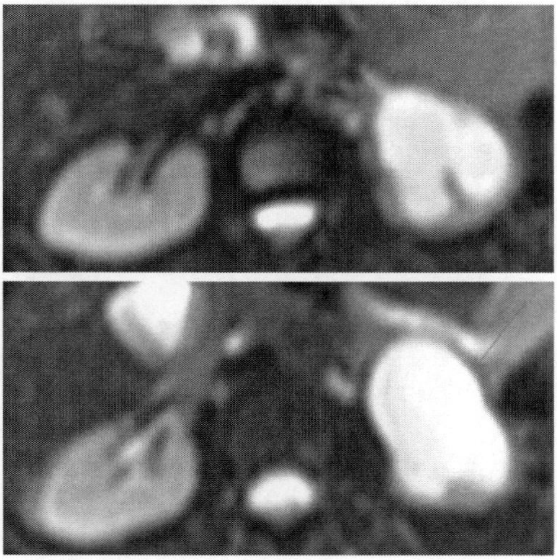

Figure 18. IgG4-related retroperitoneal fibrosis in a 49-year-old woman. Axial diffusion-weighted MR images show severe left hydronephrosis (arrows).

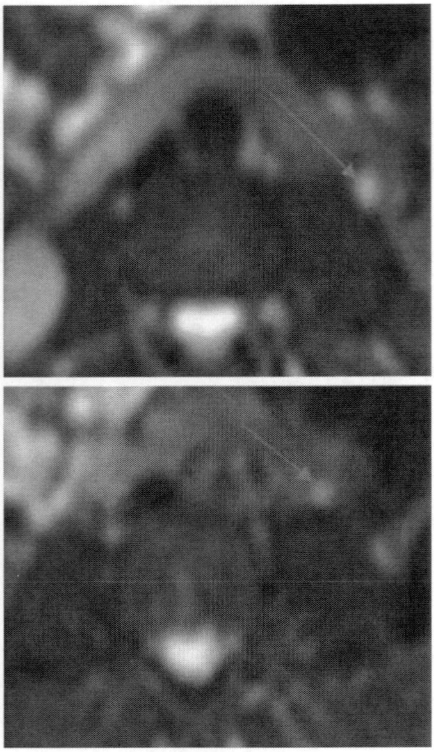

Figure 19. IgG4-related retroperitoneal fibrosis in a 49-year-old woman. Axial diffusion-weighted MR images show left hydroureter (arrows).

MRCP

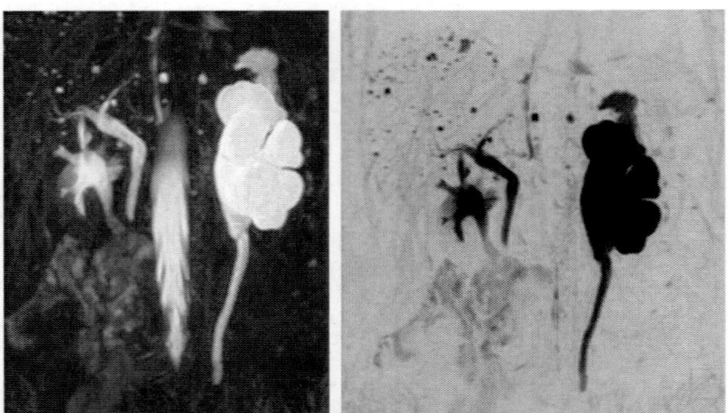

Figure 20. IgG4-related disease in a 49-year-old woman. MR cholangiopancreatographic (MRCP) images show severe left hydroureteronephrosis.

Gadolinium-Enhanced T1-Weighted MR Imaging

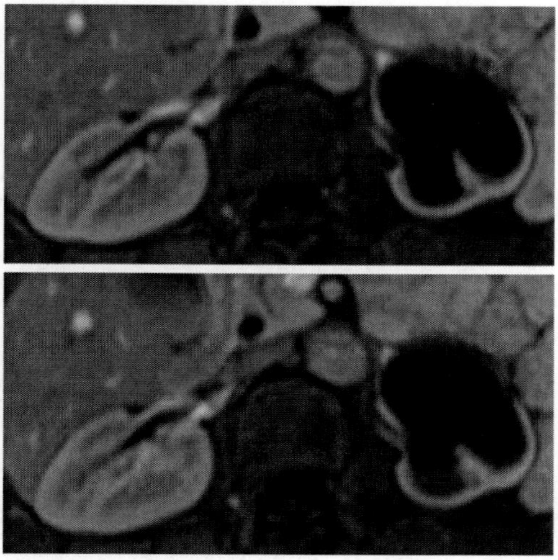

Figure 21. IgG4-related retroperitoneal fibrosis in a 49-year-old woman. Axial gadolinium-enhanced T1-weighted MR images of the abdomen show severe left hydronephrosis.

Gallium Scan

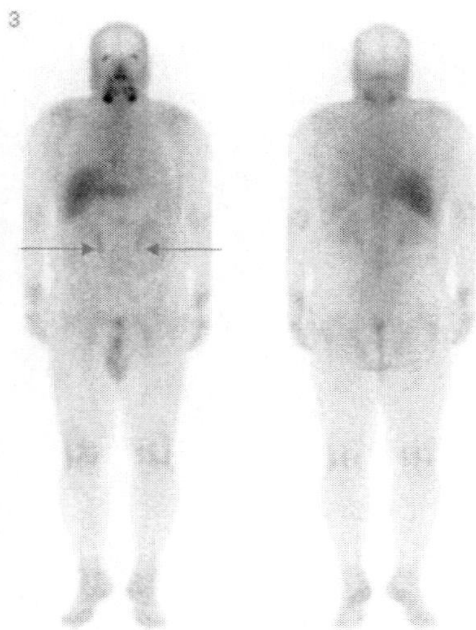

Figure 22. IgG4-related retroperitoneal fibrosis in a 66-year-old man. Gallium scan shows abnormal uptake of bilateral periureteral tissue.

FDG-PET/CT

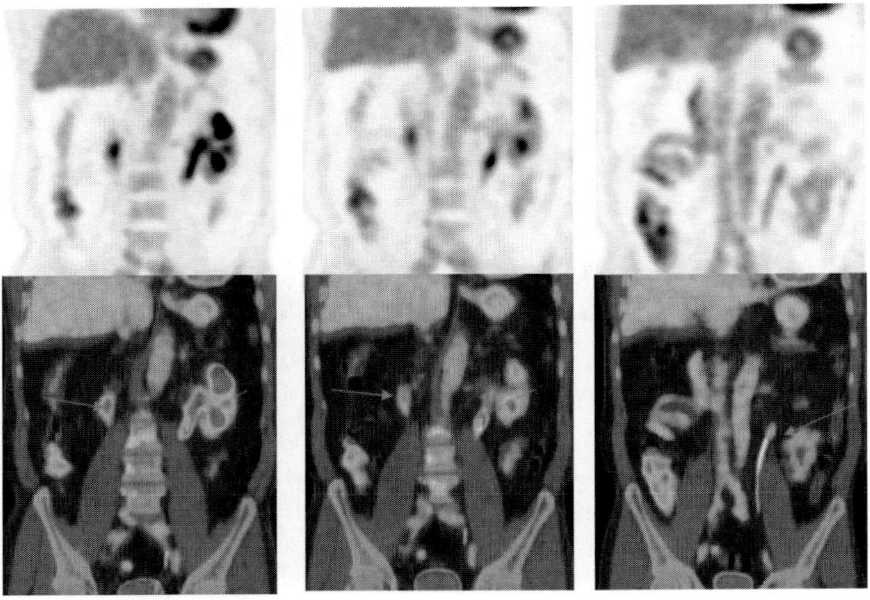

Figure 23. IgG4-related retroperitoneal fibrosis in a 67-year-old man. Coronal FDG-PET/CT images show positive lesions of bilateral periureteral tissue.

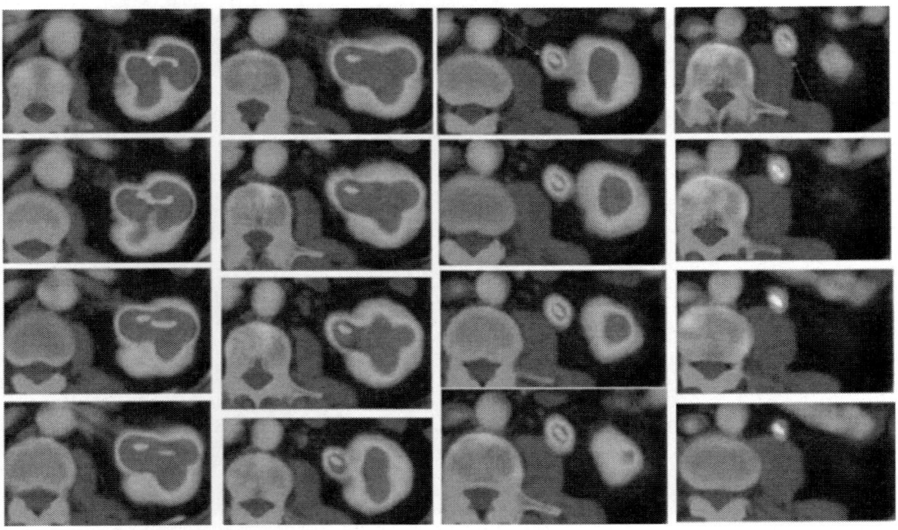

Figure 24. IgG4-related retroperitoneal fibrosis in a 67-year-old man. Axial FDG-PET/CT images show positive lesions of the left periureteral tissue.

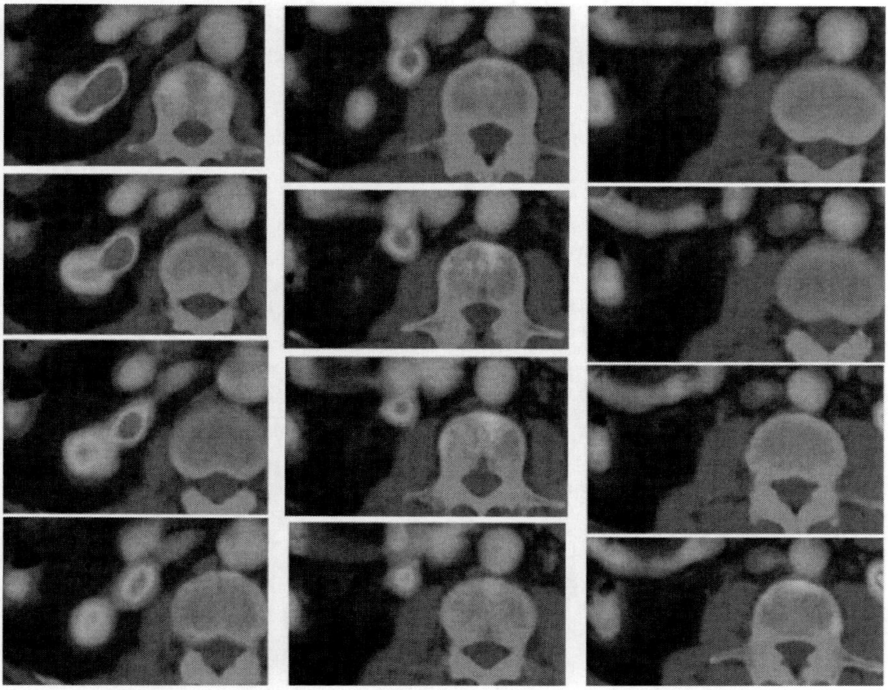

Figure 25. IgG4-related retroperitoneal fibrosis in a 67-year-old man. Axial FDG-PET/CT images show positive lesions of the right periureteral tissue.

Treatment

Hydronephrosis and irreversible renal failure may be caused by a periureteral mass, and usually responds well to corticosteroid treatment.

IgG4-Related Prostate Disease

Patients diagnosed with benign prostatic hyperplasia (BPH) may have IgG4-related disease, but their frequency is unknown. Usually, a prostate lesion is accidentally noticed while searching for other systemic IgG4-related disease.

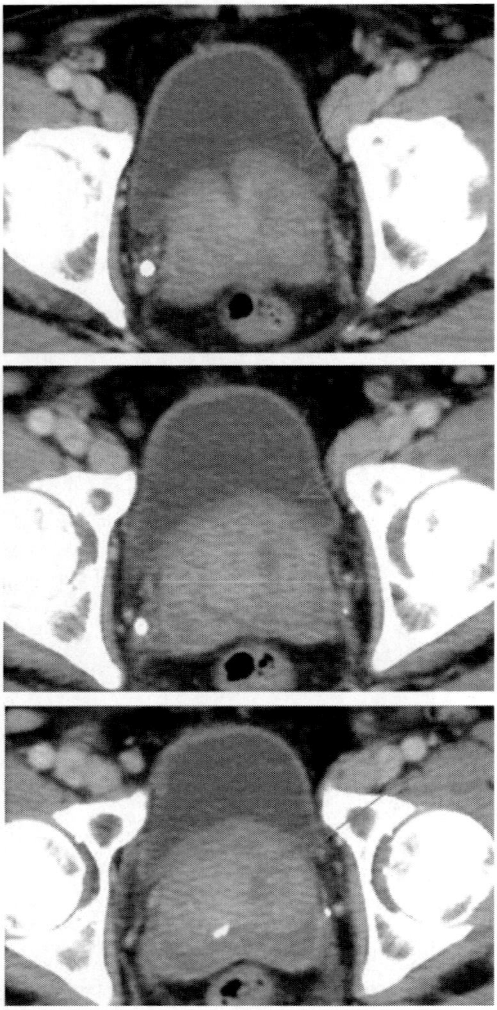

Figure 26. IgG4-related prostate disease in a 73-year-old man. Axial contrast enhanced abdominal CT images show enlarged prostate (arrows).

A male patient with an IgG4-related disease who has dysuria and accumulation by 18F-fiuorodeoxyglucose (18-FDG) positron emission tomography (PET) or 67Ga scan is suspected to be an IgG4-Related Prostate Disease.

The age of onset of IgG4-related prostate lesions is relatively old and it needs to be differentiated from prostate cancer.

IgG4-Related Renal Disease

IgG4-related renal disease is characterized by tubulointerstitial nephritis and/or membranous glomerulonephritis. In some patients, renal damage may be the first symptom of IgG4-RD.

Most patients are diagnosed on the basis of imaging studies and have only minor urinary dysfunction, but some patients may develop acute or progressive renal failure (Saeki T 2010) (Kawano M 2016) (Mizushima I 2016).

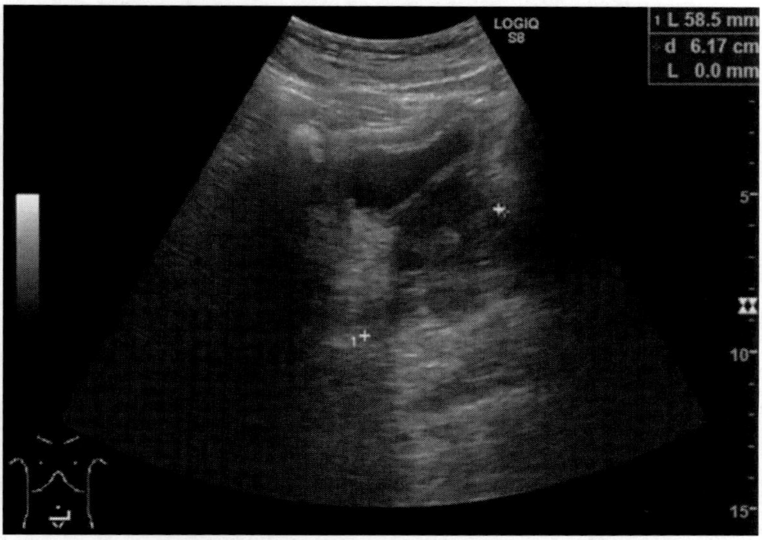

Figure 27. IgG4-related prostate disease in a 73-year-old man. Transverse ultrasound image shows enlarged prostate.

Five patterns of IgG4-related kidney disease have been reported: diffuse patchy lesions, a rim of soft tissue swelling around the kidney, most common in multifocal round or wedge-shaped peripheral cortical lesions, bilateral nodules in the renal sinuses and diffuse wall thickening of the renal pelvis.

Imaging of Renal Lesions

Diffuse Patchy Lesions

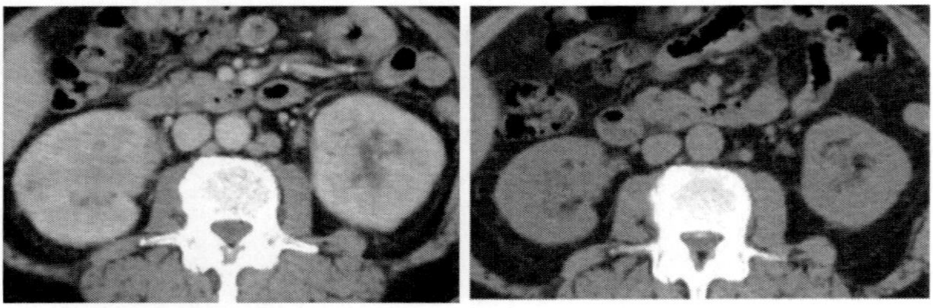

Figure 28. IgG4-related disease in a 72-year-old man. Axis abdominal CT images indicate that the renal parenchyma is generally swollen. There is no defined standard for kidney size of IgG4-related kidney disease.

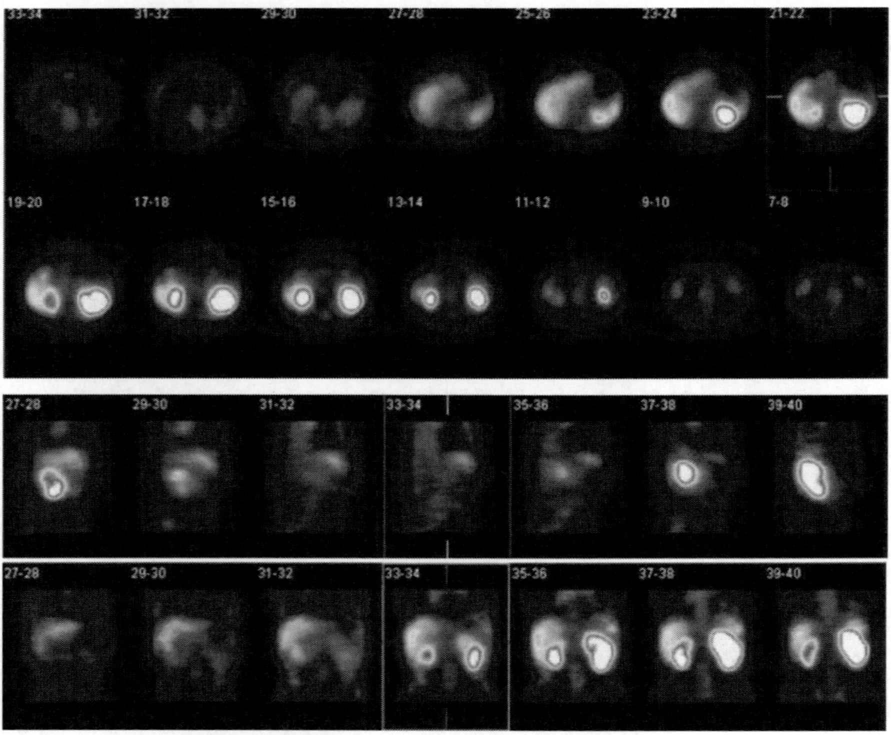

Figure 29 (Continued).

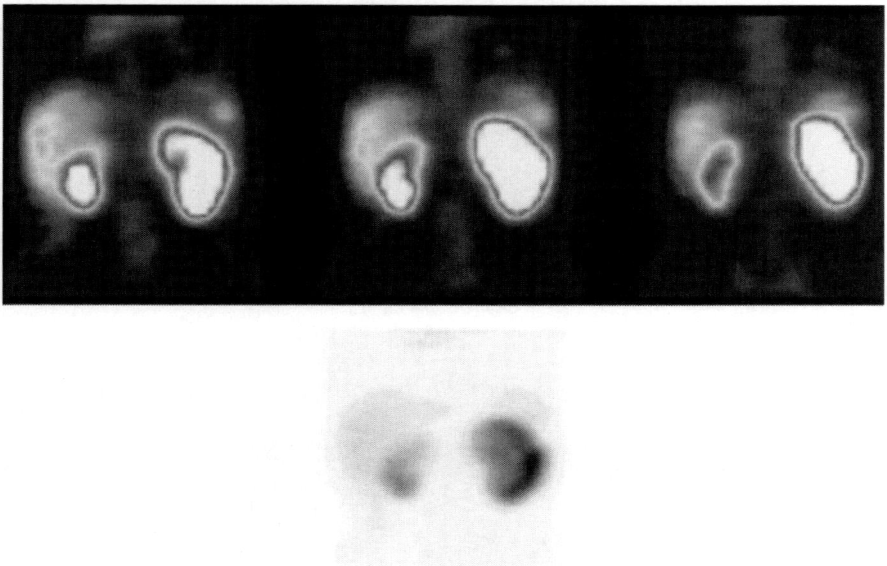

Figure 29. IgG4-related renal disease in a 64-year-old man. Axial (the upper panel), sagittal (the middle panel), and coronal gallium scan (the lower panel) show abnormal uptake in the left kidney.

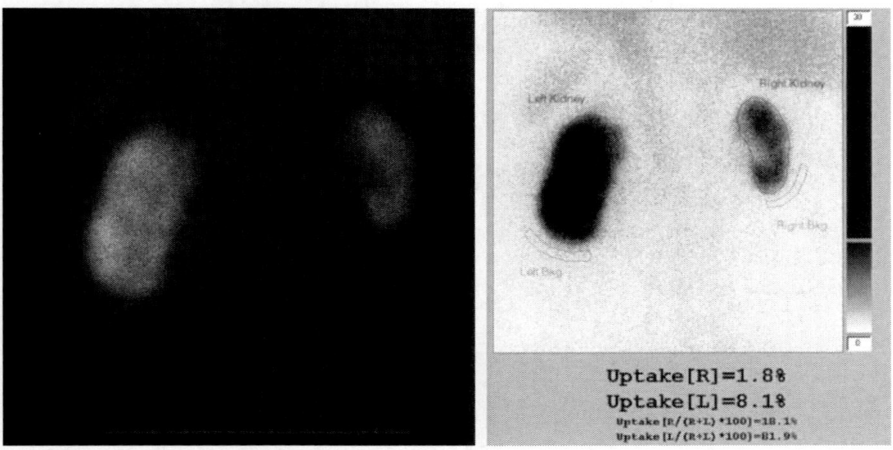

RI uptake.

Right kidney = 1.8%.

Left kidney = 8.1%.

Figure 30. 99mTc- DMSA renal scintigraphy (the left panel) shows atrophy of the right kidney. Moreover, renal scintigram (the right panel) shows reduced uptake on the right kidney. The left kidney has normal uptake.

Rims of Soft Tissue Swelling around the Kidney

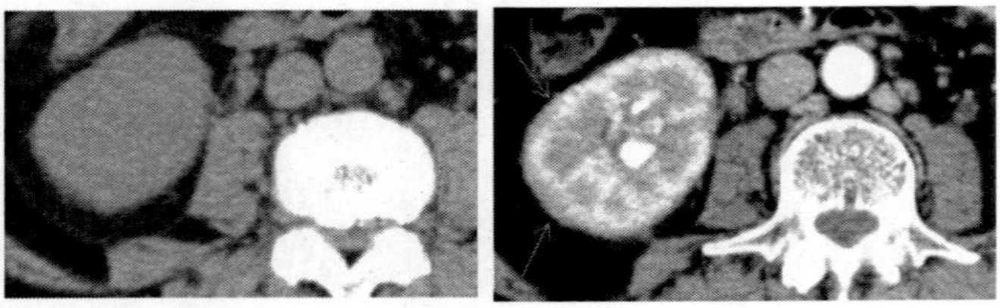

Figure 31. IgG4-related disease in a 72-year-old man. Axial abdominal NCECT and CECT images show rims of soft tissue swelling around the right kidney.

Multifocal Round or Wedge-Shaped Peripheral Cortical Lesions

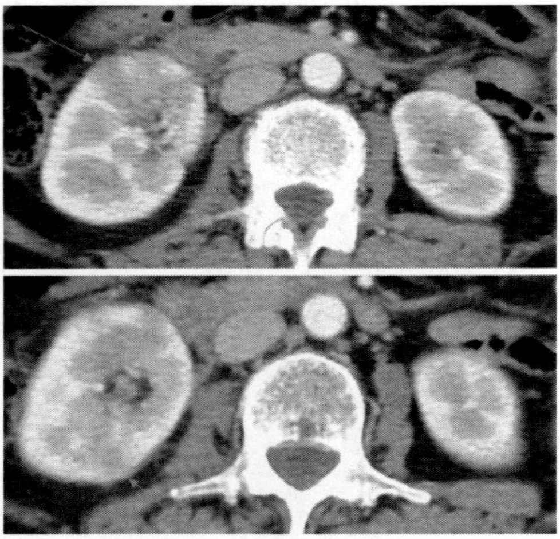

Figure 32. IgG4-related renal disease in a 76-year-old woman. Axial contrast enhanced corticomedullary phase CT images show multiple well-defined, wedge-shaped, low-attenuation lesions in the right kidney (arrows).

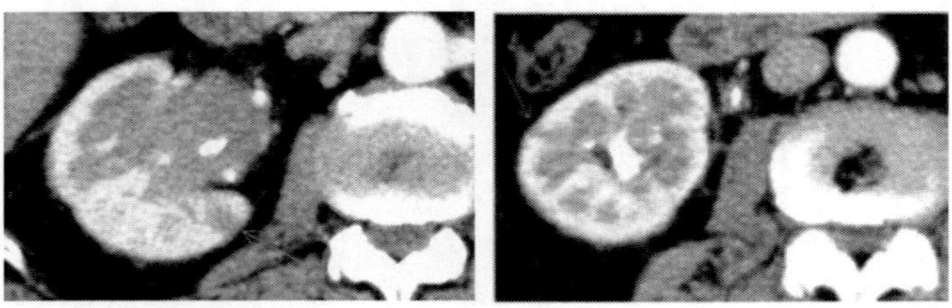

Figure 33. IgG4-related renal disease (multifocal type) in a 72-year-old man. Axial contrast enhanced corticomedullary phase CT images show multiple well-defined, wedge-shaped, low-attenuation lesions in the kidney (arrows).

Bilateral Nodules/Masses in the Renal Sinuses

CT

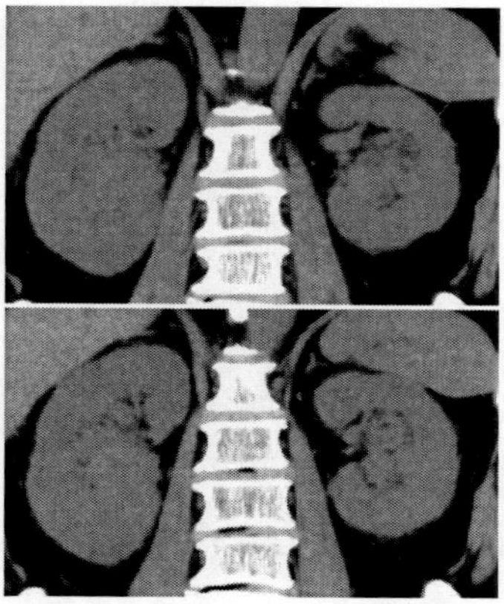

Figure 34. IgG4-related renal disease in a 72-year-old man. Coronal non-contrast enhanced abdominal CT images show bilateral masses of the renal sinuses (arrows).

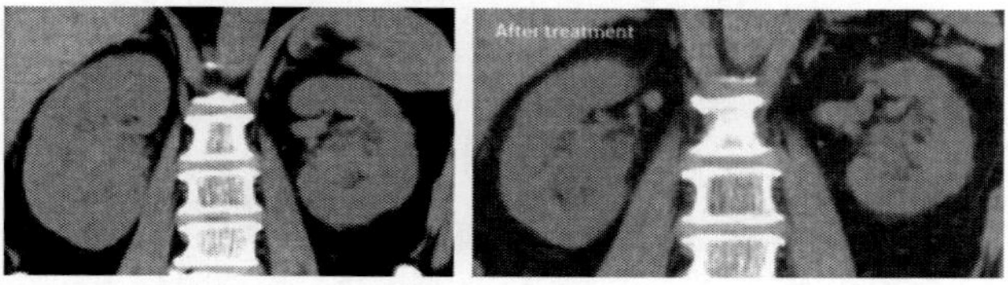

Figure 35. IgG4-related renal disease in a 72-year-old man. Non-contrast enhanced abdominal CT images show large masses in bilateral renal sinuses and slight improvement after treatment.

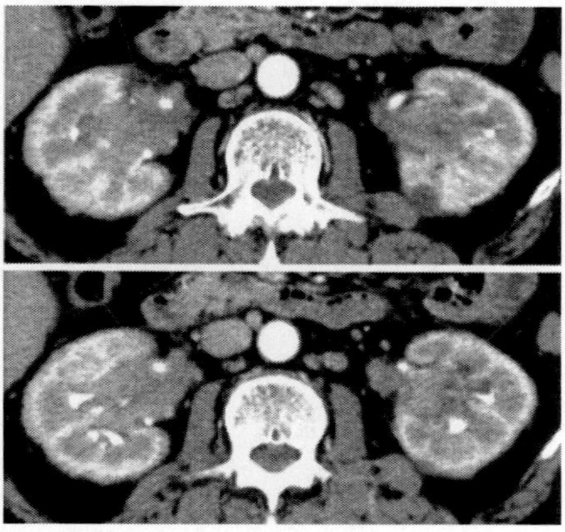

Figure 36. IgG4-related renal disease in a 73-year-old man. Axial contrast enhanced abdominal CT images show bilateral masses of the renal sinuses (arrows).

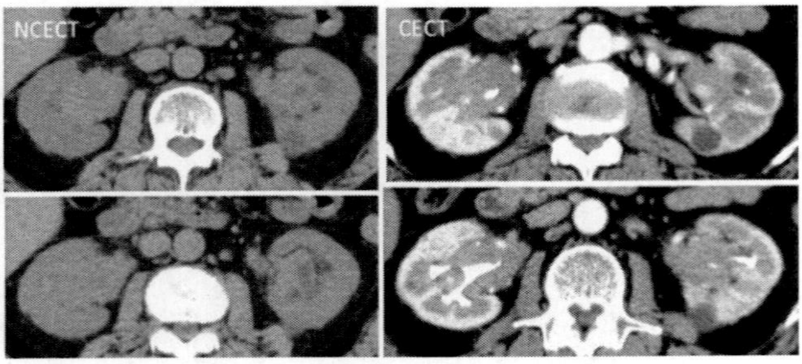

Figure 37. IgG4-related renal disease in a 73-year-old man. The panels show a comparison of NCECT and CECT of the renal sinuses.

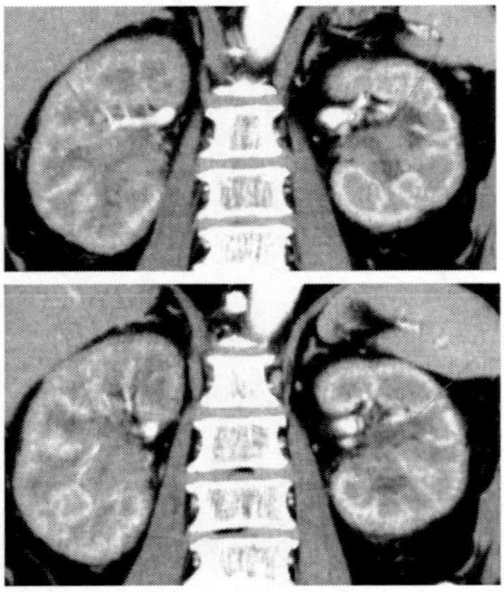

Figure 38. IgG4-related disease in a 72-year-old man. Coronal contrast enhanced abdominal CT images show bilateral masses of the renal sinuses (arrows).

MRI

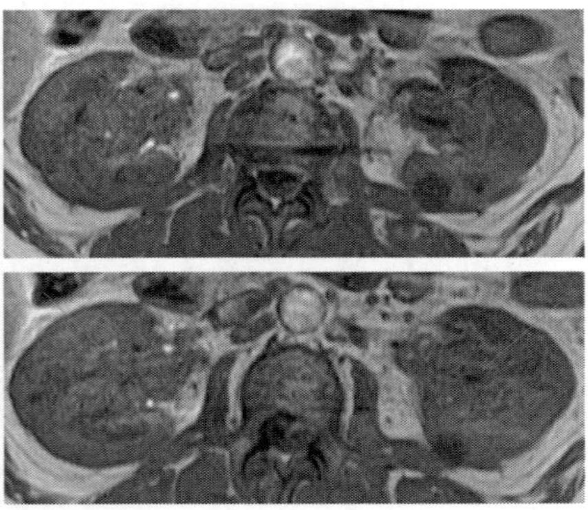

Figure 39. IgG4-related renal disease in a 73-year-old man. Axial T1-weighted MR images show bilateral masses of the renal sinuses (arrows).

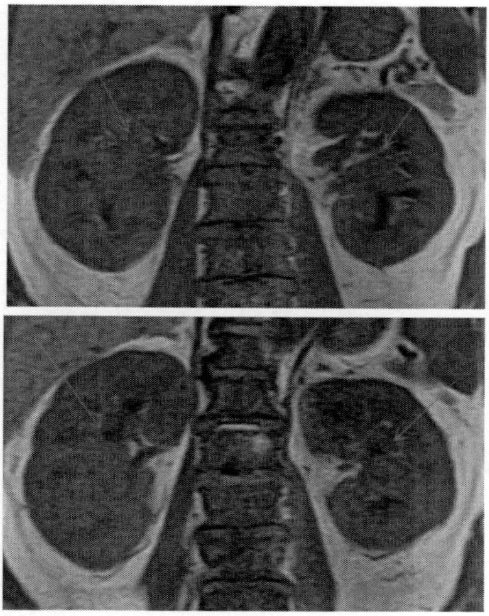

Figure 40. IgG4-related renal disease in a 73-year-old man. Coronal T1-weighted MR images show bilateral masses of the renal sinuses (arrows).

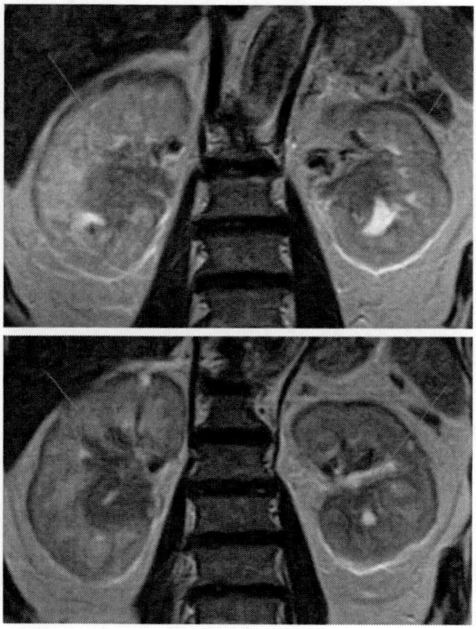

Figure 41. IgG4-related renal disease in a 73-year-old man. Coronal T2-weighted MR images of the abdomen show bilateral masses of the renal sinuses (arrows).

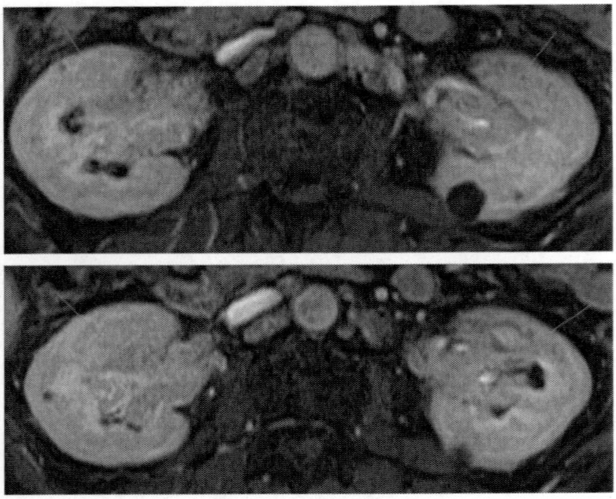

Figure 42. IgG4-related renal disease in a 73-year-old man. Axial gadolinium-enhanced T1-weighted MR images of the abdomen show bilateral masses of the renal sinuses (arrows).

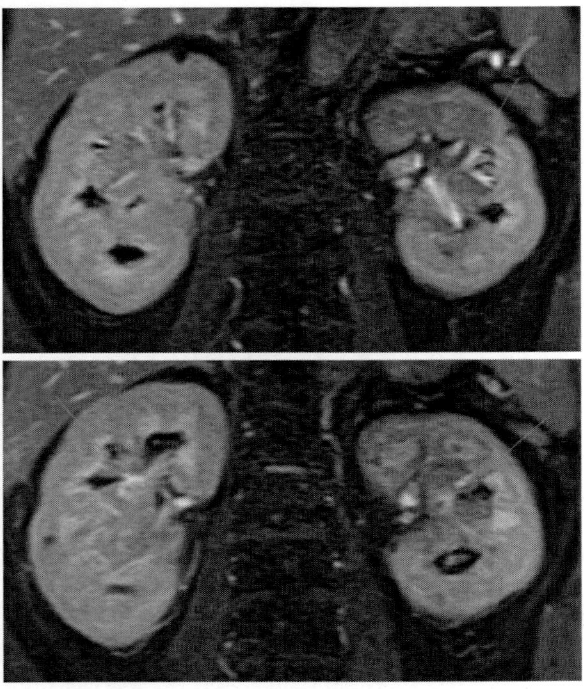

Figure 43. IgG4-related renal disease in a 73-year-old man. Coronal gadolinium-enhanced T1-weighted MR images of the abdomen show bilateral masses of the renal sinuses (arrows).

Ultrasound Imaging

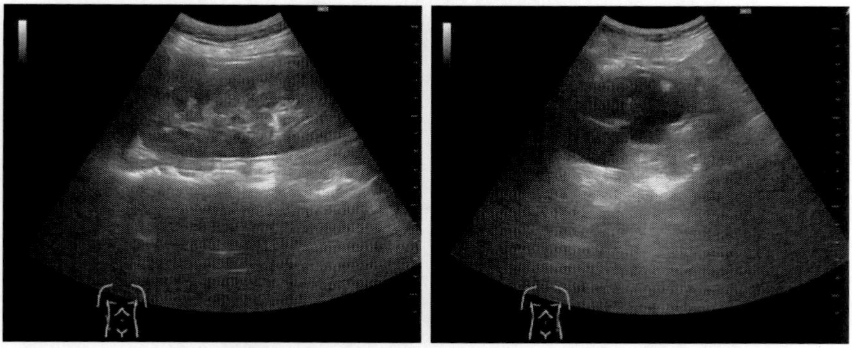

Figure 44. IgG4-related renal disease in a 55-year-old woman. The longitudinal ultrasound image of the right kidney (left panel) shows that parenchyma is normal in thickness. The longitudinal ultrasound image of the left kidney shows a large hypoechoic area (right panel) in the center of the kidney. The normal hyperechoic area in the center of the kidney (the hilum) is replaced by the large hydronephrotic renal pelvis. The kidney has hydronephrosis due to obstruction of the lower ureter.

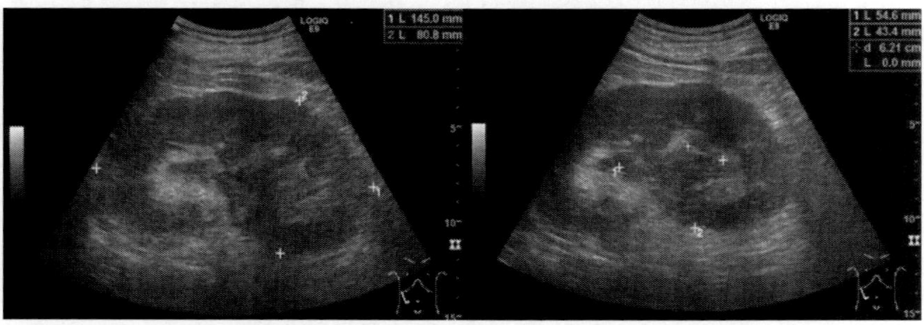

Figure 45. IgG4-related renal disease in a 72-year-old man. The longitudinal ultrasound images of the right kidney show enlargement of the kidney (left panel) and a large hypoechoic area (right panel) in the center of the kidney.

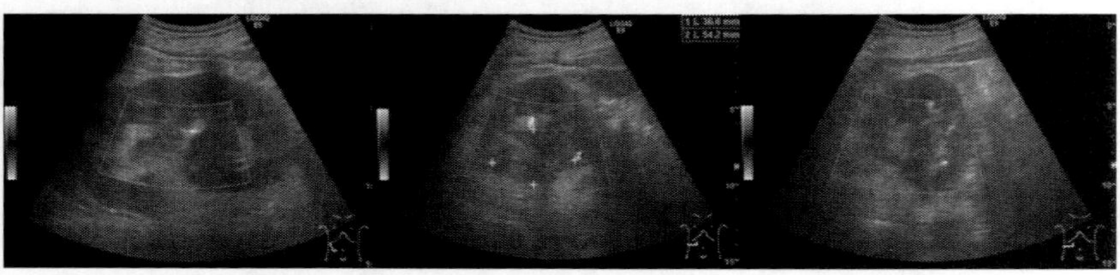

Figure 46. IgG4-related renal disease in a 72-year-old man. The longitudinal and transverse color Doppler ultrasound images of the right kidney show a mass in the center of the kidney.

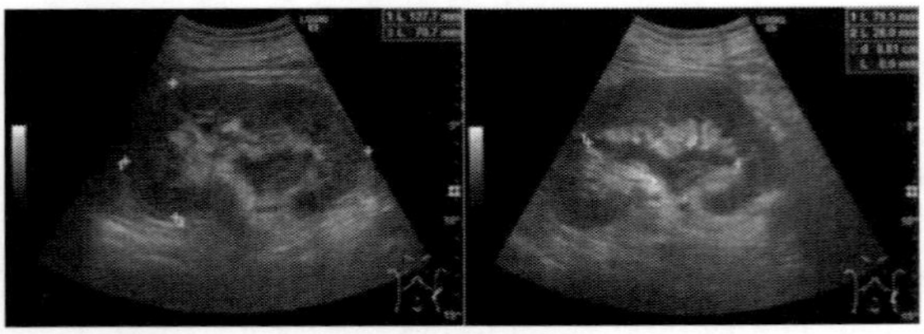

Figure 47. IgG4-related renal disease in a 72-year-old man. The longitudinal ultrasound images of the left kidney show enlargement of the kidney (left panel) and a large hypoechoic area (right panel) in the center of the kidney.

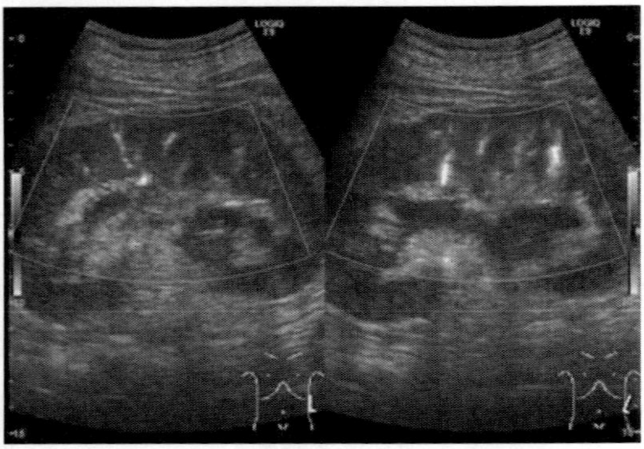

Figure 48. IgG4-related renal disease in a 72-year-old man. The longitudinal and transverse color Doppler ultrasound images of the left kidney show a mass in the center of the kidney.

Diffuse Wall Thickening of the Renal Pelvis

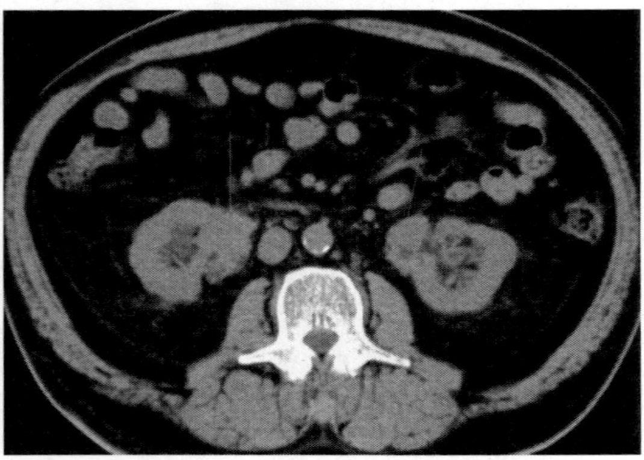

Figure 49. IgG4-related disease in a 66-year-old man. Axial non-contrast enhanced abdominal CT image shows bilateral mass-like diffuse wall thickening of the renal pelvises and the proximal ureters (arrows).

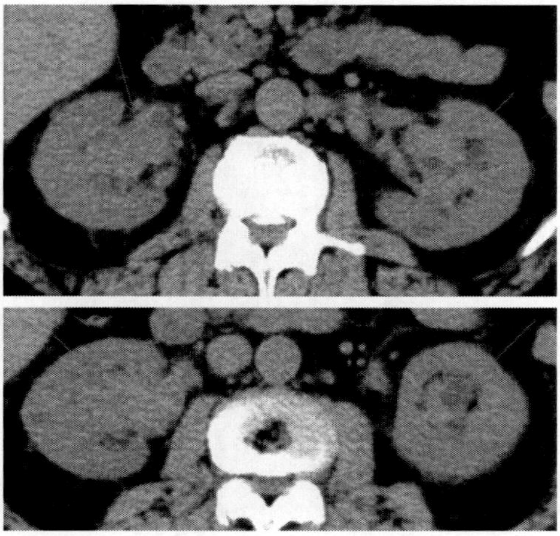

Figure 50. IgG4-related renal disease in a 72-year-old man. Axial non-contrast enhanced abdominal CT images show bilateral diffuse wall thickening of the renal pelvises and masses of the renal sinuses (arrows).

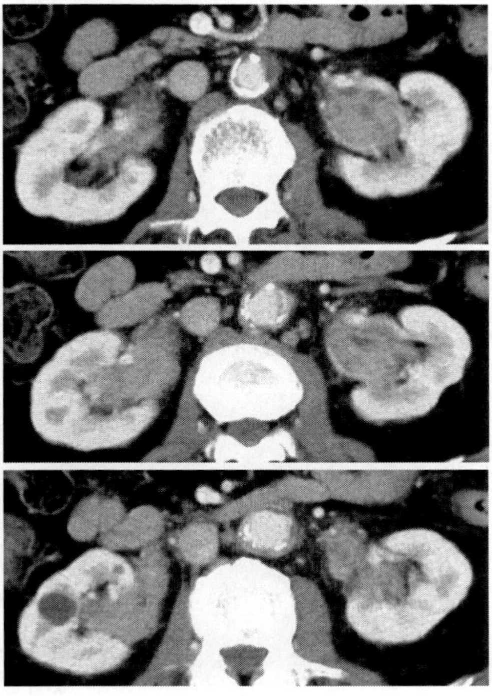

Figure 51. IgG4-related renal disease in a 67-year-old man. Axial contrast enhanced abdominal CT images show bilateral mass-like wall thickening of the renal pelvises and the proximal ureters.

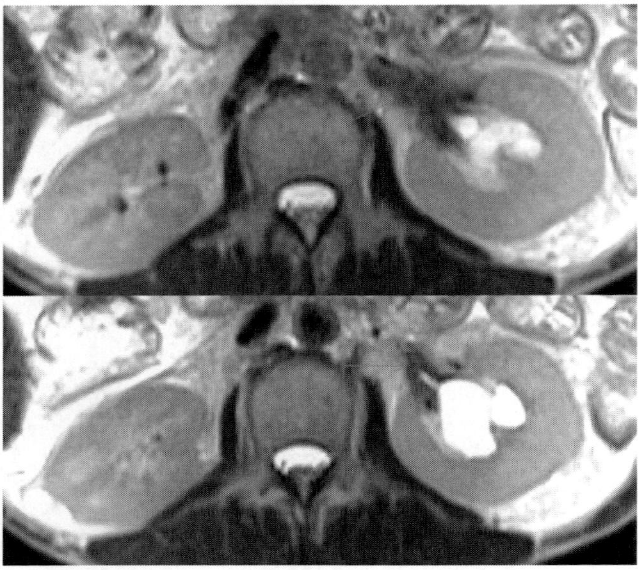

Figure 52. IgG4-related renal disease in a 56-year-old man. T2-weighted (HASTE) images of the abdomen show unilateral mass of the left renal sinuses (arrows). In some cases, there may be unilateral mass-like lesion of IgG4-related disease.

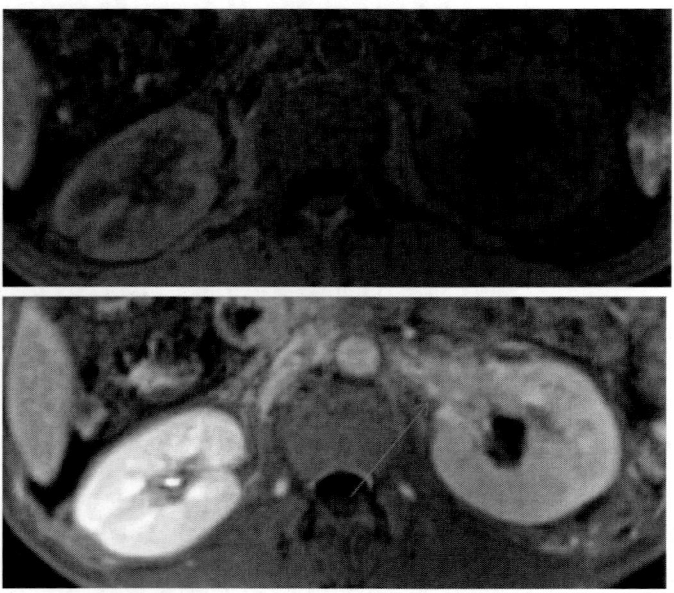

Figure 53. IgG4-related renal disease in a 56-year-old man. Axial gadolinium-enhanced T1-weighted MR images of the abdomen show unilateral mass-like lesion of the pelvis with delayed enhancement.

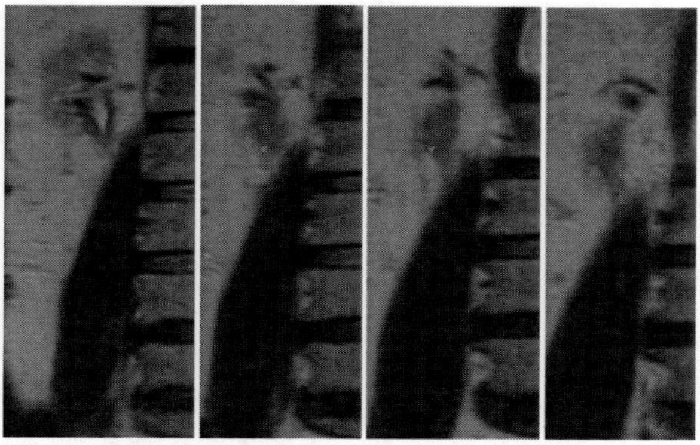

Figure 54. IgG4-related renal disease in a 67-year-old man. Coronal T2-weighted MR images through the right renal pelvis show a hypointense mass-like thickening of the right pelvis and ureter wall at the ureteropelvic junction (UPJ) (arrows). No irregularities on the luminal surface of the thickened right ureter.

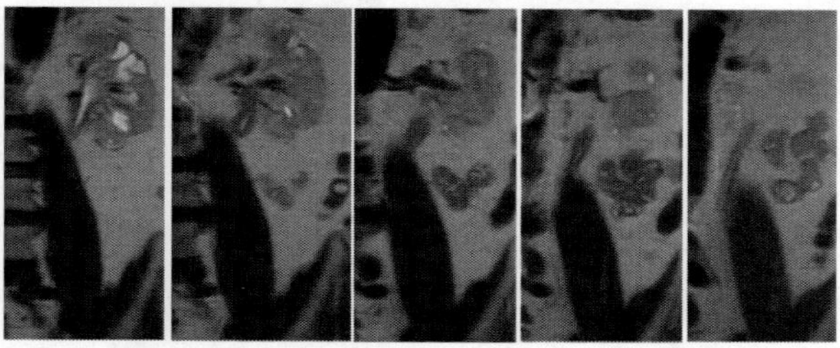

Figure 55. IgG4-related renal disease in a 67-year-old man. Coronal T2-weighted MR images show a hypointense diffuse wall thickening from the left renal pelvis to the middle part of ureter (arrows). No irregularities on the luminal surface of the thickened left ureter.

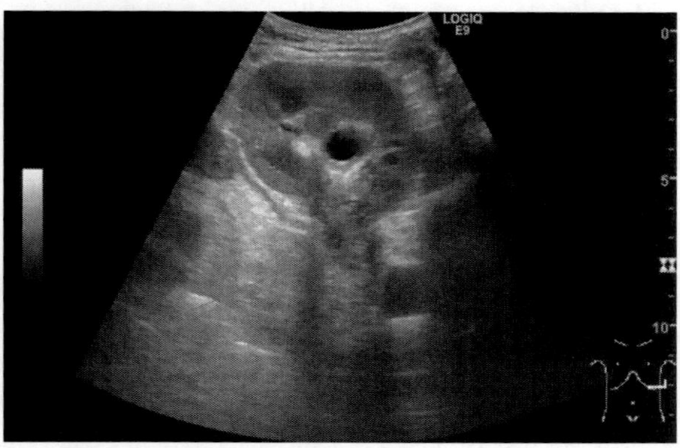

Figure 56. The transverse ultrasound image shows a hypointense diffuse wall thickening of the left renal pelvis (arrows).

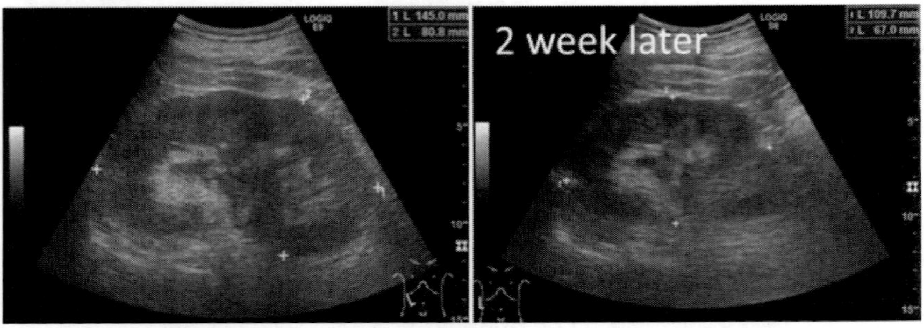

Figure 57. IgG4-related renal disease in a 72-year-old man. The longitudinal ultrasound images of the right kidney show enlargement of the kidney (left panel). Ultrasound image two weeks after treatment shows improvement in renal swelling (14.5 cm to 11.0 cm) and in size of the mass in the center of the kidney (5.5x4.3 cm to 3.6x3.4 cm) (right panel).

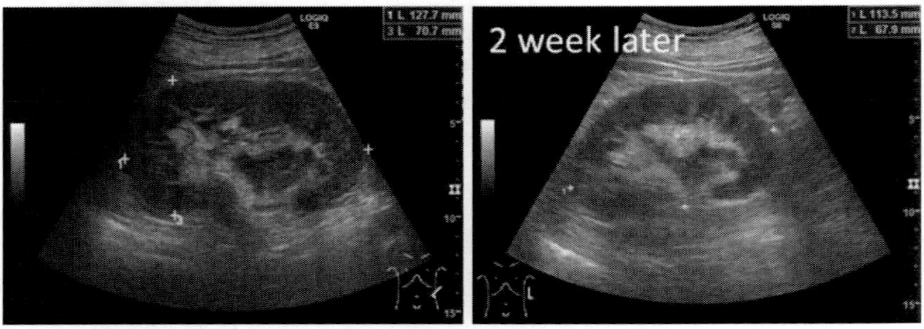

Figure 58. IgG4-related renal disease in a 72-year-old man. The longitudinal ultrasound images of the left kidney show enlargement of the kidney (left panel). Ultrasound image two weeks after treatment shows improvement in renal swelling and in size of the mass (right panel).

Histopathology

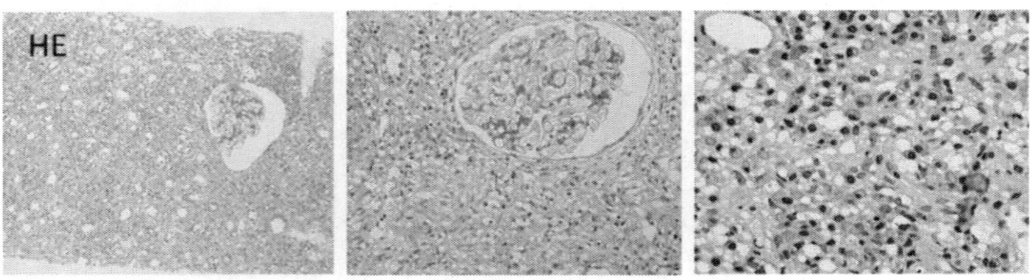

Figure 59. Histological findings of the kidney in a patient with IgG4-related renal disease reveal normal unchanged nephrons (glomeruli) and vessels. However, biopsy reveals tubulointerstitial nephritis.

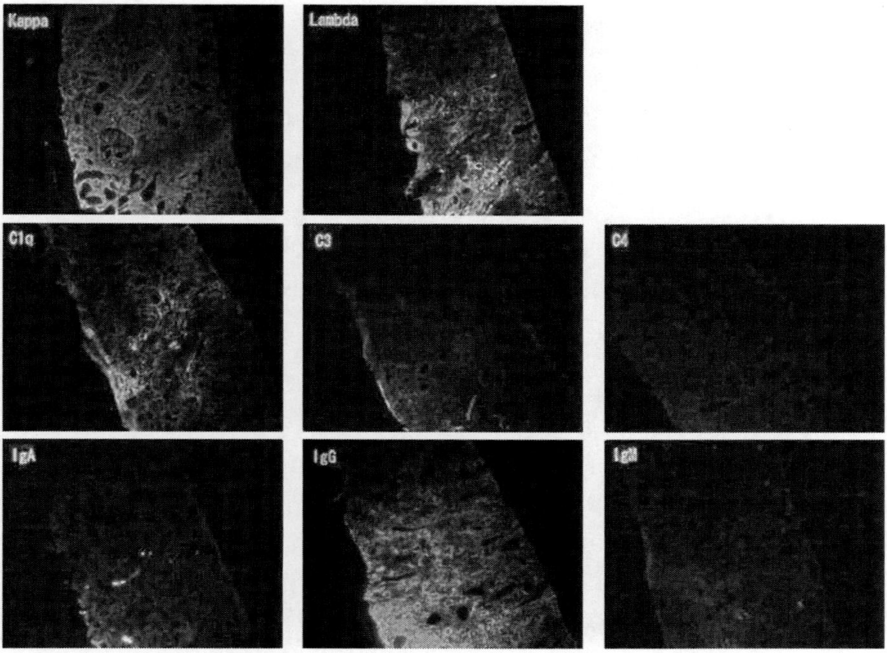

Figure 60. Immunofluorescent staining of in the kidney sections of a patient with IgG4-related renal disease is normal.

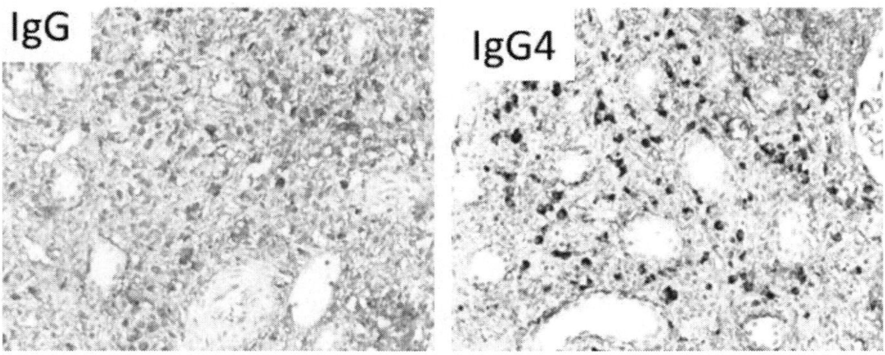

Figure 61. Immunohistochemistry of specimens for total IgG (left panel) and IgG4 (right panel) shows markedly increased IgG secreting plasma cells, a majority of which are positive for IgG4. Renal biopsy reveals tubulointerstitial nephritis with abundant IgG4-positive plasma cell infiltration.

References

Hamano, H., Kawa, S., Ochi, Y. et al. "Hydronephrosis associated with retroperitoneal fibrosis and sclerosing pancreatitis". *Lancet,* 359 (2002): 1403 - 4.

Kawano, M., Yamada, K. "IgG4-Related Kidney Disease and IgG4-Related Retroperitoneal Fibrosis". *Semin. Liver Dis.,* 36 (2016): 283 - 90.

Mizushima, I., Yamamoto, M., Inoue, D. et al. "Factors related to renal cortical atrophy development after glucocorticoid therapy in IgG4-related kidney disease: a retrospective multicenter study". *Arthritis Res. Ther.,* 18 (2016): 273.

Saeki, T., Nishi, S., Imai, N. et al. "Clinicopathological characteristics of patients with IgG4-related tubulointerstitial nephritis". *Kidney Int.,* 78 (2010): 1016 - 23.

In: IgG4 Related Disease
Editor: Syuichi Koarada
ISBN: 978-1-53618-050-3

Chapter 5

CARDIOVASCULAR MANIFESTATIONS OF IGG4-RELATED DISEASE

Syuichi Koarada** and Yuri Shirahama
Division of Rheumatology, Faculty of Medicine,
Saga University, Nabeshima, Saga, Japan

ABSTRACT

Cardiovascular lesions of IgG4-related disease include various pathologies and are diverse. IgG4-related cardiovascular lesions include aortitis, periaortitis, inflammatory aortic aneurysm, coronary periarteritis, pericarditis and pericardial effusion. However, the lesions may not only extend to the heart and aorta but also the branched vessels from the aorta, the iliac arteries, and the venous system. In addition, lymph node swelling may be accompanied around the aorta.

---

* Corresponding Author's Email: koarada@cc.saga-u.ac.jp.

INTRODUCTION

IgG4-related cardiovascular lesions include aortitis, periaortitis, inflammatory aortic aneurysms (IAAA), coronary periarteritis, pericarditis, and peri-aortic lymphadenopathy (Arao K. 2019).

AORTITIS AND PERIAORTITIS

Among IgG4-related retroperitoneal fibrosis, there is a condition in which the arteries are mainly affected, especially in infrarenal aorta and the iliac arteries. IgG4-related aortitis is characterized by adventitial arterial wall thickening that responds well to corticosteroid therapy. Therefore, IgG4-related cardiovcular disease is a condition that should be considered as one of the causes of non-infectious aortitis (Stone 2011). Inflammatory abdominal aortitis may also be associated with retroperitoneal fibrosis (Stone 2011).

CT (NCECT)

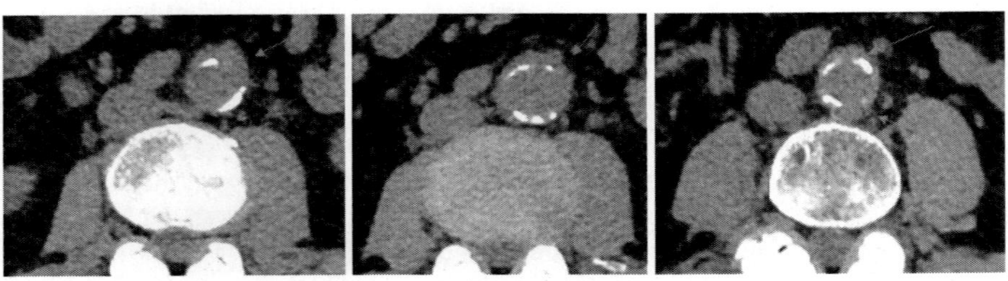

Figure 1. IgG4-related periaortitis in a 66-year-old man. Axial non-contrast enhanced CT images of the abdomen show thickening of the abdominal aortic wall (arrows) with surrounding inflammatory changes.

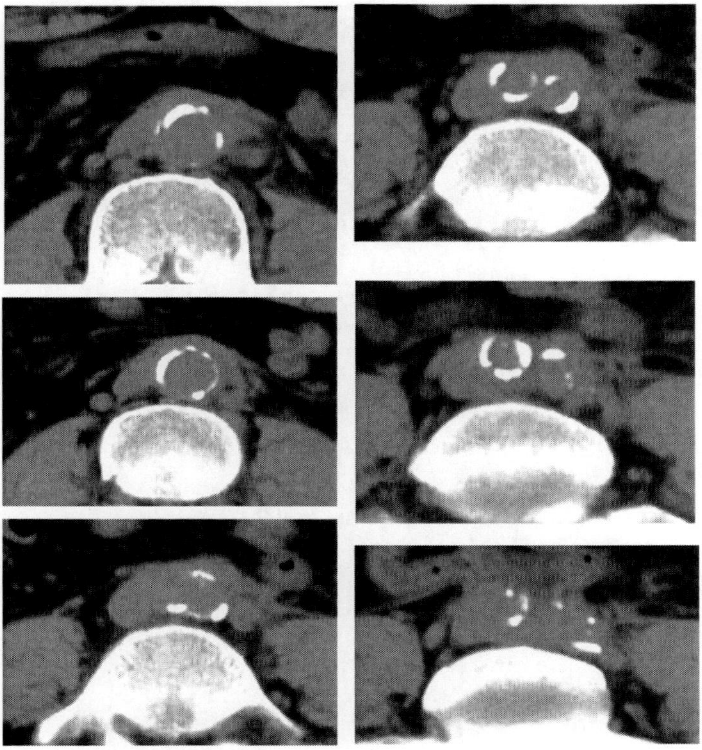

Figure 2. IgG4-related retroperitoneal fibrosis in a 69-year-old man. Abdomen axial non-contrast enhanced CT images show the periarterial masses of the iliac arteries.

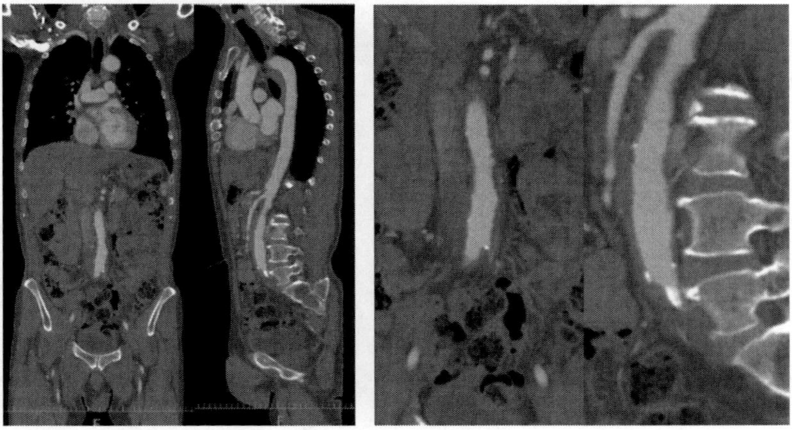

Figure 3. IgG4-related periaortitis in a 60-year-old man. Coronal and sagittal abdominal CT images show thickening of the abdominal aortic wall (arrows) with surrounding inflammatory changes.

Contrast Enchanced Abdominal CT (CECT)

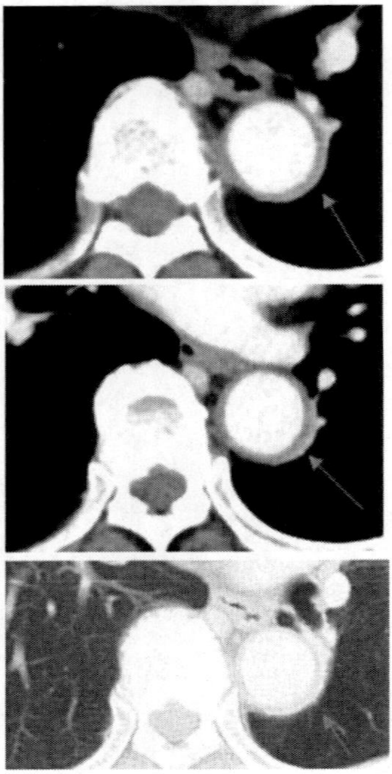

Figure 4. IgG4-related periaortitis in a 76-year-old woman. Axial contrast enhanced chest CT images show thickening of the thoracic aortic wall (arrows) with surrounding inflammatory changes.

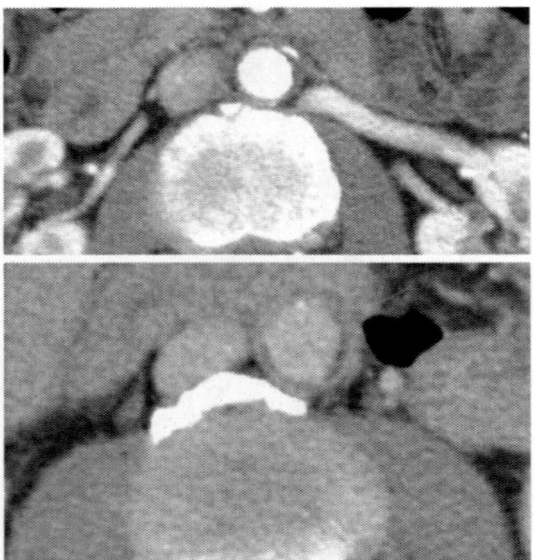

Figure 5. IgG4-related periaortitis in a 60-year-old man. Axial contrast enhanced abdominal CT images show thickening of the abdominal aortic wall (arrows) with surrounding inflammatory changes.

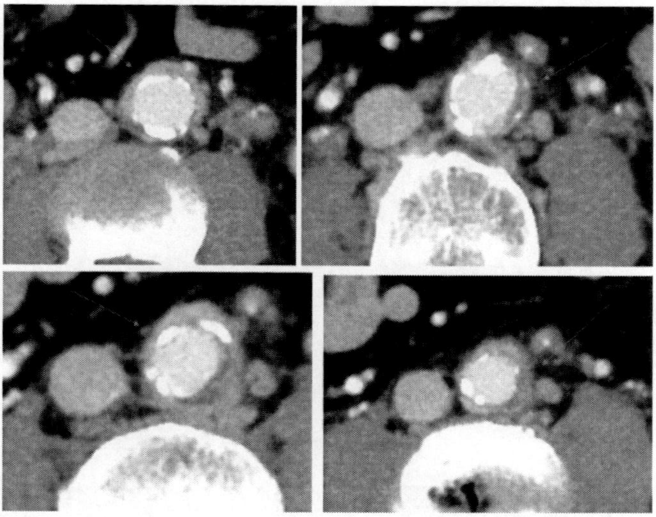

Figure 6. IgG4-related periaortitis in a 67-year-old man. Axial contrast enhanced abdominal CT images show thickening of the abdominal aortic wall (arrows) with surrounding inflammatory changes, calcification and enhancement.

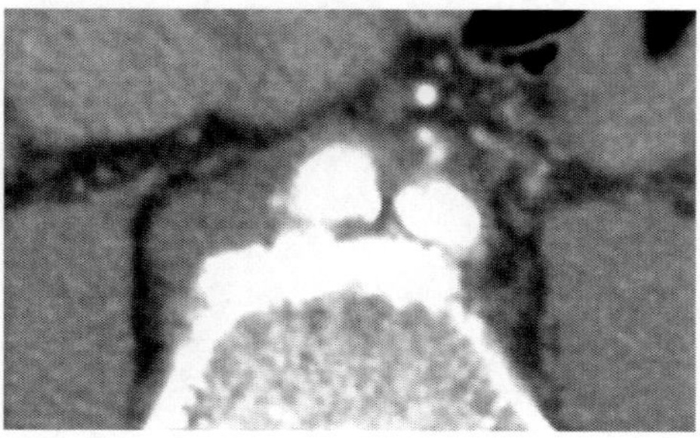

Figure 7. IgG4-related retroperitoneal fibrosis in a 60-year-old man. Axial contrast enhanced abdominal CT image shows thickening of the wall of iliac arteries (arrows) with surrounding inflammatory changes.

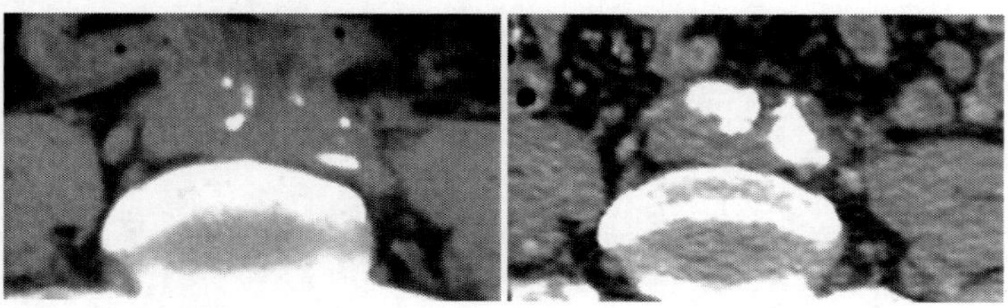

Figure 8. IgG4-related retroperitoneal fibrosis in a 69-year-old man. Abdomen axial non-contrast enhanced (left panel) and contrast enhanced CT images (right panel) show the periarterial masses of the iliac arteries. In the non-contrast enhanced CT image, there is patchy calcification typical of atherosclerosis.

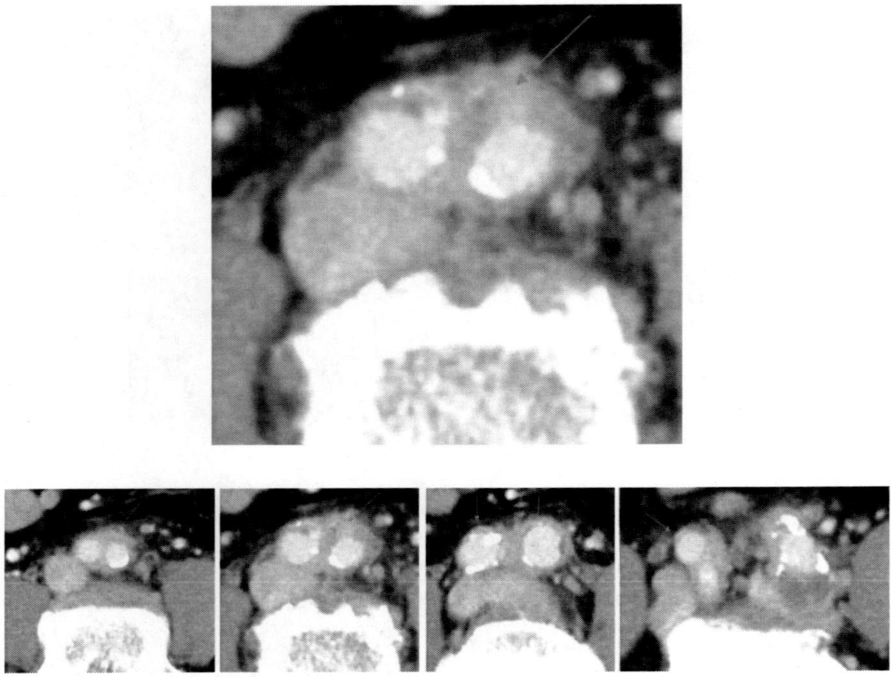

Figure 9 (a, b). IgG4-related disease in a 69-year-old man. Axial contrast enhanced abdominal CT images show thickening of the wall of the iliac arteries (arrows) with surrounding inflammatory changes.

MRI

Gadolinium-Enhanced T1-Weighted MRI

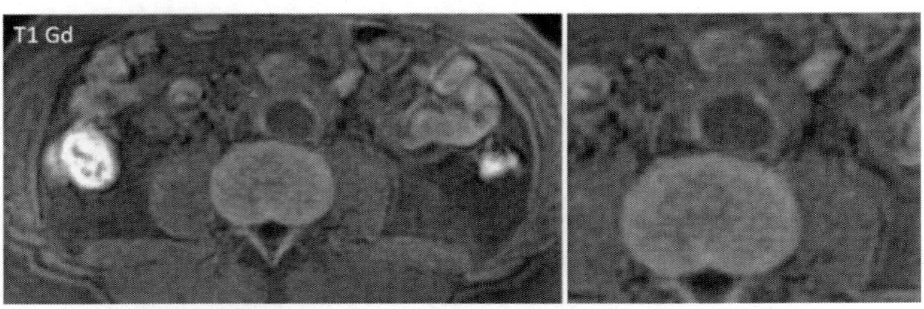

Figure 10. IgG4-related periaortitis in a 40-year-old man. Axial gadolinium-enhanced T1-weighted MR images of the abdomen show a ring-like enhancement in the periaortic area (arrows).

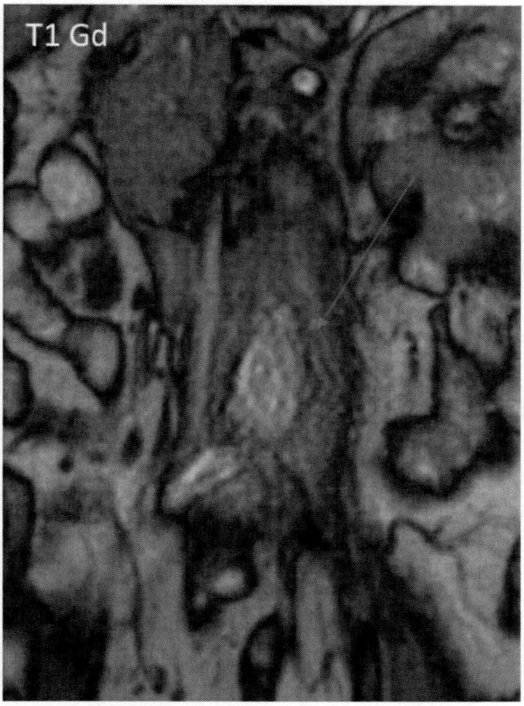

Figure 11. IgG4-related periaortitis in a 40-year-old man. Coronal gadolinium-enhanced T1-weighted MR image of the abdomen shows an enhanced mass-like lesion in the periaortic area (arrow).

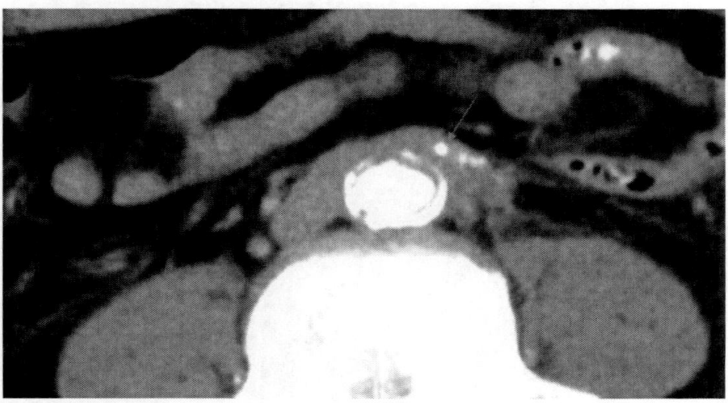

Figure 12. IgG4-related periaortitis in a 69-year-old man. Axial contrast enhanced CT image reveals a low intensity area surrounding the aorta at the level of the inferior mesenteric artery. The lower mesenteric artery is surrounded by an IgG4-related mass-like lesion.

Ultrasound Images

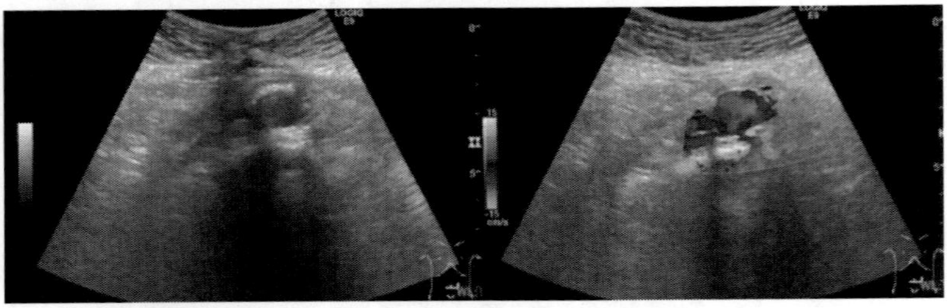

Figure 13. IgG4-related retroperitoneal fibrosis in a 60-year-old man. Abdominal ultrasound images (left panel: B-mode US, right panel: color Doppler US) demonstrate a thin hypoechoic structure that covers the front of the aorta below the renal artery.

IgG4-Related Periarteritis and Coronary Luminal Narrowing

IgG4-related disease may involve the cardiovascular system (Zen Y. 2009). IgG4-related perivascular inflammation has been observed in small vessels, including coronary arteries (Matsumoto Y 2008) (Maturen KE 2012). It has been pointed out that IgG4-related inflammation may be involved in the development of periarteritis and luminal atherosclerosis (Sakamoto A 2017).

Contrast Enhanced Chest CT

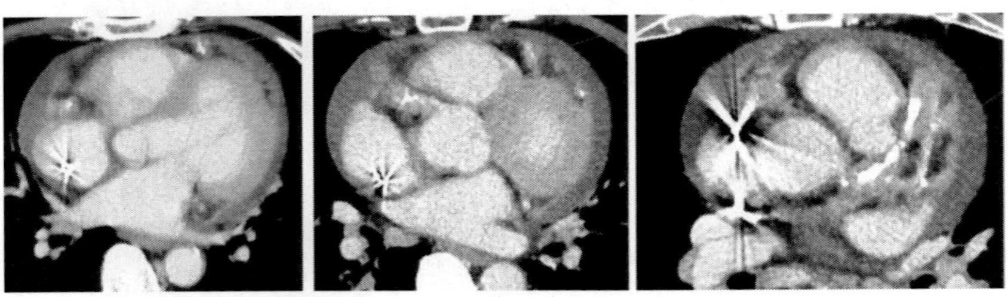

Figure 14. IgG4-related coronary periarteritis in a 67-year-old man. Axial contrast enhanced chest CT images. Soft tissue swelling (arrows) was observed around the left anterior descending artery (LAD) and left main coronary artery (LMCA), suggesting coronary periarteritis.

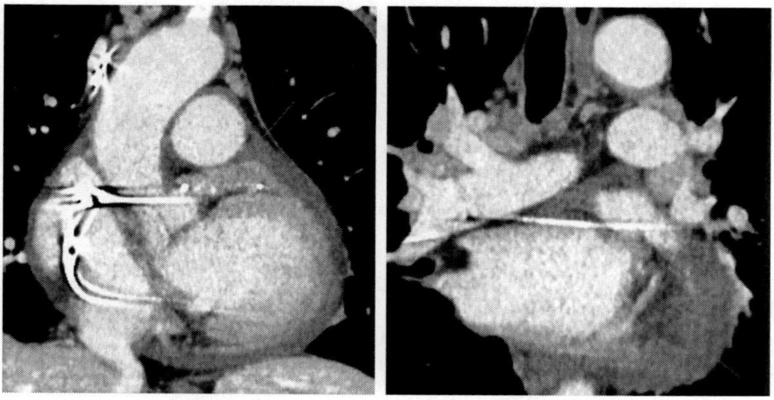

Figure 15. IgG4-related coronary periarteritis in a 67-year-old man. Coronal contrast enhanced chest CT images show soft tissue swelling (arrows) around the left anterior descending artery (LAD) and left main coronary artery (LMCA), suggesting coronary periarteritis.

ECG

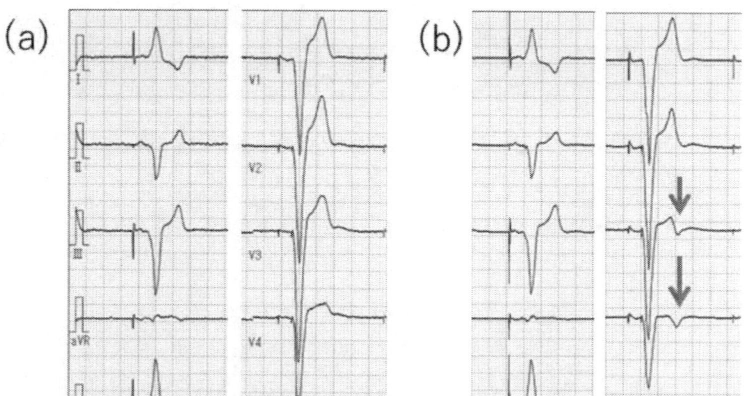

Figure 16. IgG4-related coronary periarteritis with around the left anterior descending artery (LAD) and left main coronary artery (LMCA) in a 67-year-old man. (a) Pre-onset electrocardiogram (ECG) shows pacemaker rhythm before disease. (b) ECG recorded at the time of the onset shows ST depression and T wave inversion in leads V3-4.

IgG4-Related Pericarditis

IgG4-related cardiovascular lesions include pericarditis (Arao K.. 2019). There are some cases involving IgG4-related pericarditis accompanied by massive effusion and soft tissue swelling. However, since most of the reports of IgG4-related periarteritis are limited to isolated cases (Kusunose K 2015) (Sugimoto T 2008), the precise frequency of these lesions is unclear. Patients with IgG4-related pericarditis usually respond to oral corticosteroid therapy.

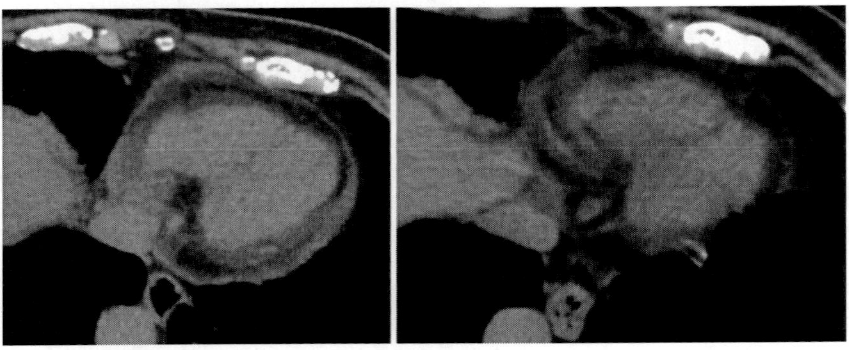

Figure 17. IgG4-related pericarditis in a 76-year-old man. Axial chest CT images show pericardial effusion.

Plain Radiograph

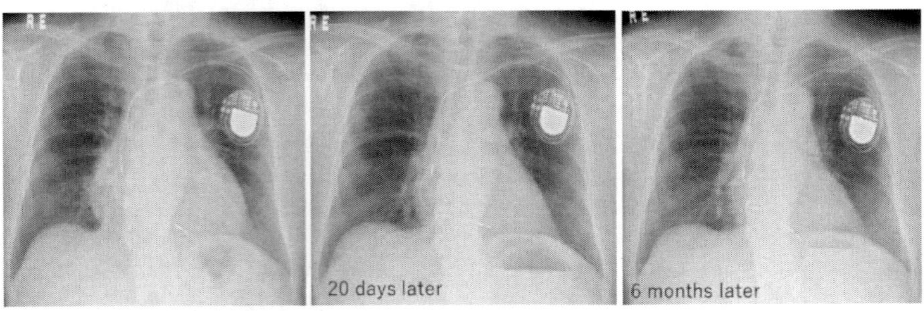

Figure 18. IgG4-related disease in a 67-year-old man. Serial chest radiographs show that massive pericardial effusion was improved after corticosteroid therapy.

Contrast Enhanced Chest CT

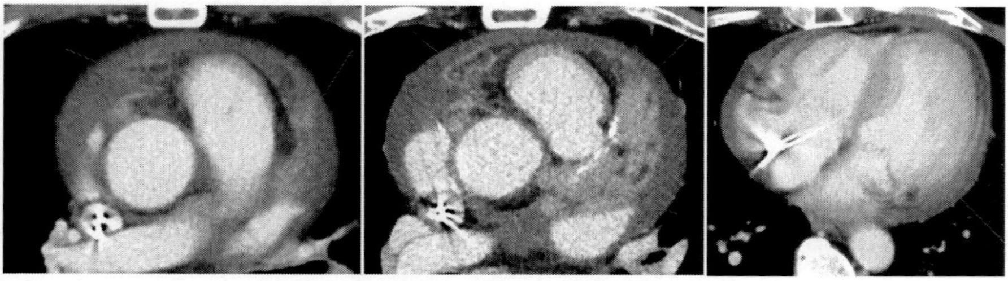

Figure 19. IgG4-related pericarditis in a 67-year-old man. Axial contrast enhanced chest CT images show pericardial thickening and effusion with soft tissue swelling (arrows).

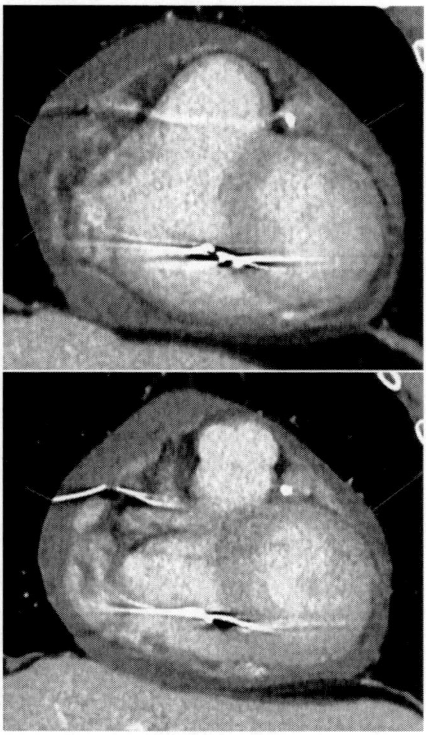

Figure 20. IgG4-related pericarditis in a 67-year-old man. Coronal reconstructed contrast enhanced chest CT images show pericardial thickening and effusion with soft tissue swelling (arrows).

IgG4-Related Periaortic Lymphadenopathy

Non-Contrast Enhanced Chest CT

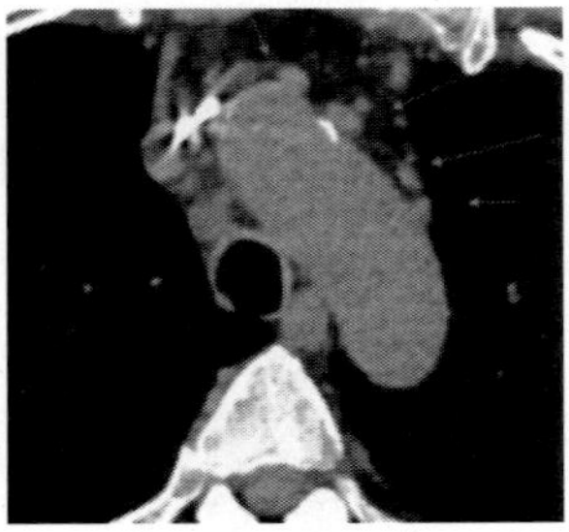

Figure 21. IgG4-related thoracic lymphadenopathy in a 66-year-old man. Axial non-contrast enhanced CT image shows multiple periaortic lymphadenopathy (arrows).

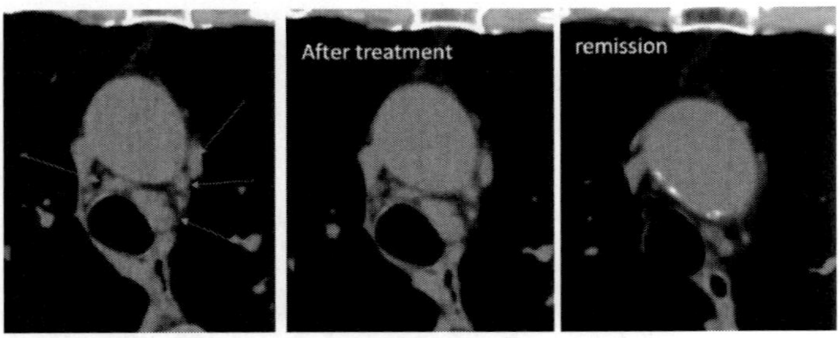

Figure 22. IgG4-related thoracic lymphadenopathy in a 76-year-old man. Axial non-contrast CT images show multiple enlarged periaortic lymph nodes (arrows). Periaortic lymphadenopathy resolved completely after corticosteroid therapy and was in remission.

Contrast Enhanced Chest CT

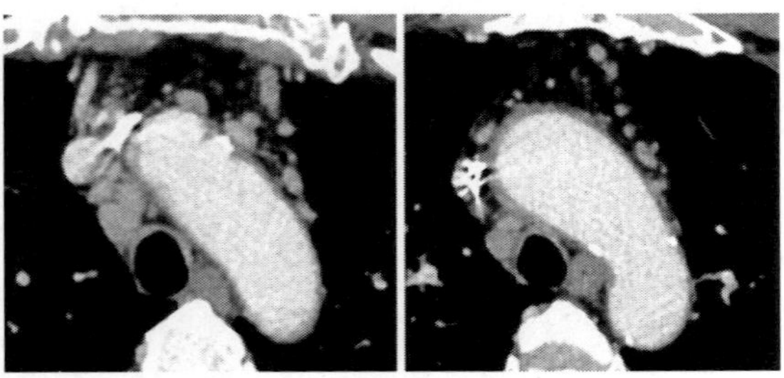

Figure 23. IgG4-related thoracic lymphadenopathy in a 67-year-old man. Axial contrast CT images show multiple enlarged periaortic lymph nodes.

References

Arao K., Mase T, Iwanami K, Nakai M, Sekiguchi H, Abe Y, Kawakami M. "IgG4-related Pericarditis in which Oral Corticosteroid Therapy Was Effective." *Intern. Med.* 58 (2019).

Arao K., Mase T, Iwanami K, Nakai M, Sekiguchi H, Abe Y, Kawakami M. "IgG4-related Pericarditis in which Oral Corticosteroid Therapy Was Effective." *Intern. Med.* 58 (2019): 1119-1122.

Kusunose K, Hotchi J, Takagawa Y, et al. "Serial imaging changes during treatment of immunoglobulin G4-related disease with multiple pseudotumors." *Circulation* 131 (2015): 1882-1883.

Matsumoto Y, Kasashima S, Kawashima A, et al. "A case of multiple immunoglobulin G4-related periarteritis: a tumorous lesion of the coronary artery and abdominal aortic aneurysm." *Hum. Pathol.* 39: 975-980, 2008. 39 (2008): 975-980.

Maturen KE, Sundaram B, Marder W, Swartz RD. "Coronary artery involvement in idiopathic retroperitoneal fibrosis: computed tomographic findings." *J. Thorac. Imaging* 27: 27 (2012): W35-W37.

Sakamoto A, Tanaka T, Hirano K, Koike K, Komuro I. "Immunoglobulin G4-related Coronary Periarteritis and Luminal Stenosis in a Patient with a History of Autoimmune Pancreatitis." *Intern. Med.* 56 (2017): 2445-2450.

Stone, JR. "Aortitis, periaortitis, and retroperitoneal fibrosis, as manifestations of IgG4-related systemic disease." *Curr. Opin. Rheumatol.* 23 (2011): 88.

Sugimoto T, Morita Y, Isshiki K, et al. "Constrictive pericarditis as an emerging manifestation of hyper-IgG4 disease." *Int. J. Cardiol.* 130 (2008): e100-e101.

Zen Y., Onodera M, Inoue D, et al. "Retroperitoneal fibrosis: a clinicopathologic study with respect to immunoglobulin G4." *Am. J. Surg. Pathol.* 33 (2009): 1833-1839.

In: IgG4 Related Disease
Editor: Syuichi Koarada
ISBN: 978-1-53618-050-3

Chapter 6

MUSCULOSKELETAL MANIFESTATIONS OF IGG4-RELATED DISEASE

Syuichi Koarada** and Satoko Tashiro
Division of Rheumatology, Faculty of Medicine,
Saga University, Nabeshima, Saga, Japan

ABSTRACT

Musculoskeletal lesions of IgG4-related disease are not uncommon and present a variety of lesions. Although arthritis is relatively common, it can also cause soft tissue enlargement in front of the thoracic spine and sacrum. In addition, patients with IgG4-related disease often have diffuse idiopathic skeletal hyperostosis (DISH-like lesions. Swelling of the lower extremity can also occur, in which case the possibility of IgG4-related myositis must be considered.

---

* Corresponding Author's Email: koarada@cc.saga-u.ac.jp.

IgG4-Related Arthropathy

Joints may be involved in IgG4-related diseases in some cases. Arthritis has been reported to occur in 10% of patients with IgG4-related disease (Masaki Y 2009). Histopathological examination of the synovium showed infiltration of IgG4-positive plasma cells in destructive arthritis of a patient with Mikulicz's disease. However, no arthropathy has been reported without infiltration of IgG4-positive plasma cells in the tissues (Umekita K 2012).

Diffuse idiopathic skeletal hyperostosis (DISH, Forestier disease) is relatively a common condition characterized by bone proliferation at sites of tendinous and ligamentous insertion of the spine. In some of our cases, DISH-like structures are found, but their association with IgG4-related disease is unknown.

Plain Radiography

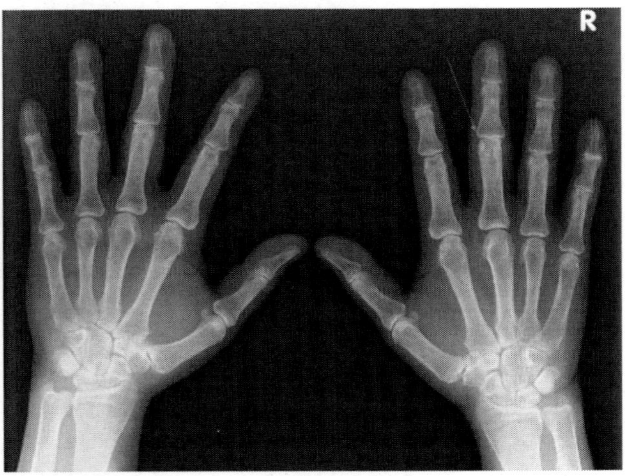

Figure 1. IgG4-related disease in a 75-year-old woman with joint pain. PA view of plain X-ray of both the hands shows mild swelling of soft tissue around the PIP joint of the right third digit and narrowing of the joint space. However, these findings are nonspecific.

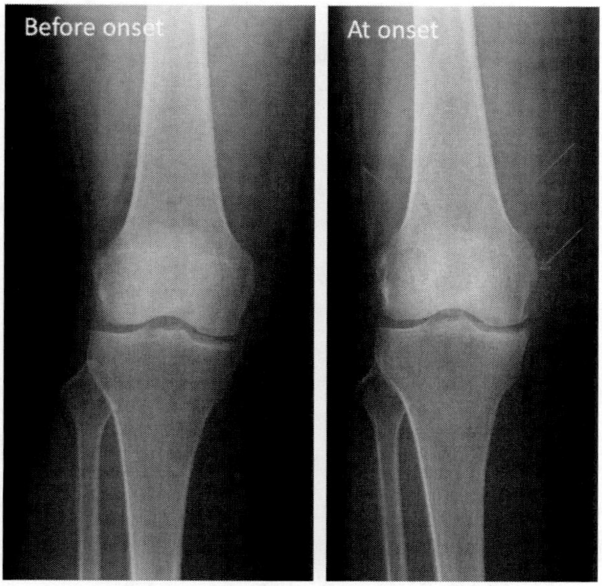

Figure 2. AP views of plain radiography of the right knee before and at onset show joint effusion and narrowing of the femorotibial joint space.

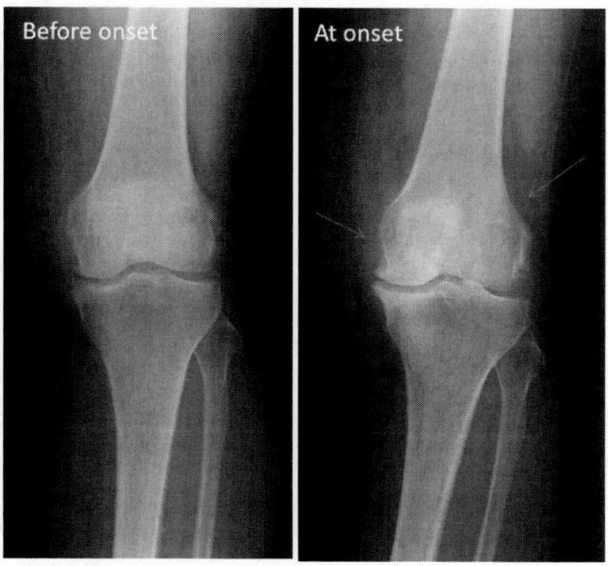

Figure 3. AP views of plain radiography of the left knee before and at onset show joint effusion and narrowing of the femorotibial joint space. Soft tissue swelling on the medial and lateral aspect of the knee is seen.

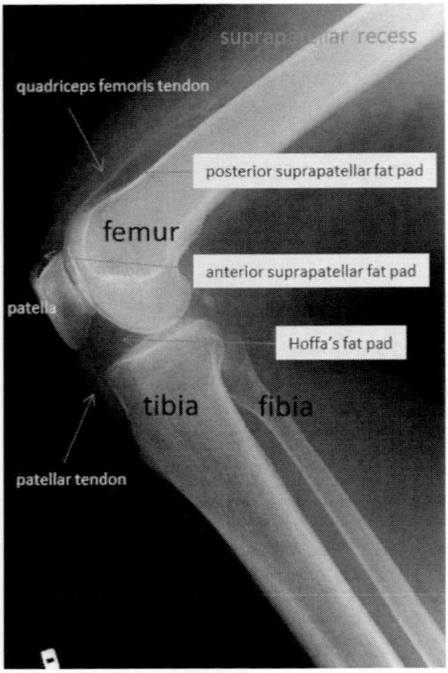

Figure 4. Lateral view of the right knee. Knee joint effusion is only reliably seen on lateral projections.

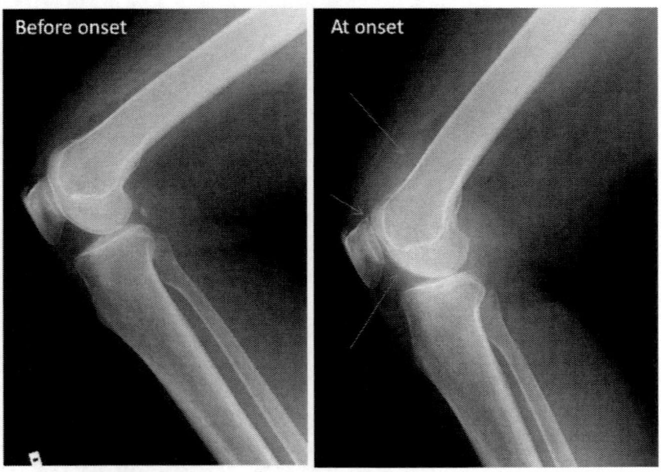

Figure 5. Lateral view of the right knee at onset (right panel) shows the fluid in the suprapatellar pouch and in Hoffa's fat pad (arrows). The patella is displaced anteriorly by the fluid in the suprapatellar pouch. Compare this image with the patient's before onset image (left panel).

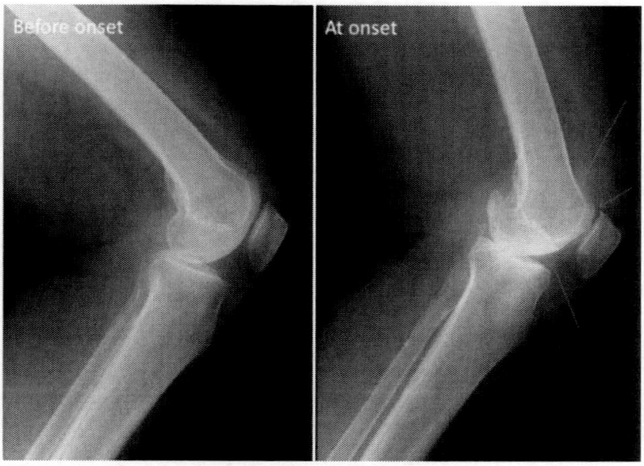

Figure 6. Lateral view of the left knee at onset shows the fluid in the suprapatellar pouch and in Hoffa's fat pad (arrows).

Estimating the size of knee Effusions (Hall 1975).

Width of Base of Suprapatellar Pouch	Knee joint Aspiration Volume (ml)
<5 mm	0
5-10mm	1-9ml
10mm or greater	10ml ≦

CT

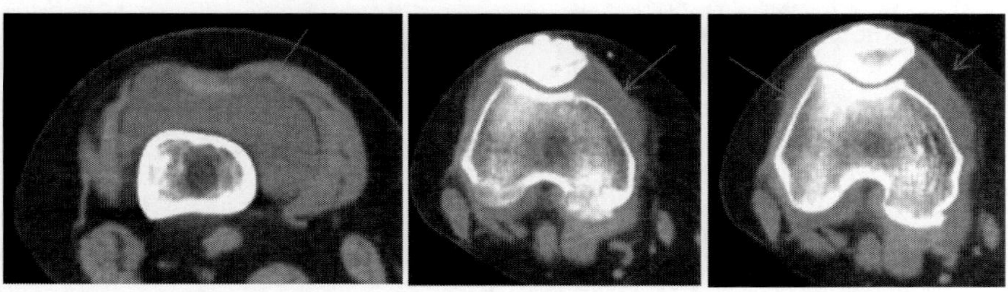

Figure 7. IgG4-related disease in a 76-year-old woman. Axial non-contrast enhanced CT images of the right knee show marked joint effusion in the suprapatellar, medial and lateral patellar recesses.

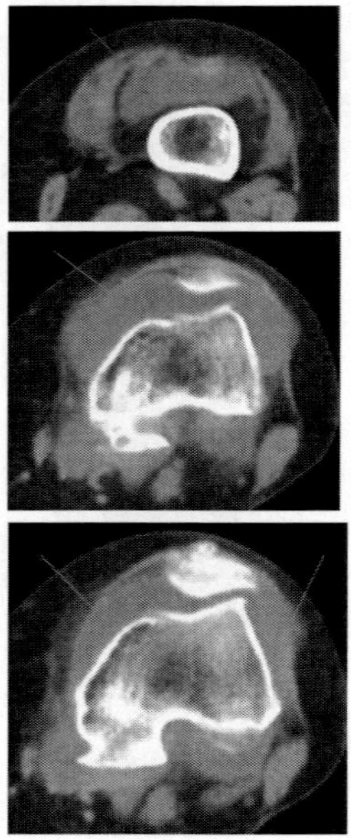

Figure 8. IgG4-related disease in a 76-year-old woman. Axial non-contrast enhanced CT images of the left knee show marked joint effusion in the suprapatellar, medial and lateral patellar recesses.

MRI

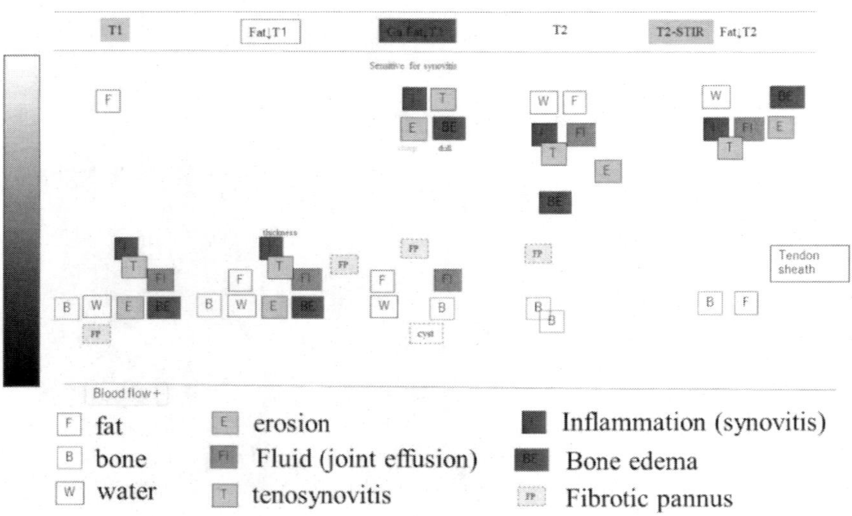

Figure 9. Musculoskeletal lesions and MRI findings.

T1-Weighted MR Images

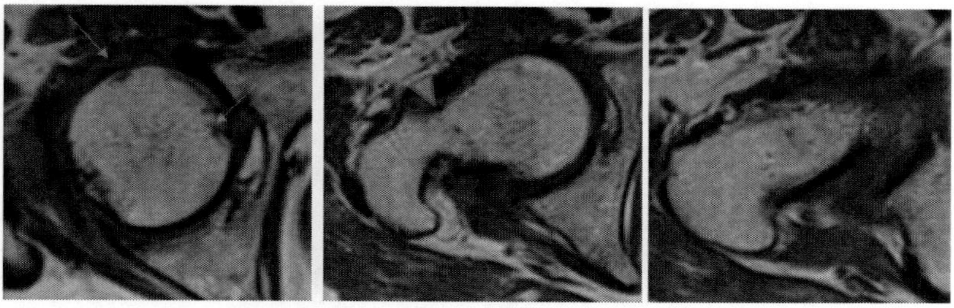

Figure 10. IgG4-related disease in a 75-year-old woman. Coronal non-contrast enhanced T1-weighted MR images of the right hip show bone erosions and subchondral vulnerable fracture (arrowhead).

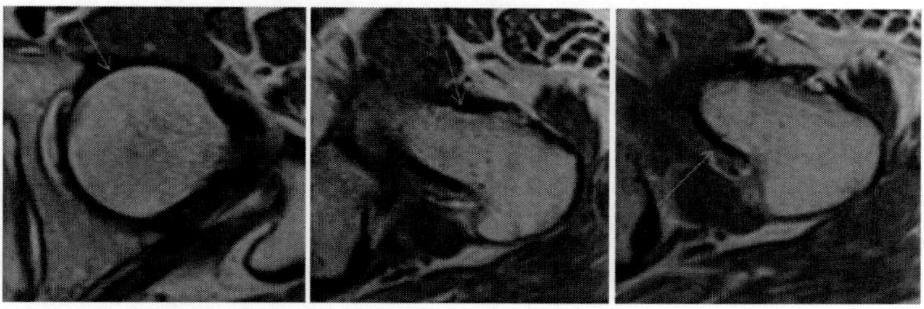

Figure 11. IgG4-related disease in a 75-year-old woman. Axial non-contrast enhanced T1-weighted MR images of the left hip show mild synovitis with low signal intensity (arrows).

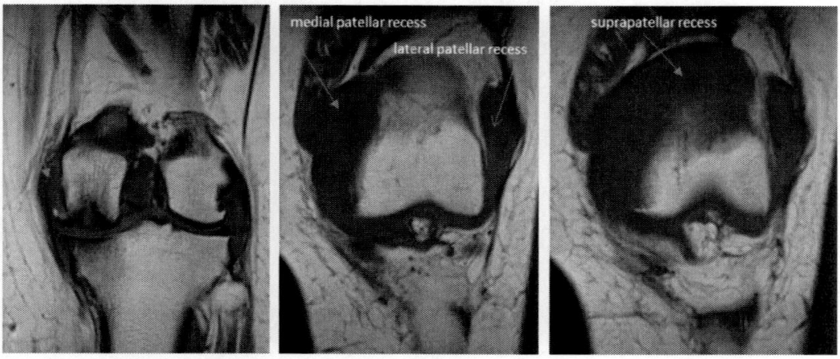

Figure 12. IgG4-related disease in a 76-year-old woman. Coronal non-contrast enhanced T1-weighted MR images of the left knee show marked joint effusion in the suprapatellar, medial and lateral patellar recesses.

T2-Weighted MR Images

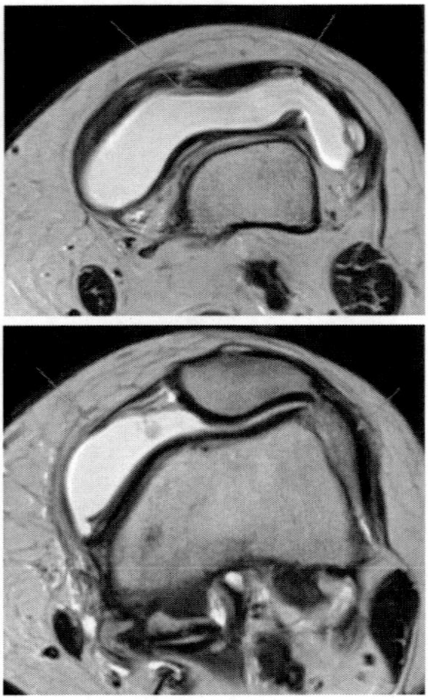

Figure 13. IgG4-related disease in a 76-year-old woman. Axial non-contrast enhanced T2-weighted MR images of the left knee show diffuse severe synovial thickening and marked joint effusion in the suprapatellar (upper panel), medial and lateral patellar recesses (lower panel) (arrows).

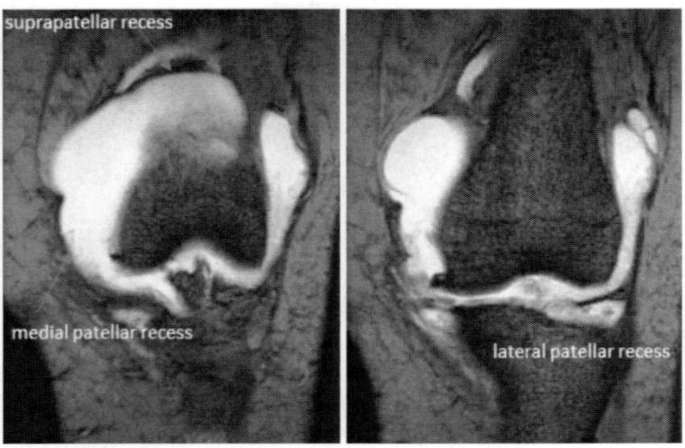

Figure 14. IgG4-related disease in a 76-year-old woman. Coronal non-contrast enhanced T2-weighted MR images of the left knee show synovial thickening and marked joint effusion in the suprapatellar, medial and lateral patellar recesses (arrows).

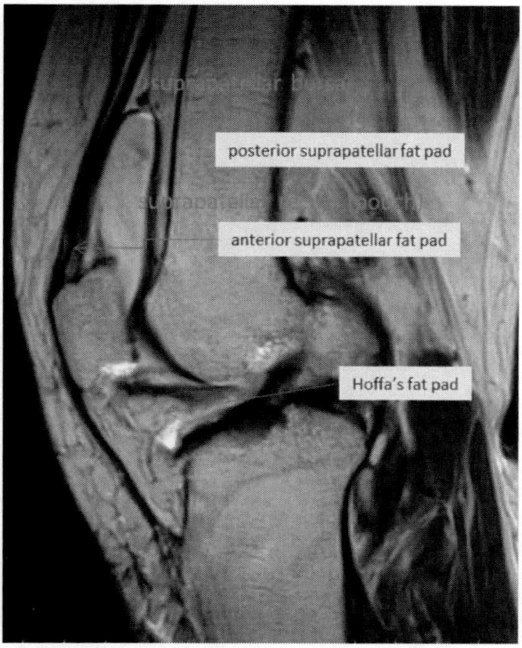

Figure 15. Anatomy of the knee joint. Sagittal non-contrast enhanced T2-weighted MR image of the knee.

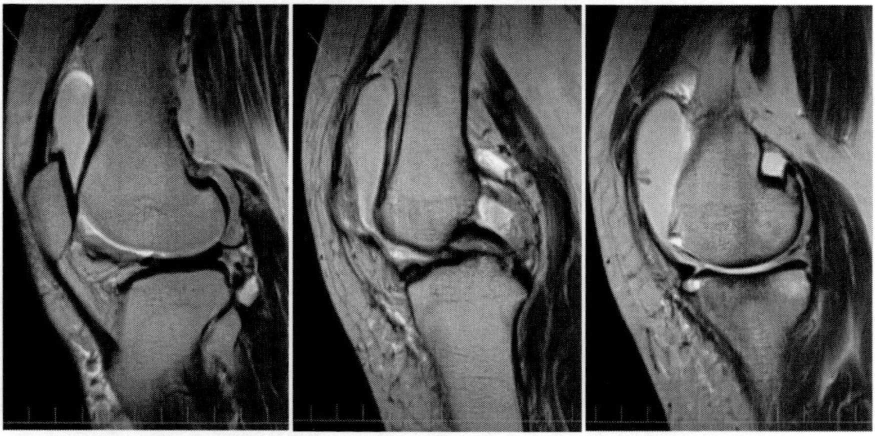

Figure 16. IgG4-related disease in a 76-year-old woman. Sagittal non-contrast enhanced T2-weighted MR images of the left knee show synovial thickening and marked joint effusion in the suprapatellar recesses (arrows).

T2-STIR MR Images

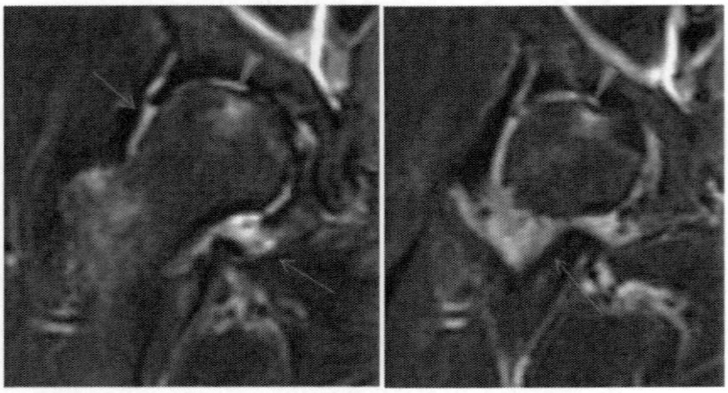

Figure 17. IgG4-related disease in a 75-year-old woman. Coronal non-contrast enhanced T2-STIR MR images of the right hip show synovitis and/or joint effusion (arrows), bone erosion and bone marrow edema (arrowheads).

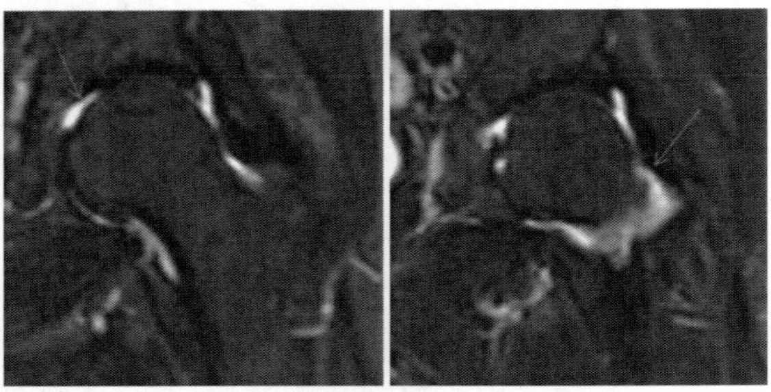

Figure 18. IgG4-related disease in a 75-year-old woman. Coronal non-contrast enhanced T2-STIR MR images of the left hip show synovitis and/or joint effusion (arrows).

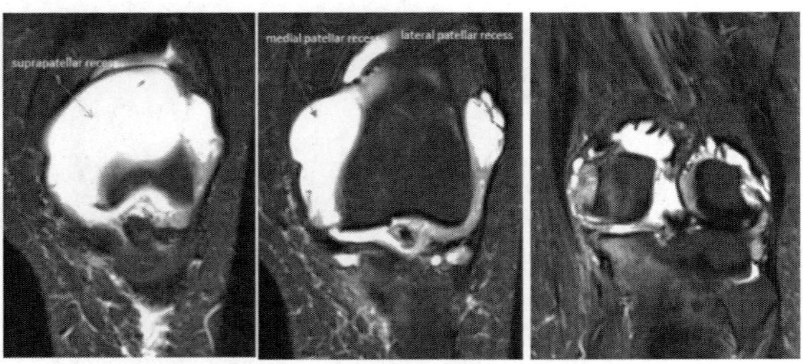

Figure 19. IgG4-related disease in a 76-year-old woman. Coronal non-contrast enhanced T2-STIR MR images of the left knee show marked joint effusion in the suprapatellar recesses, medial and lateral patellar recesses (arrows).

Normal bone marrow shows low signal intensity on both T1- and T2-weighted MR images, reflecting fatty bone marrow. On the other hand, bone marrow edema is recognized as an abnormal signal intensity with an unclear boundary indicating low signal intensity on T1-weighted images, iso-signal intensity on T2-weighted images, and high signal intensity on fat-suppressed T2-weighted MR images and STIR images. A contrast-enhanced MR image shows a contrast effect. Although bone marrow edema on MRI is a nonspecific imaging finding, bone marrow edema observed in arthritis including rheumatoid arthritis reflects bone marrow inflammation (infiltration of inflammatory cells mainly by lymphocytes).

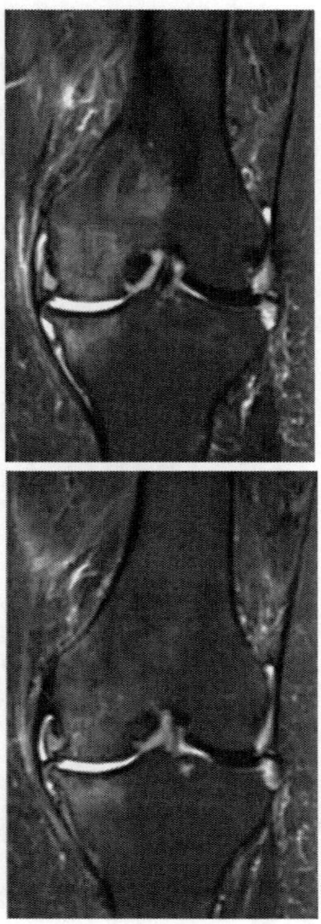

Figure 20. IgG4-related disease in a 76-year-old woman. Coronal non-contrast enhanced T2-STIR MR images of the left knee show bone marrow edema (changes of osteitis) in tibial and femoral condyles. There is also thinning with loss of articular cartilage seen at the medial tibiofemoral joint space. Narrowing of the tibiofemoral joint space is observed. These changes may also be affected by existing osteoarthritis.

Gadolinium-Enhanced T1-Weighted MR Images

Synovitis and Effusion

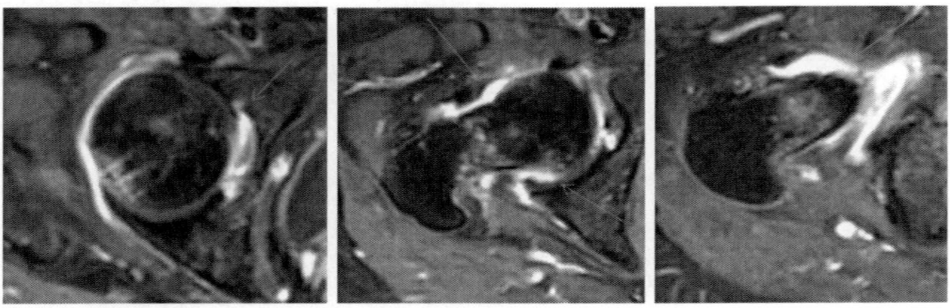

Figure 21. IgG4-related disease in a 75-year-old woman. Axial gadolinium-enhanced T1-weighted FS MR images of the right hip show synovial proliferation (arrows).

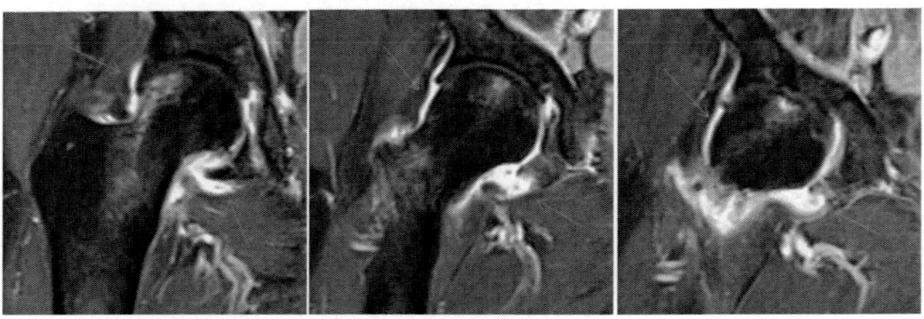

Figure 22. IgG4-related disease in a 75-year-old woman. Coronal gadolinium-enhanced T1-weighted FS MR images of the right hip show synovial proliferation (arrows).

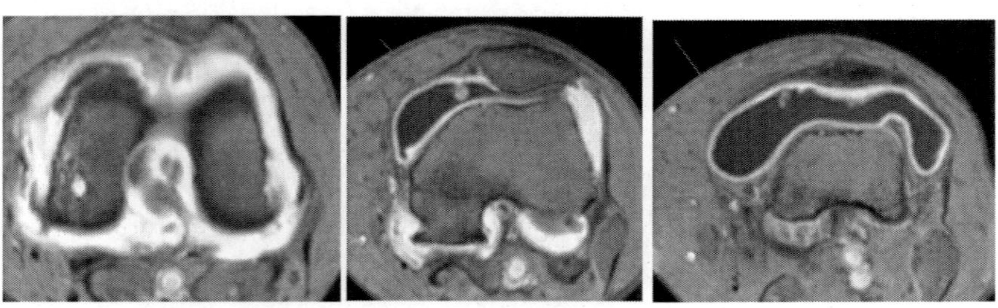

Figure 23. IgG4-related disease in a 76-year-old woman. Axial gadolinium-enhanced T1-weighted MR (T1 vibe) images of the left knee show synovial hypertrophy and contrast enhancement in hypertrophied synovium and marked joint effusion in the suprapatellar, medial and lateral patellar recesses (arrows).

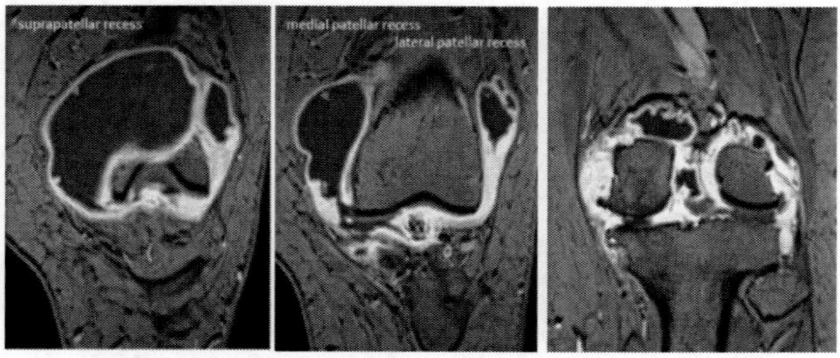

Figure 24. IgG4-related disease in a 76-year-old woman. Coronal gadolinium-enhanced T1-weighted MR (T1 vibe) images of the left knee show synovial hypertrophy and contrast enhancement in hypertrophied synovium and marked joint effusion in the suprapatellar, medial and lateral patellar recesses (arrows).

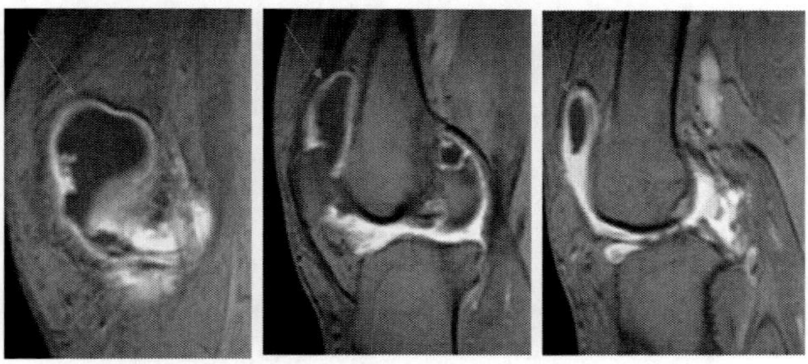

Figure 25. IgG4-related disease in a 76-year-old woman. Sagittal gadolinium-enhanced T1-weighted MR (T1 vibe) images of the left knee show synovial hypertrophy and contrast enhancement in hypertrophied synovium and marked joint effusion in the suprapatellar recess (arrows).

Bone Marrow Edema

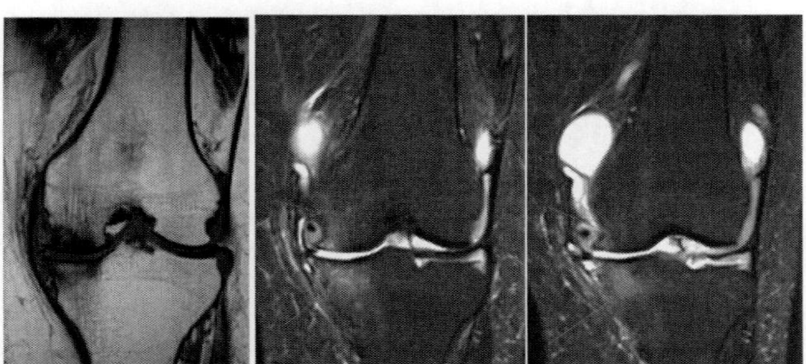

Figure 26. IgG4-related disease in a 76-year-old woman. Coronal gadolinium-enhanced T1-weighted MR (T1 vibe) images of the left knee show bone marrow edema in the tibial and the femoral condyles.

Bursitis

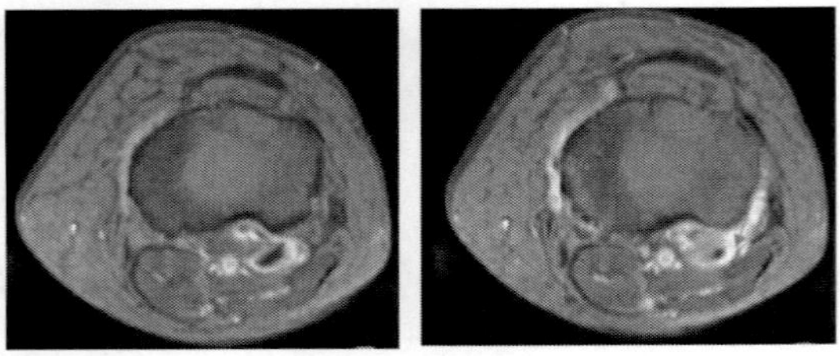

Figure 27. IgG4-related disease in a 76-year-old woman. Axial gadolinium-enhanced T1-weighted MR (T1 vibe) images of the left knee show synovial hypertrophy and contrast enhancement in hypertrophied synovium and effusion of the subpopliteal recess (arrows).

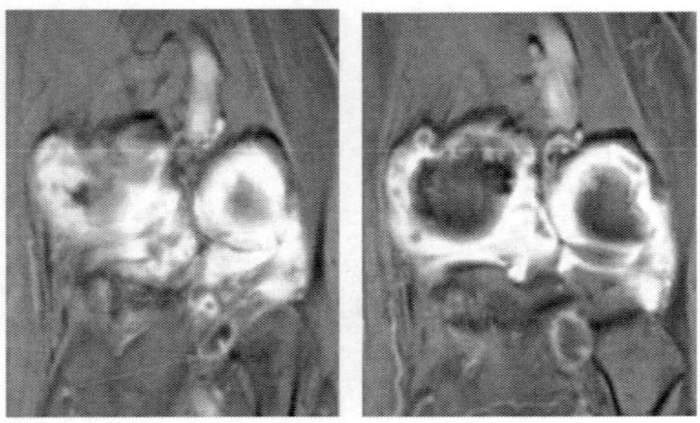

Figure 28. IgG4-related disease in a 76-year-old woman. Coronal gadolinium-enhanced T1-weighted MR (T1 vibe) images of the left knee show synovial hypertrophy and contrast enhancement in hypertrophied synovium and effusion of the subpopliteal recess (arrows).

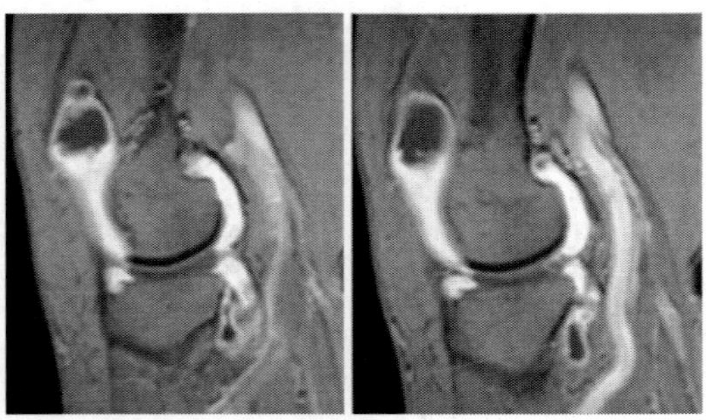

Figure 29. IgG4-related disease in a 76-year-old woman. Sagittal gadolinium-enhanced T1-weighted MR (T1 vibe) images of the left knee show synovial hypertrophy and contrast enhancement in hypertrophied synovium and effusion of the subpopliteal recess (arrows).

Gallium Scintigraphy

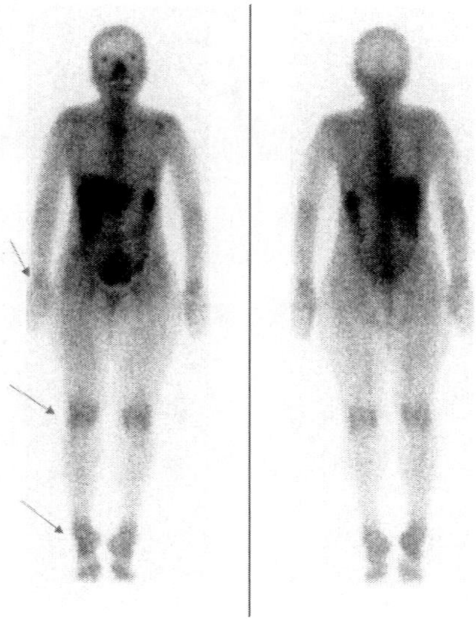

Figure 30. IgG4-related disease in a 49-year-old woman. Gallium scintigraphy shows uptake in the wrists, knees and ankles.

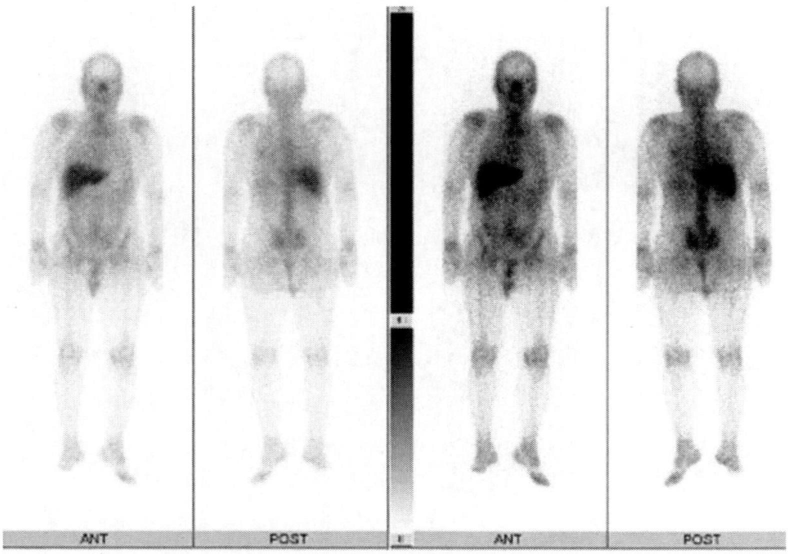

Figure 31. IgG4-related disease in a 63-year-old man. Gallium scintigraphy shows abnormal uptake in the multiple joints.

PET/CT Images

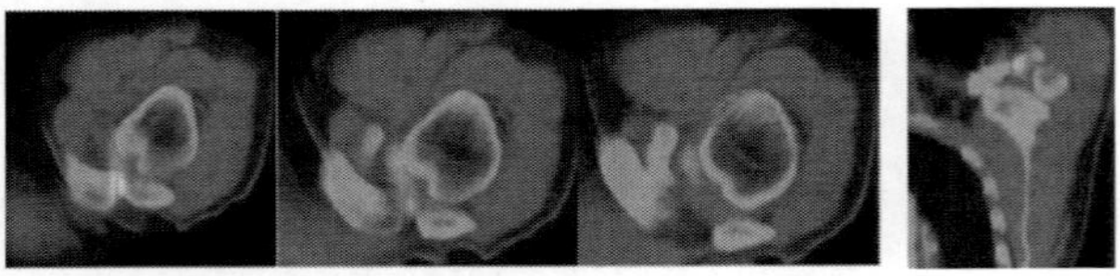

Figure 32. IgG4-related arthropathy in a 67-year-old man with joint pain. FDG-PET/CT images show uptake in the left acromioclavicular joint.

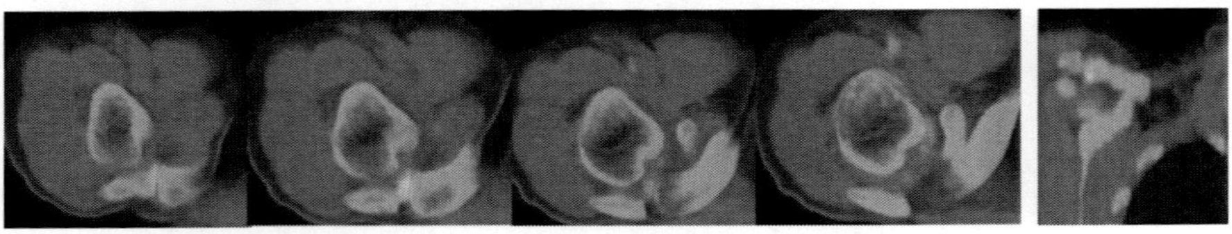

Figure 33. IgG4-related arthropathy in a 67-year-old man with joint pain. FDG-PET/CT images show uptake in the right acromioclavicular joint.

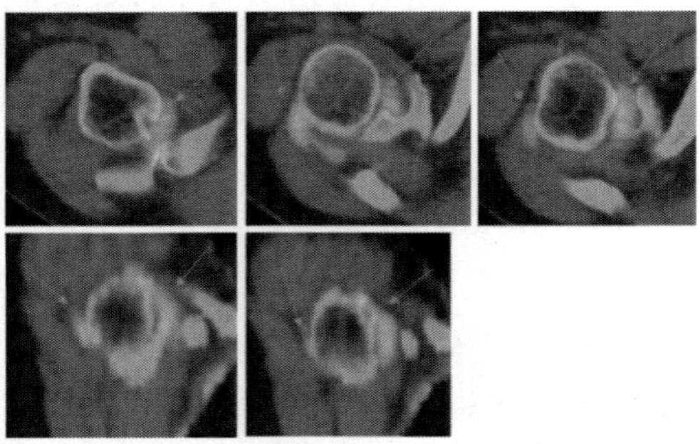

Figure 34. IgG4-related disease in a 75-year-old woman. FDG-PET/CT images show uptake in the right shoulder (arrows).

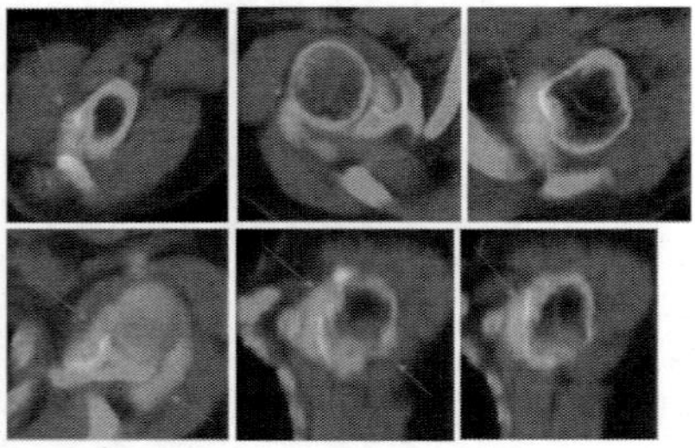

Figure 35. IgG4-related disease in a 75-year-old woman. FDG-PET/CT images show uptake in the left shoulder (arrows).

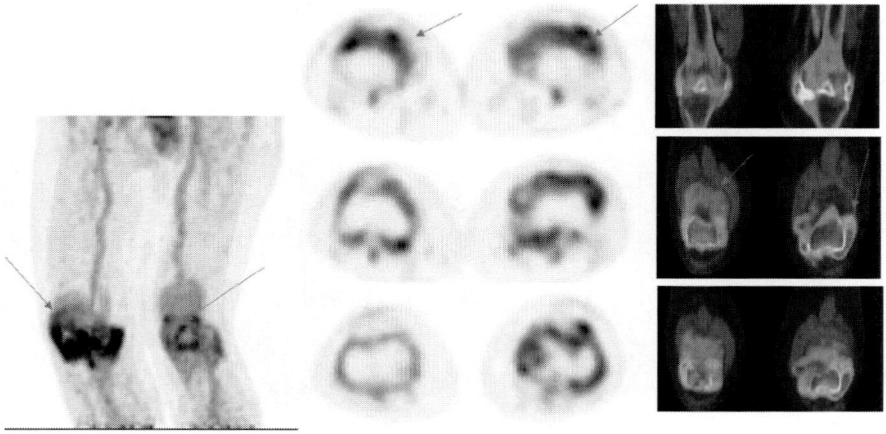

Figure 36. IgG4-related disease in a 75-year-old woman. Various FDG-PET/CT images show uptake in bilateral knees (arrows).

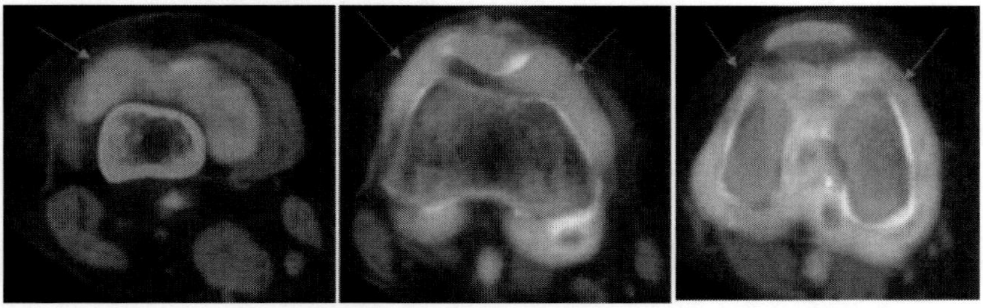

Figure 37. IgG4-related disease in a 75-year-old woman. Axial FDG-PET/CT images show uptake in the right knee (arrows).

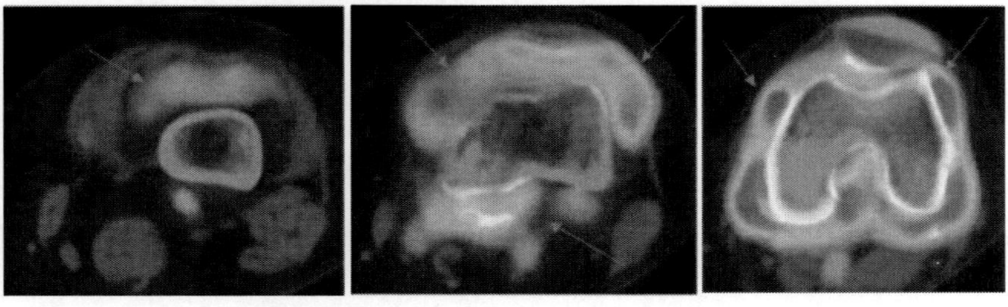

Figure 38. IgG4-related disease in a 75-year-old woman. Axial FDG-PET/CT images show uptake in the left knee (arrows).

Technetium 99m-Bisphosphonate Bone Scan

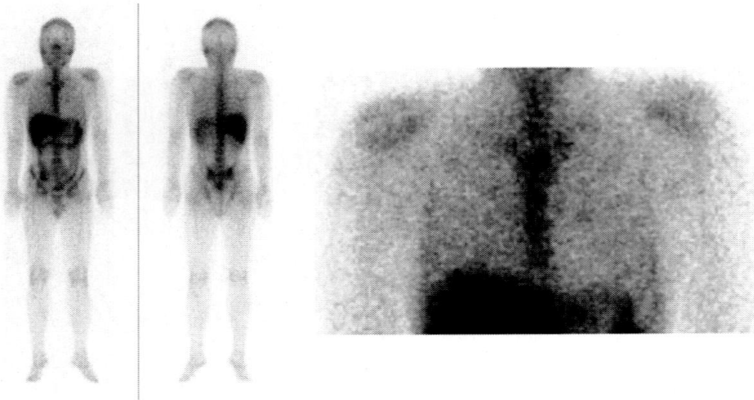

Figure 39. Technetium 99m-bisphosphonate bone scan of a patient with IgG4-related arthropathy. Bone scan images reveal uptake in the shoulder joints.

Clinical Photography

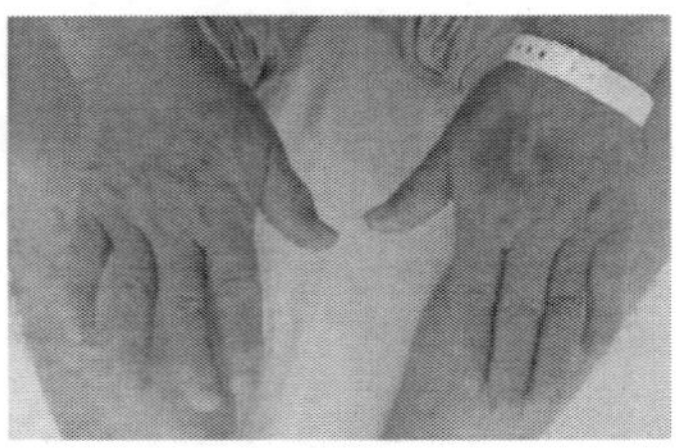

Figure 40. IgG4-related arthropathy in a 71-year-old man. The photographic image shows mild swelling of the hands and the wrists.

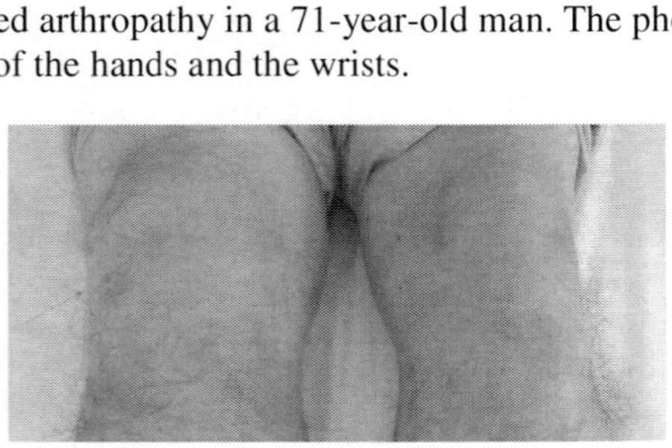

Figure 41. IgG4-related arthropathy in a 71-year-old man. The photographic image shows swelling of the right knee.

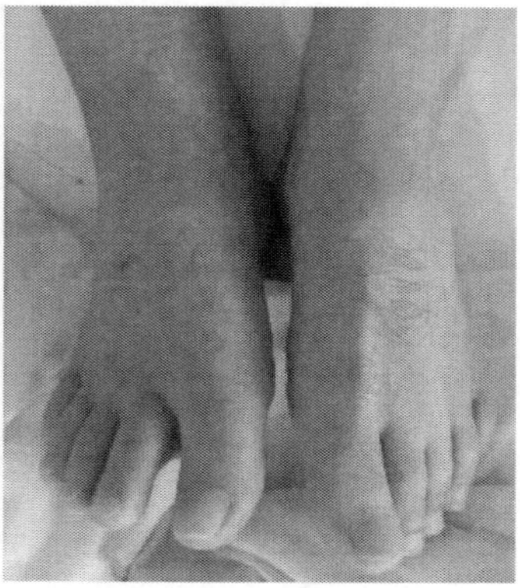

Figure 42. IgG4-related arthropathy in a 71-year-old man. The photographic image shows swelling of the right ankle.

Spinal Lesions

DISH (Diffuse Idiopathic Skeletal Hyperostosis)

Plain Radiography

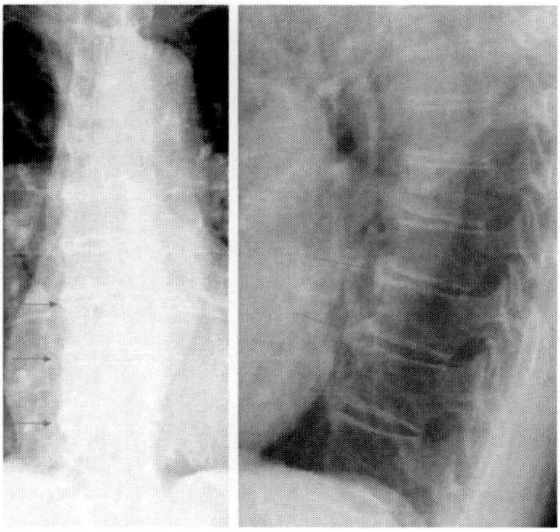

Figure 43. IgG4-related disease with DISH-like ossification in a 55-year-old woman. PA and lateral views of thoracic spine show the flowing ossification along the anterolateral aspect of at least 4 contiguous vertebrae.

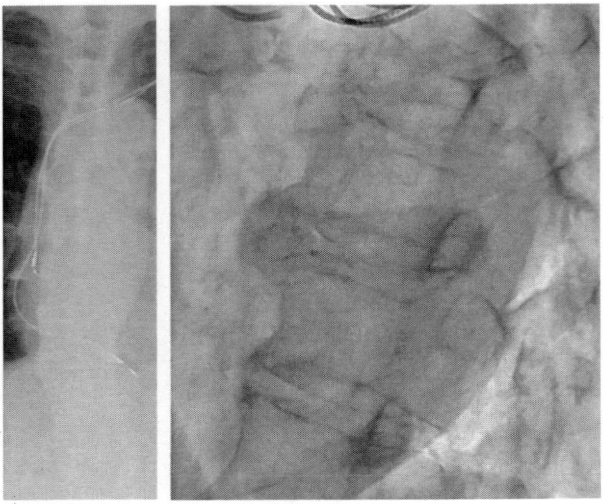

Figure 44. IgG4-related disease in a 67-year-old man. Plain radiographs of thoracic spine show flowing ossification of DISH.

CT

Non-Contrast Enhanced Chest CT

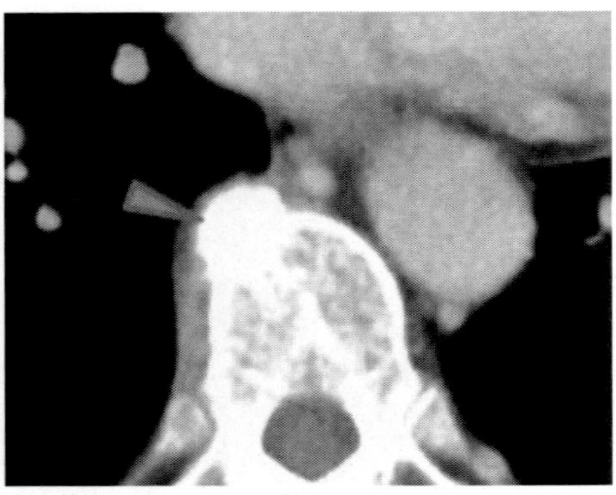

Figure 45. IgG4-related disease with DISH (diffuse idiopathic skeletal hyperostosis)-like ossification in a 55-year-old woman. Axial chest non-contrast enhanced CT (NCECT) image shows focal calcification and ossification of the right side of the anterior longitudinal ligament (arrowhead). In addition, CT image shows soft tissue swelling of the right side of the para-vertebra near the ossified lesion.

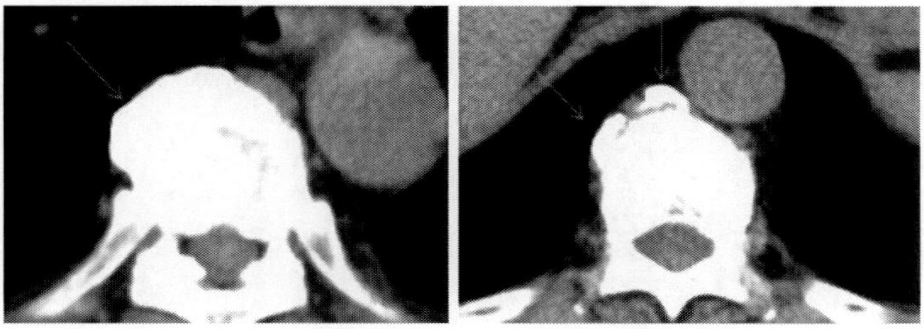

Figure 46. IgG4-related disease in a 72-year-old man. Axial non-contrast enhanced chest CT (CECT) images show focal calcification and ossification of the right side and the front of the anterior longitudinal ligament (arrows).

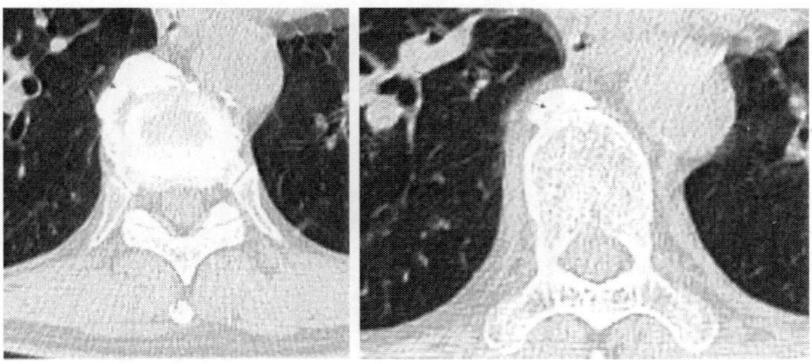

Figure 47. IgG4-related disease with ossification due to DISH (diffuse idiopathic skeletal hyperostosis) in a 66-year-old man. Axial chest non-contrast enhanced CT (NCECT) images show focal calcification and ossification of the right side of the anterior longitudinal ligament (arrows). CT images show swelling of the soft tissue of the right side of the vertebra.

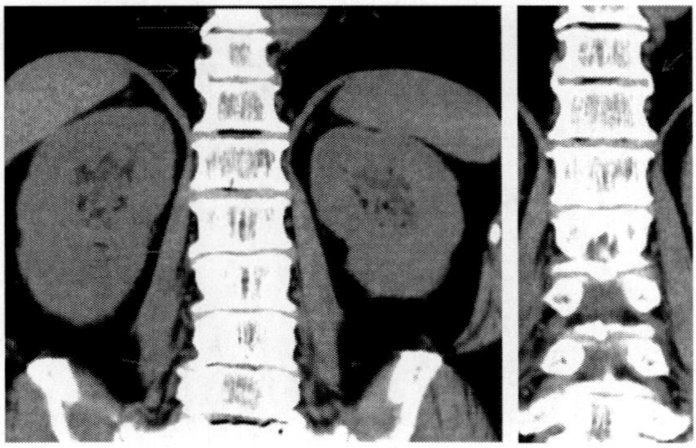

Figure 48. IgG4-related disease with ossification due to DISH (diffuse idiopathic skeletal hyperostosis) in a 72-year-old man. Coronal non-contrast enhanced chest CT (NCECT) images show ossification of the spine (arrows).

Contrast Enhanced Chest CT

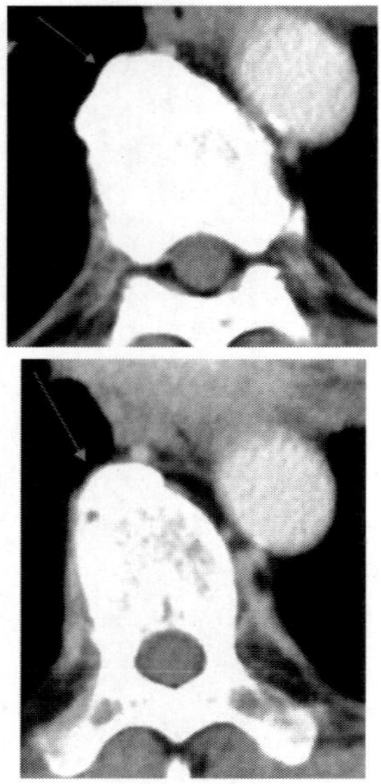

Figure 49. IgG4-related disease in a 67-year-old man. Axial contrast enhanced chest CT (CECT) images show focal calcification and ossification of the anterior longitudinal ligament (arrows).

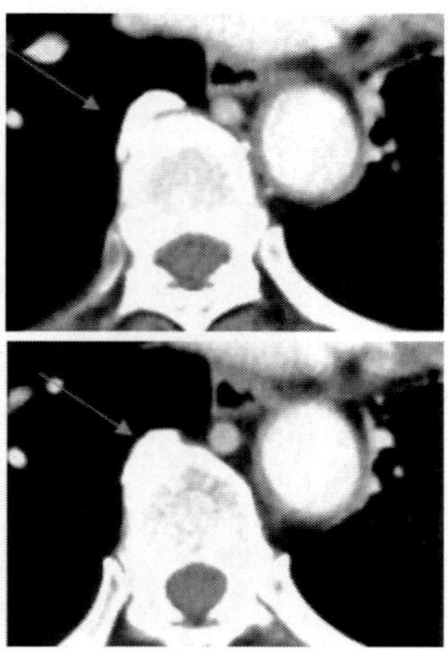

Figure 50. IgG4-related disease in a 76-year-old woman. Axial contrast enhanced chest CT images show focal calcification and ossification of the anterior longitudinal ligament (arrows) with periaortitis.

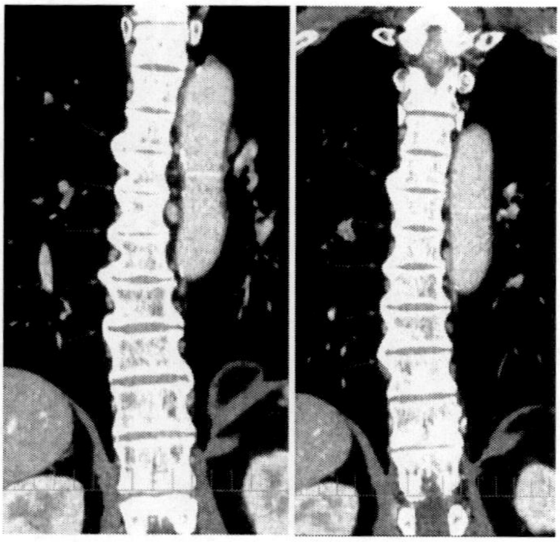

Figure 51. IgG4-related disease in a 67-year-old man. Coronal contrast enhanced chest CT (CECT) reconstructed images show ossification of the thoracic spine at least 4 contiguous vertebrae (arrows).

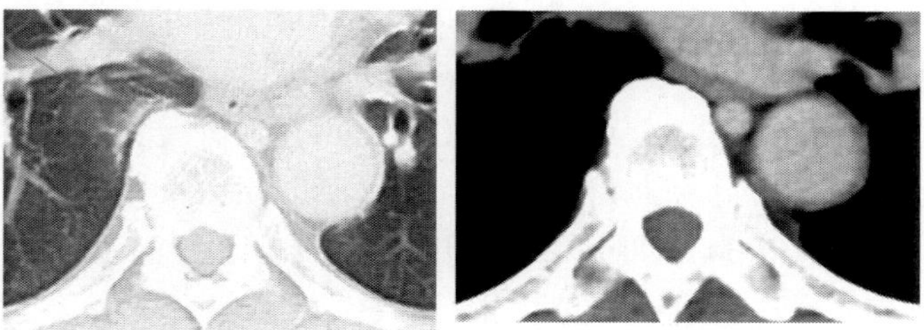

Figure 52. IgG4-related disease with ossification due to DISH (diffuse idiopathic skeletal hyperostosis) in a 72-year-old man. Axial contrast enhanced chest CT (NCECT) images show focal calcification and ossification of the right side and the front of the anterior longitudinal ligament. Lung window CT image (left panel) shows lung inflammation adjacent to the DISH lesion.

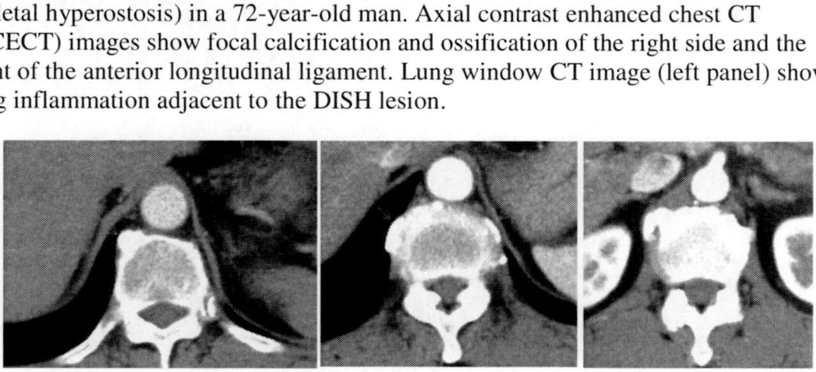

Figure 53. IgG4-related disease in a 63-year-old man. Axial contrast enhanced chest CT images show calcification and ossification of bilateral sides of the anterior longitudinal ligament.

Paravertebral Lesions in IgG4-Related Disease

IgG4-related paravertebral lesions appear as part of a systemic disorder usually associated with classic symptoms of IgG4-related disease such as pancreatitis, sialadenitis, and periaortitis (Inoue D. 2019) (Inoue D 2015) (Fujinaga Y 2009) (Flanagan EP 2015). IgG4-related paravertebral involvement was first described in 2010 (Zen Y. 2010). IgG4-related paravertebral lesions are asymptomatic and are often found incidentally on images.

IgG4-related paravertebral lesions primarily occur on the right side of the lower thoracic vertebrae. The lesions are present as well-demarcated band-like soft tissue masses due to plasma cell-rich sclerosing inflammation (Inoue D. 2019). On contrast-enhanced CT, IgG4-related paravertebral lesions have patent small arteries in early phase and show a homogeneous enhancement in late phase, corresponding to the sclerosing inflammatory process. IgG4-related paravertebral lesions respond well to corticosteroid therapy.

Inoue and colleagues reported that 29 patients had IgG4-related paravertebral involvement in 326 cases with IgG4-related disease (Inoue D. 2019). The 30 patients with IgG4-related para-spinal disease consisted of 25 men and 5 women, with a median age of 69.5 years and a range of ages from 47 to 87 years.

Anatomy of Vertebra

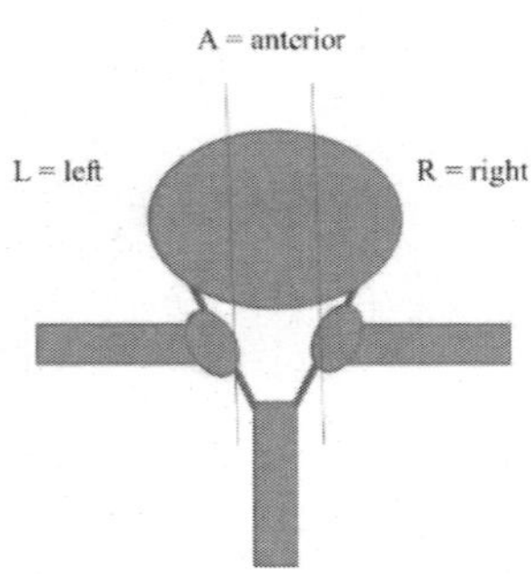

Figure 54. Definitions of sites of involvement in IgG4-related paravertebral lesions.

CT

Non-Contrast Enhanced Chest CT

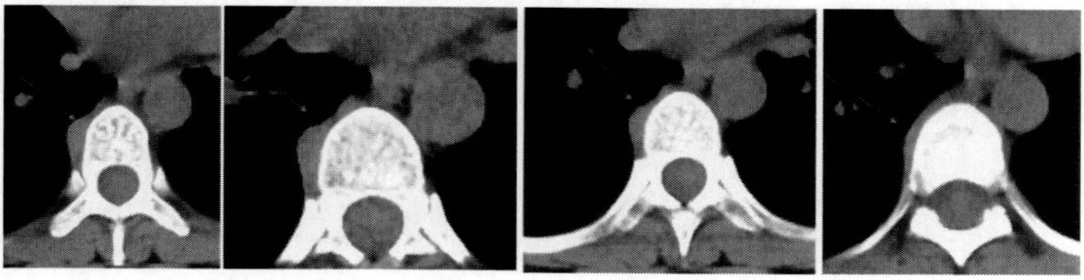

Figure 55. IgG4-related paravertebral lesion in a 44-year-old woman. Axial non-contrast enhanced chest CT (NCECT) images show soft tissue thickening along the right side of the lower thoracic vertebra (arrows).

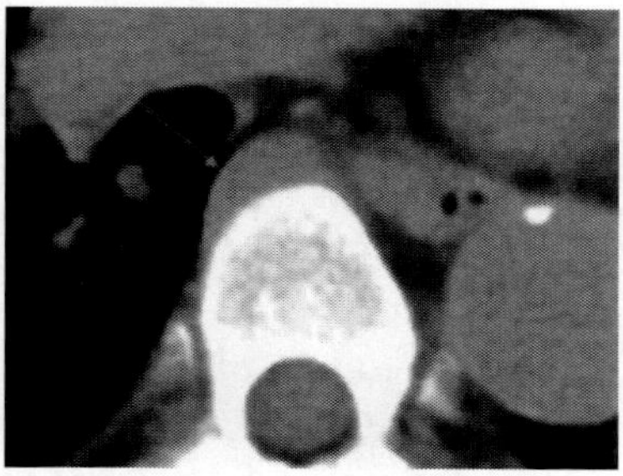

Figure 56. IgG4-related paravertebral lesion in a 67-year-old man. Axial non-contrast enhanced chest CT (NCECT) image shows paravertebral soft tissue thickening along the anterior of the lower thoracic vertebra (arrow).

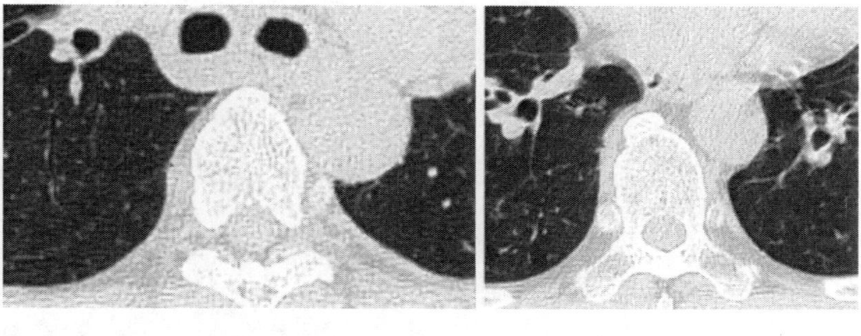

Figure 57. IgG4-related paravertebral lesion in a 66-year-old man. Axial chest non-contrast enhanced CT (NCECT) images show band-like masses of soft tissue on the right side of the thoracic vertebrae.

Contrast Enhanced Chest CT

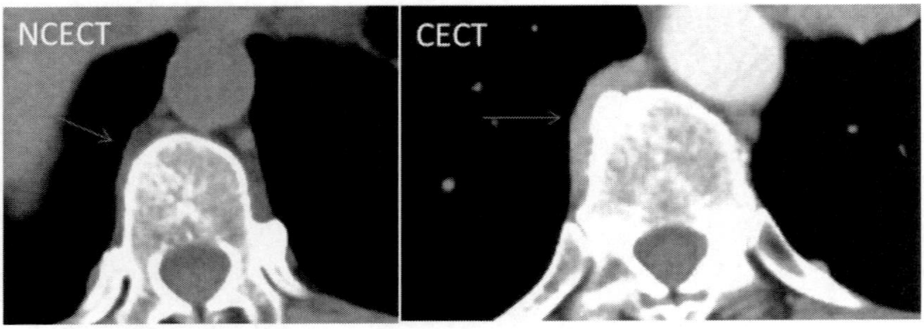

Figure 58. IgG4-related paravertebral lesion in a 55-year-old woman. Axial non-contrast enhanced chest CT (NCECT) image (left panel) shows soft tissue thickening along the anterior and right side of the lower thoracic vertebra (arrow). Axial contrast enhanced chest CT (CECT) image (right panel) shows homogeneously enhanced soft tissue (arrow).

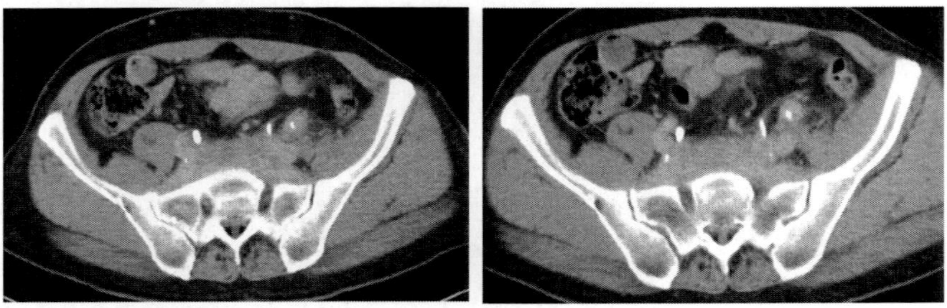

Figure 59. IgG4-related disease in a 63-year-old man. Non-contrast enhanced abdominal CT images show a soft mass in front of the sacrum. The internal structure of the mass is uniform.

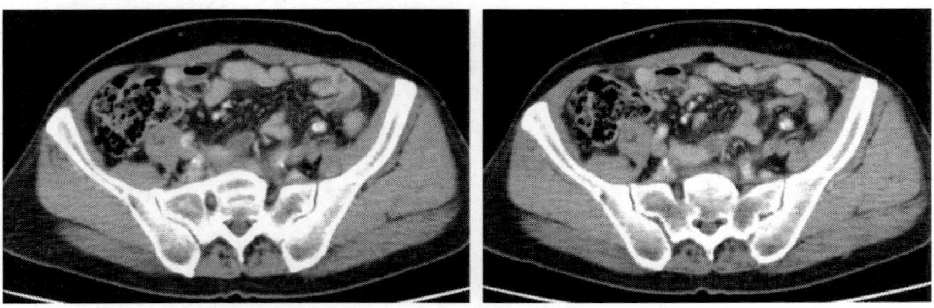

Figure 60. IgG4-related disease in the same patient as in previous figure. The soft mass in front of the sacrum was resolved after corticosteroid therapy.

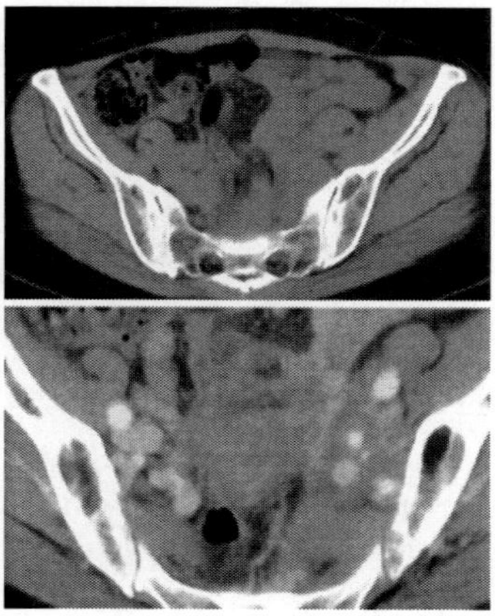

Figure 61. IgG4-related disease in a 59-year-old woman. Non-contrast enhanced and contrast-enhanced abdominal CT images show a soft mass that is relatively poor contrast enhancement surrounding the left common iliac artery and the internal iliac artery in front of the sacrum. The internal structure of the mass is relatively uniform. In the same area, the left internal iliac artery and left ureter are narrowed. The left ureter, the renal pelvis and the renal calyx, which is upstream of the same area, expand.

MRI

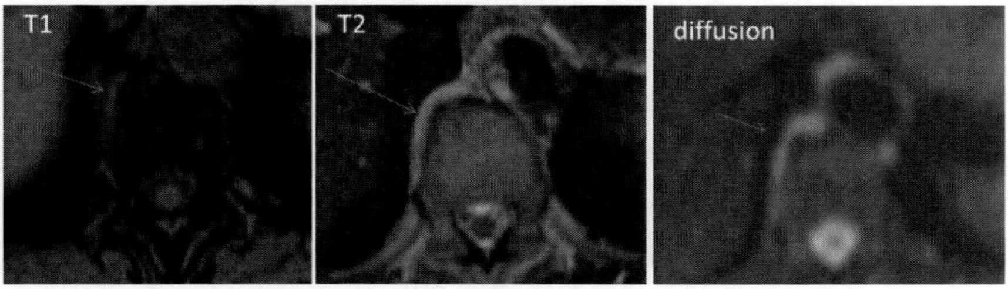

Figure 62. IgG4-related paravertebral lesion in a 49-year-old woman. Axial MR images (T1, T2 and diffusion-weighted images) show soft tissue thickening along the anterior and right side of the lower thoracic vertebra (arrows).

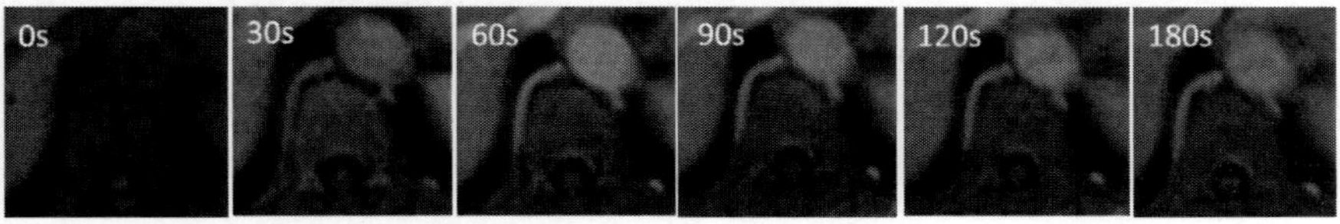

Figure 63. IgG4-related disease in a 49-year-old woman. Gadolinium-enhanced T1-weighted MR images depict a paravertebral lesion with enhancement in the delayed phase.

PET/CT

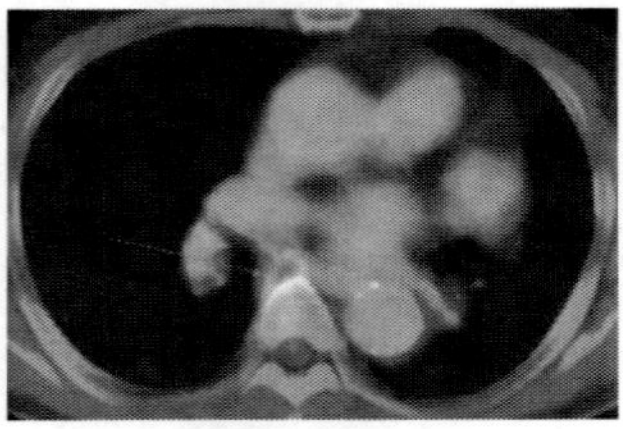

Figure 64. IgG4-related paravertebral lesions in a 67-year-old man. FDG PET/CT images show uptake in the paravertebral soft tissue (arrow).

Swelling of the Lower Limbs

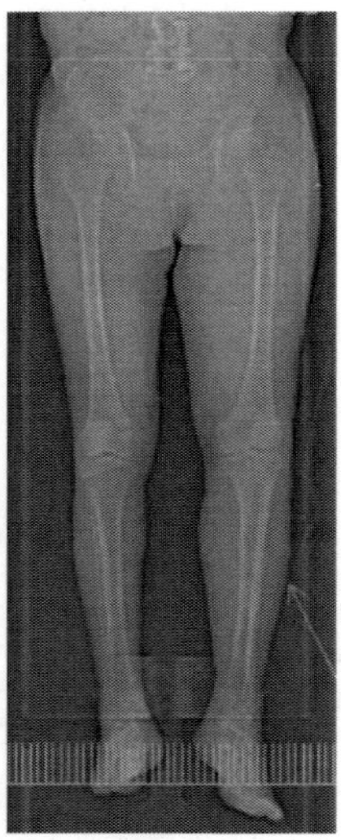

Figure 65. IgG4-related disease in a 63-year-old man. Conventional X-ray image shows swelling and edematous changes in the left lower limb (arrow).

IgG4-Related Myositis

Patients with IgG4-related myositis showing elevated serum IgG4, high ratio of IgG4 to total IgG (20%), IgG4 plasma cell infiltration of the muscular tissue, and a good response to glucocorticoid therapy have been reported (Tsai MK 2019). There are many conditions that can mimic IgG4-related myositis, such as cellulitis, necrotizing fasciitis, pyomyositis, deep venous thrombosis (DVT), and post-thrombotic syndrome. Histopathology is the gold standard for the diagnosis of IgG4-related disease.

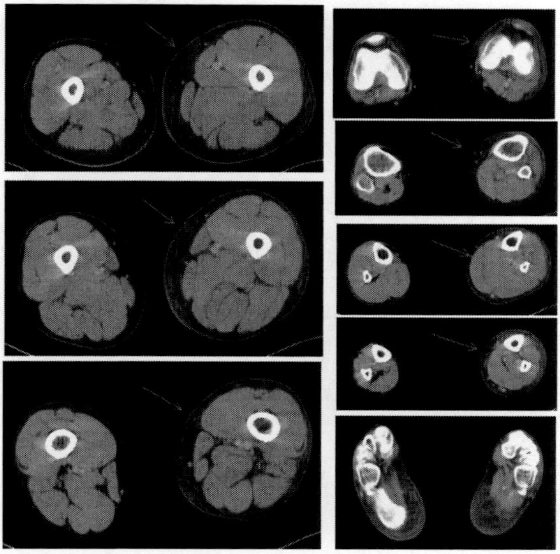

Figure 66. IgG4-related disease in a 63-year-old man. Axial non-contrast enhanced CT images show swelling and edematous changes of the subcutaneous tissue and muscles of the left lower limb (arrows). These lesions may be caused by IgG4-related inflammation and obstruction of veins and lymphatic vessels, and/or myositis.

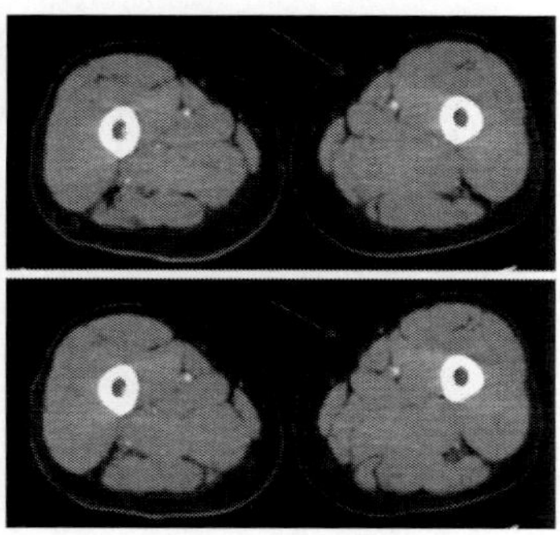

Figure 67. IgG4-related disease in the same patient as in previous figure. Swelling of the muscles of the left lower limb was resolved after corticosteroid therapy.

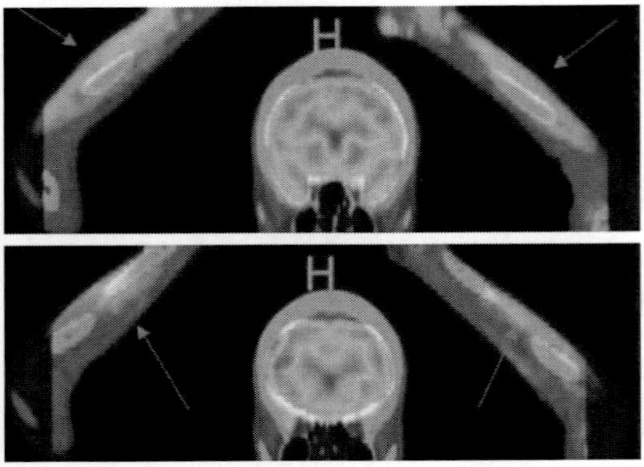

Figure 68. IgG4-related disease in a 66-year-old woman. Coronal PET/CT images show uptake in the muscles of bilateral upper limbs (arrows) caused by IgG4-related myositis.

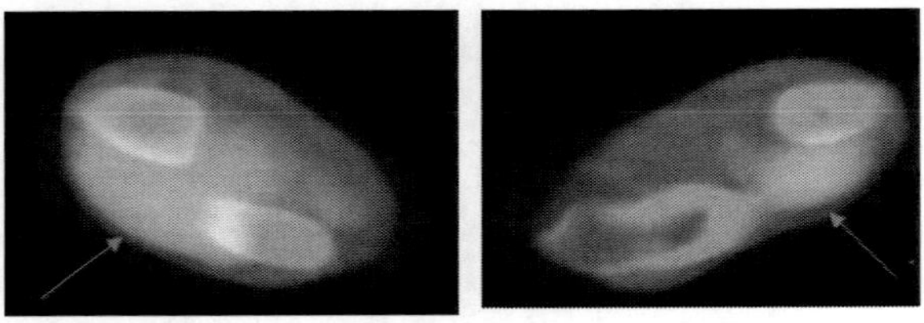

Figure 69. IgG4-related disease in a 66-year-old woman. Axial PET/CT images show uptake in the muscles of bilateral upper limbs (arrows) caused by IgG4-related myositis.

References

Flanagan EP, Chowdhary VR, McCarthy JT, Smyrk TC, Chari ST, Kumar N. "IgG4-related (neurologic) disease: diagnostic challenges, clinical clues and expanding spectrum." *Int J Rheum Dis* 18 (2015): 807-809.

Fujinaga Y, Kadoya M, Kawa S, et al. "Characteristic findings in images of extra-pancreatic lesions associated with autoimmune pancreatitis." *Eur J Radiol* 76 (2009): 228-238.

Hall, FM. "Radiographic diagnosis and accuracy in knee joint effusions." *Radiology* 15 (1975): 49-54.

Inoue D, Yoshida K, Yoneda N, et al. "IgG4-related disease: dataset of 235 consecutive patients." *Medicine (Baltimore)* 94 (2015): e680.

Inoue D., Zen Y, Komori T, Yoshida K, Yoneda N, Kitao A, Kozaka K, Izumozaki A, Matsumoto J, Toshima F, Kobayashi S, Gabata T. "CT Findings of Thoracic Paravertebral Lesions in IgG4-Related Disease." *AJR Am J Roentgenol* 213 (2019): W99-W104.

Masaki Y, Dong L, Kurose N, et al. "Proposal for a new clinical entity, IgG4-positive multiorgan lymphoproliferative syndrome: analysis of 64 cases of IgG4-related disorders." *Ann Rheum Dis* 68 (2009): 1310-5.

Tsai MK, Kuo CW, Chang LC. "IgG4-related myositis." *QJM: An International Journal of Medicine.* 112 (2019): 872-873.

Umekita K, Kaneko Y, Yorita K, Hashiba Y, Matsuda M, Miyauchi S, Ueno S, Takajo I, Kusumoto N, Nagatomo Y, Marutsuka K, Okayama A. "Arthropathy with infiltrate IgG4-positive plasma cells in synovium." *Rheumatology (Oxford)* 51 (2012): 580-2.

Zen Y., Nakanuma Y. "IgG4-related disease: a cross-sectional study of 114 cases." *Am J Surg Pathol* 34 (2010): 1812-1819.

In: IgG4 Related Disease
Editor: Syuichi Koarada
ISBN: 978-1-53618-050-3

Chapter 7

ABDOMINAL MANIFESTATIONS OF IGG4-RELATED DISEASE

Syuichi Koarada* and Akihito Maruyama
Division of Rheumatology, Faculty of Medicine,
Saga University, Nabeshima, Saga, Japan

ABSTRACT

IgG4-related disease is known to cause various abdominal lesions. The most famous lesion, however, is autoimmune pancreatitis. Autoimmune pancreatitis is a chronic pancreatitis characterized by elevated serum IgG4 and radiographically enlarged sausage-like pancreas that responds well to corticosteroids. Abdominal lesions of IgG4-related disease include various pathologies such as sclerosing cholangitis, peritoneal lesions, gastrointestinal tract lesions, enlarged lymph nodes, liver lesions, and splenomegaly.

---

* Corresponding Author's Email: koarada@cc.saga-u.ac.jp.

Pancreas: IgG4-Related Autoimmune Pancreatitis: Type 1 (IgG4-Related) Autoimmune Pancreatitis (AIP)

Autoimmune pancreatitis, a pancreatitis that often begins with obstructive jaundice and sometimes forms a pancreatic mass, is characterized by a high degree of lymphoplasmacytic infiltration, obstructive phlebitis, storiform fibrosis, and IgG4-bearing plasma cell infiltration, and a favorable response to corticosteroid therapy. Autoimmune pancreatitis (AIP) is a rare but specific form of chronic pancreatitis that occurs secondary to an immune-mediated fibrotic inflammatory process associated with elevated serum IgG4 levels in elderly male preponderance (Okazaki K. 2011). Pancreas is the most affected organ in IgG4-related disease.

The prevalence of autoimmune pancreatitis in Japan has been estimated at 0.82 per 100,000 persons, which may be underestimated (Nishimori I 2007) (Shimosegawa T 2009). IgG4-related autoimmune pancreatitis has been estimated to account for 2%-8% of patients with chronic pancreatitis (Nishimori I 2007) (Kamisawa T. 2006). Focal lesions account for 33%-41% of all cases with autoimmune pancreatitis (Muhi A 2012). There is also a report that an estimated 3% -9% of patients who have been resected for presumed pancreatic cancer have autoimmune pancreatitis (Abraham SC 2003).

Middle-aged and older men are predominantly affected, with 95% of patients aged 45 years or older (Cheuk W. 2010) (Nishimori I 2007). The ratio of men and women with autoimmune pancreatitis is of 3 to 7: 1.

Classification

There are two subtypes of autoimmune pancreatitis, type 1 (lymphoplasmacytic sclerosing pancreatitis) and type 2 (idiopathic duct-centric chronic pancreatitis) (Sah RP 2010). Type 2 autoimmune pancreatitis is not associated with elevated serum IgG4 levels and autoantibodies and has different histological and clinical characteristics from type 1 (Okazaki K. 2011). Patients with type 1 autoimmune pancreatitis have elevated serum IgG4 levels and show infiltration of IgG4-positive plasma cells in pancreatic specimens (Hamano H. 2001).

Clinical Features

There are no specific symptoms of type 1 autoimmune pancreatitis. Abdominal pain is absent or mild and presents with obstructive jaundice, diabetes, and accompanying extra-pancreatic symptoms. Abdominal pain is common in type 2 autoimmune pancreatitis, often accompanied by acute pancreatitis. In some cases, acute pancreatitis or severe pancreatitis occurs. Obstructive jaundice is observed in 1/3 to half of patients, and back pain and weight loss are also observed. Some patients have anorexia, general malaise, and stool abnormality.

Many patients consult a physician for mild abdominal pain, general malaise, jaundice, and thirst, while others have no apparent subjective symptoms. In urinalysis and blood biochemistry, pancreatic enzymes and hepatobiliary enzymes are abnormal, and sometimes the patient is referred for a high CA19-9 level. In the process of differential diagnosis from pancreatic cancer and bile duct cancer, autoimmune pancreatitis is often pointed out by pancreatic imaging such as abdominal ultrasonography, CT, and MRI.

Systemic lesions of autoimmune pancreatitis include sclerosing cholangitis (60%), sialadenitis (14%), retroperitoneal fibrosis (10%), interstitial pneumonia (8%), and tubular interstitial nephritis (8%). Many other organs are also recognized as targets for IgG4-related disease and type 1 autoimmune pancreatitis (Matsubayashi H 2014).

Table 1. Extrapancreatic lesions associated with type 1 autoimmune pancreatitis (Matsubayashi H 2014)

Close association
Lachrymal gland inflammation
Sialadenitis
Hilar lymphadenopathy
Interstitial pneumonitis
Sclerosing cholangitis
Retroperitoneal fibrosis
Tubulointerstitial nephritis
Possible association
Hypophysitis
Autoimmune neurosensory hearing loss
Uveitis
Chronic thyroiditis
Pseudotumor (breast, lung, liver)
Gastric ulcer
Swelling of Papilla of Vater
IgG4 hepatopathy
Periaortitis
Prostatitis
IgA vasculitis
Autoimmune thrombocytopenia

Laboratory Findings

There are no disease-specific laboratory findings for autoimmune pancreatitis. However, blood pancreatic enzymes, hepatobiliary enzymes, and total bilirubin are often elevated. In autoimmune pancreatitis, elevated serum IgG4 levels are of diagnostic value, but are not disease specific. In autoimmune pancreatitis, the sensitivity of elevated serum IgG4 levels is 80%, and the specificity is 98% when pancreatic cancer is used as a control group. Some non-specific autoantibodies are positive for IgG4-RD-related autoimmune pancreatitis, while other disease-specific antibodies, such as anti-SSA /

Ro, anti-SSB/La, and anti-mitochondrial antibodies, are negative (Kawa S 2019). Many cases of autoimmune pancreatitis have exocrine pancreatic insufficiency and pancreatic endocrine dysfunction (diabetes).

Diagnosis

After excluding malignant neoplasms, a comprehensive diagnosis is made based on pancreatic imaging findings, blood tests, histopathological findings, extrapancreatic lesions, and responsiveness to glucocorticoids. Although pathological diagnosis is important, obtaining tissue samples from specific organs such as the pancreas is difficult (Shimosegawa T. 2011).

Classification criteria are standardized definitions aimed at creating clear and homogeneous cohorts for clinical research. A classification criteria for IgG4-related disease are needed to distinguish between IgG4-related disease and similar diseases.

The International Consensus Diagnostic Criteria (ICDC), diagnostic criteria for autoimmune pancreatitis proposed by the international consensus, can diagnose type 1 and type 2 autoimmune pancreatitis (Shimosegawa T. 2011). In Japan, Clinical diagnostic criteria for autoimmune pancreatitis in 2011 by Japan Pancreas Society are used (JPS 2011).

When a patient with a focal/segmental image of AIP on CT/MRI without ERCP findings fulfill more than one of III, IVb and V (a/b) ERP criteria, he/she can be diagnosed as probable AIP only after the negative workup for malignancy by EUS-FNA, and confirmed as definitive one by an optional steroid response. 1Possible diagnosis: A case may possibly be type 2, although it is extremely rare in Japan. AIP: Autoimmune pancreatitis; CT: Computed tomography; MRI: Magnetic resonance image.

Table 2. Diagnosis of definitive and probable type 1 autoimmune pancreatitis using international consensus diagnostic criteria

Diagnosis	Primary basis for diagnosis	Imaging evidence	Collateral evidence
Definitive type 1 AIP	Histology	Typical/indeterminate	Histologically confirmed LPSP (level 1 H)
	Imaging	Typical	Any non-D level 1/level 2
		Indeterminate	Two or more from level 1 (+ level 2 D1)
	Response to steroid	Indeterminate	level 1 S/OOI + Rt or level 1 D + level 2 S/OOI/H + Rt
Probable type 1 AIP		Indeterminate	level 2 S/OOI/H + Rt

Criterion	Level 1	Level 2
P: Parenchymal imaging	Typical: Diffuse enlargement with delayed enhancement (sometimes associated with rim-like enhancement)	Indeterminate (including atypical3): Segmental/focal enlargement with delayed enhancement
D: Ductal imaging (ERP)	long (> 1/3 length of the main pancreatic duct) or multiple strictures without marked upstream dilatation	Segmental/focal narrowing without marked upstream dilatation (duct size, < 5 mm)
S: Serology	IgG4, > 2 × upper limit of normal value	IgG4, 1-2 × upper limit of normal value
OOI:Other organ involvement a or b		a or b
	a: Histology of extrapancreatic organs Any three of the following: (1) Marked lymphoplasmacytic infiltration with fibrosis and without granulocytic infiltration (2) Storiform fibrosis (3) Obliterative phlebitis (4) Abundant (> 10 cells/HPF) IgG4-positive cells	a: Histology of extrapancreatic organs including endoscopic biopsies of bile duct4: Both of the following: (1) Marked lymphoplasmacytic infiltration without granulocytic infiltration (2) Abundant (> 10 cells/HPF) IgG4-positive cells
	b: Typical radiological evidence At least one of the following: (1) Segmental/multiple proximal (hilar/intrahepatic) or proximal and distal bile duct stricture (2) Retroperitoneal fibrosis	b: Physical or radiological evidence At least one of the following (1) Symmetrically enlarged salivary /lachrymal glands (2) Radiological evidence of renal involvement described in association with AIP
H: Histology of the pancreas	IPSP (core biopsy/resection) At least 3 of the following: (1) Periductal lymphoplasmacytic infiltrate without granulocytic infiltration (2) Obliterative phlebitis (3) Storiform fibrosis (4) Abundant (> 10 cells/HPF) IgG4-positive cells	IPSP (core biopsy) Any 2 of the following: (1) Periductal lymphoplasmacytic infiltrate without granulocytic infiltration (2) Obliterative phlebitis (3) Storiform fibrosis (4) Abundant (> 10 cells/HPF) IgG4-positive cells
Response to steroid (Rt)2	Diagnostic steroid trial Rapid (≤ 2 wk) radiologically demonstrable resolution or marked improvement in pancreatic/extrapancreatic manifestations	

1level 2 D is counted as level 1 in this setting; 2Diagnostic steroid trial should be conducted carefully by pancreatologists with caveats (see text) only after negative workup for cancer including endoscopic ultrasound-guided fine needle aspiration; 3Atypical: Some AIP cases may show low-density mass, pancreatic ductal dilatation, or distal atrophy. Such atypical imaging findings in patients with obstructive jaundice and/or pancreatic mass are highly suggestive of pancreatic cancer. Such patients should be managed as pancreatic cancer unless there is strong collateral evidence for AIP, and a thorough workup for cancer is negative (see algorithm); 4Endoscopic biopsy of duodenal papilla is a useful adjunctive method because ampulla often is involved pathologically in AIP. AIP: Autoimmune pancreatitis; ICDC: International consensus diagnostic criteria; HPF: High power field; LPSP: Lymphplasmacytic sclerosing; OOI: Other organ involvement.

Table 3. Clinical diagnostic criteria for autoimmune pancreatitis in 2011 by Japan Pancreas Society (JPS-2011)

A: Diagnostic items

I: Enlargement of the pancreas:

(a) Diffuse enlargement

(b) Segmental/focal enlargement

II: ERP (endoscopic retrograde pancreatography) shows irregular narrowing of the main pancreatic duct

III: Serological findings

Elevated level of serum IgG4 ($\geq$ 135 mg/dl)

IV: Pathological findings: Among (1)-(4) listed below

(a) Three or more are observed

(b) Two are observed

(1) Prominent infiltration of lymphocytes and plasmacytes and fibrosis

(2) More than 10 IgG4-positive plasmacytes per high-power microscope field

(3) Storiform fibrosis

(4) Obliterative phlebitis

V: Extra-pancreatic lesions: sclerosing cholangitis, sclerosing dacryoadenitis/ sialoadenitis/ retroperitoneal fibrosis

(a) Clinical lesions

Extrapancreatic sclerosing cholangitis, sclerosing dacryoadenitis/ sialoadenitis (Mikulicz's disease) or/retroperitoneal fibrosis

(b) Pathological lesions

Pathological examination shows characteristic features of sclerosing cholangitis, sclerosing dacryoadenitis sialoadenitis or/retroperitoneal fibrosis

<Option>

Effectiveness of steroid therapy

A specialized facility may include in its diagnosis the effectiveness of steroid therapy, once pancreatic or bile duct cancers have been ruled out. When it is difficult to differentiate from malignant conditions, it is desirable to perform cytological examination using an endoscopic ultrasound-guided fine needle aspiration (EUS-FNA). Facile therapeutic diagnosis by steroids should be avoided unless the possibility of malignant tumor has been ruled out by pathological diagnosis.

B: Diagnosis

I: Definite diagnosis

(1). Diffuse type

  Ia + III/IVb/V (a/b)

(2). Segmental/focal type

  Ib + II + two or more of < III/IVb/V (a/b) >

  Or

  Ib + II + < III/IVb/V (a/b) > + Option

(3). Definite diagnosis by histopathological study

  IVa

II: Probable diagnosis

  Segmental/focal type: Ib + II + < III/IVb/V(a/b) >

III: Possible diagnosis1

  Diffuse type: Ia + II + Option

  Segmental/focal type: Ib + II + Option

Patients who respond to treatment with glucocorticoids may be autoimmune pancreatitis but cannot rule out pancreatic cancer.

Imaging of Pancreatic Lesions

Imaging of pancreatic lesions includes abdominal ultrasound (US), computed tomography (CT), and magnetic resonance imaging (MRI), which are useful for morphological diagnosis of the pancreatic parenchyma, MR cholangiopancreatographic imaging (MRCP) and endoscopic retrograde cholangiopancreatography (ERCP) are useful for morphological diagnosis of pancreatic duct.

The radiological specific features of autoimmune pancreatitis are diffuse enlargement of the pancreas ("sausage-like"), capsule-like rims (halo) surrounding the organ, and irregular narrowing of the main pancreatic duct (Kawa 2016).

There are two main patterns of autoimmune pancreatitis, diffuse and focal distribution (Sahani DV 2004) (Yang DH 1996).

Computed Tomography (CT)

Non-Contrast Enhanced Abdominal CT (NCECT) Image

On non-contrast enhanced abdominal CT images, the diffuse enlarged pancreas loses its normal pancreatic lobulations and shows smooth, sausage-like form.

Pancreatic lesions are usually hypoattenuating compared to normal parenchyma on CT, and the fat planes around the pancreas are preserved without vascular encasement, but stenosis of the peri-pancreatic vein may occur. Nonspecific enlargement of regional lymph nodes is also seen on CT.

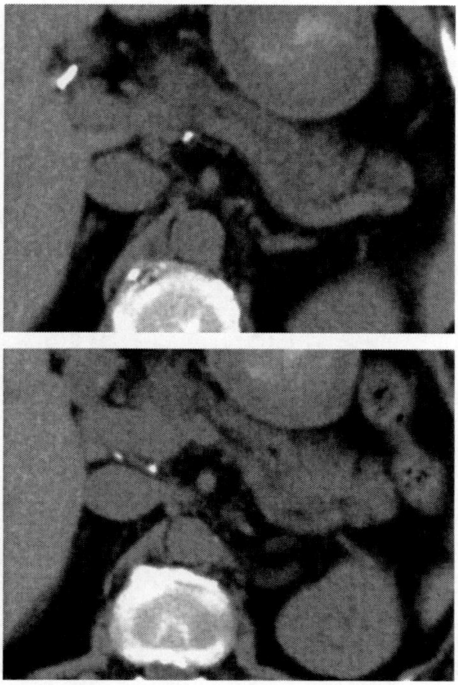

Figure 1. IgG4-related disease in an 80-year-old woman. Axial non-contrast enhanced CT images. The pancreas is enlarged. Inflammation in both pancreatic parenchyma and peri-pancreatic adipose tissue is involved.

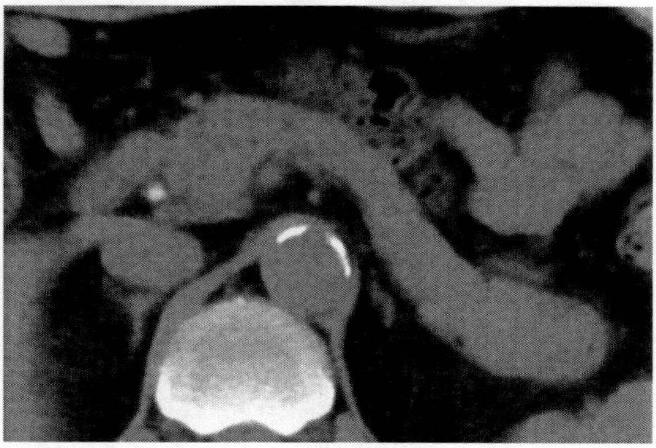

Figure 2. Autoimmune pancreatitis in a 70-year-old man. Axial non-contrast enhanced abdominal CT image. The pancreatic tail is suspected to have localized enlargement.

Contrast Enhanced CT (CECT)

Contrast enhanced CT (CECT) is an important imaging for diagnosis of autoimmune pancreatitis and shows findings such as diffuse or focal enlargement of the pancreas.

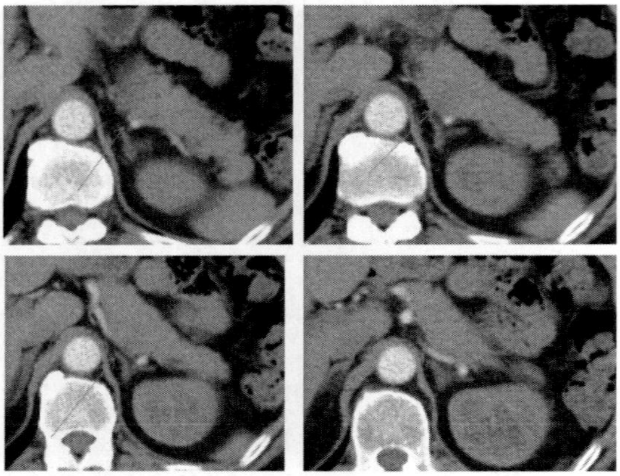

Figure 3. IgG4-related disease in a 63-year-old man. Axial contrast enhanced CT images. Post contrast, in very early phase imaging there is slightly decreased enhancement within a tumor on the dorsal side of the pancreatic body (arrows) relative to normal pancreatic parenchyma.

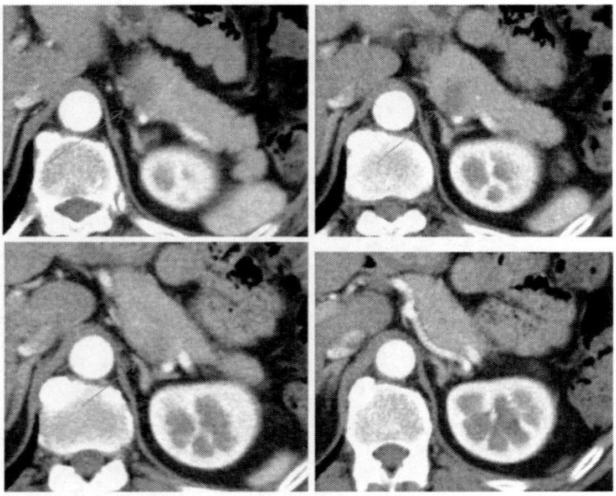

Figure 4. IgG4-related disease in a 63-year-old man. Axial contrast enhanced CT images. Post contrast, in early phase imaging there is clearly decreased enhancement within a tumor on the dorsal side of the pancreatic body (arrows) relative to normal pancreatic parenchyma.

The low attenuation capsule around the pancreas (the so-called "halo"), which is a combination of fibrosis, fluid collection and phlegmon, is a characteristic finding. This finding is unique and is not seen in other pancreatic disorders. Halo is observed in 12% -48% of patients on CT (Sahani DV 2004) (Suzuki K 2010) (Ishigami K 2010) (Kim HJ 2015). The presence of a halo is a useful finding in differentiating autoimmune pancreatitis from pancreatic cancer (Zaheer A 2014).

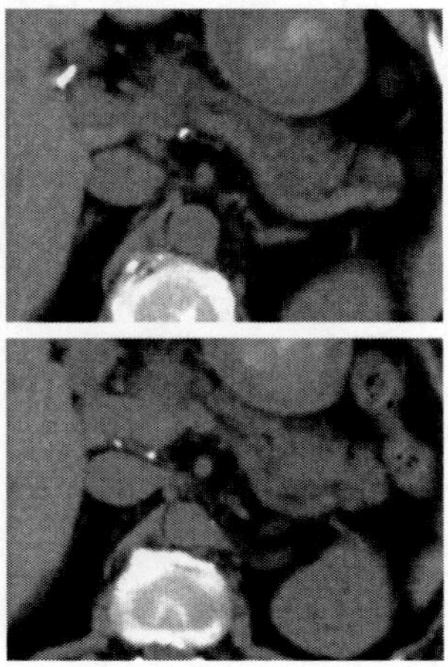

Figure 5. IgG4-related autoimmune pancreatitis in an 80-year-old woman. Axial non-contrast enhanced abdominal CT images. The pancreas is bulky.

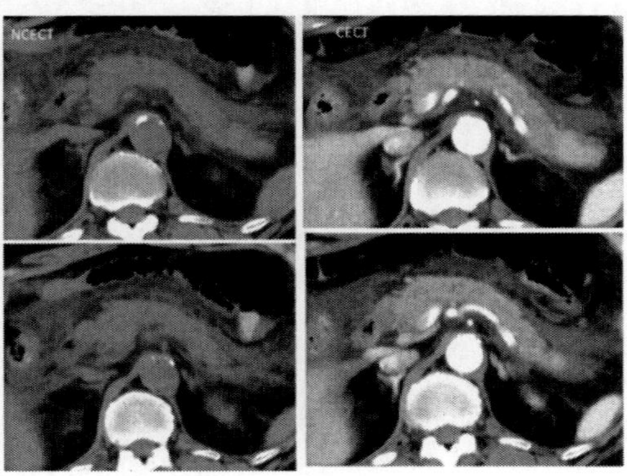

Figure 6. IgG4-related autoimmune pancreatitis in a 70-year-old man. Acute pancreatitis on chronic pancreatitis. The pancreas is bulky and the density of adipose tissue around pancreas is increased.

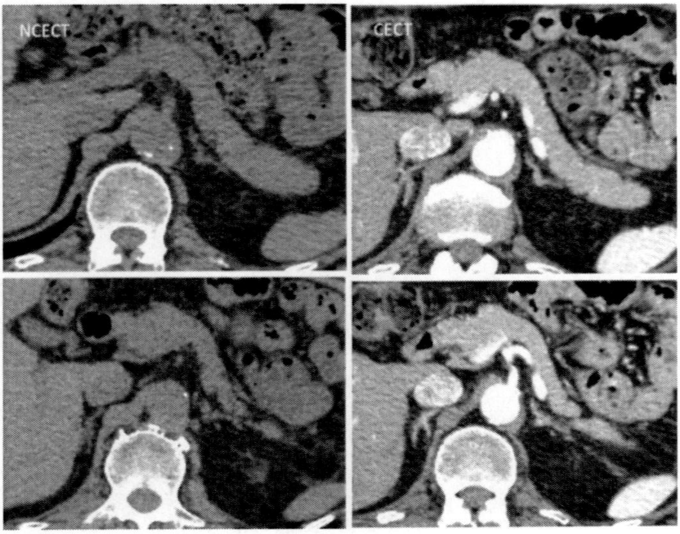

Figure 7. IgG4-related disease with acute pancreatitis in the same patient as in previous figure. The swelling of the pancreas due to pancreatitis was resolved after corticosteroid therapy.

In early phase, the enhanced effect within the affected area decreases post contrast compared with in the normal pancreatic parenchyma, but in the later delayed phase, persistent enhancement is observed (Tang CSW 2018).

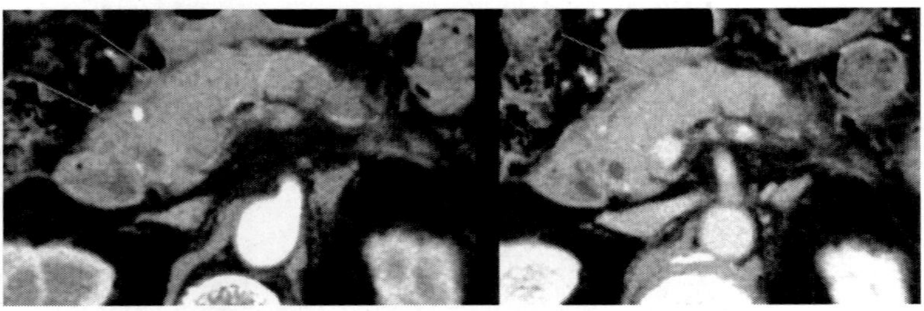

Figure 8. Autoimmune pancreatitis in a 75-year-old woman. Axial contrast enhanced abdominal CT (CETC) images. Left: early phase, Right: later delayed phase. The head of the pancreas is focally enlarged (sausage-like appearance) with a subtle peri-pancreatic halo of low attenuation (arrows). In the later delayed phase, persistent enhancement is observed. Loss of fat cleft in the pancreas is also seen. A rim surrounding the pancreatic head (halo) is thought to represent fibrous tissue.

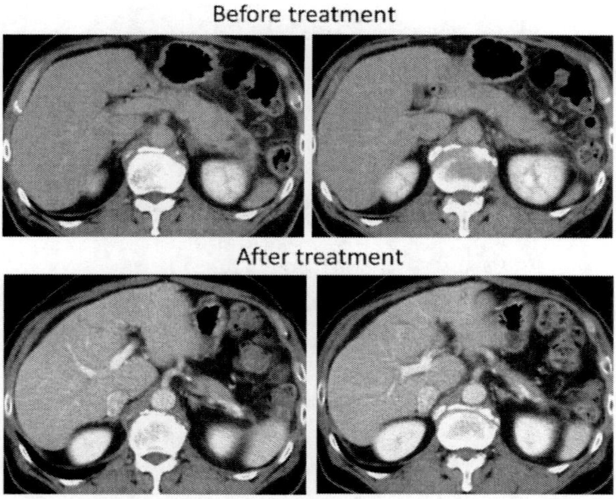

Figure 9. IgG 4-related pancreatitis in a 66-year-old man. Axial contrast enhanced abdominal CT images obtained before and after corticosteroid treatment show improved of enlargement and cystic changes of the pancreas.

MRI

Halo is observed in 18% -47% of patients on MRI (Sahani DV 2004) (Suzuki K 2010) (Ishigami K 2010) (Kim HJ 2015).

T1-Weighted MRI

Halo, surrounding fibrotic tissue, is observed as a hypointense rim in T1-weighted MRI, which is better depicted on MRI than on CT (Sangha Brar JS 2018).

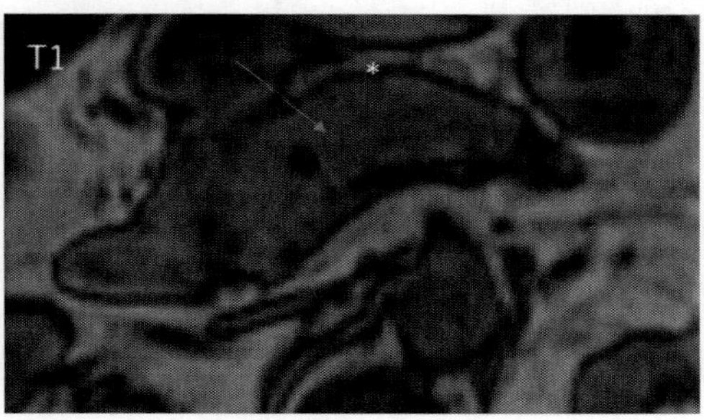

Figure 10. Autoimmune pancreatitis in a 75-year-old woman. Axial T1-weighted abdominal MR image shows a hypointense enlargement of the pancreatic head and body (arrow), loss of fat cleft and a hypointense halo of fibrosis (*).

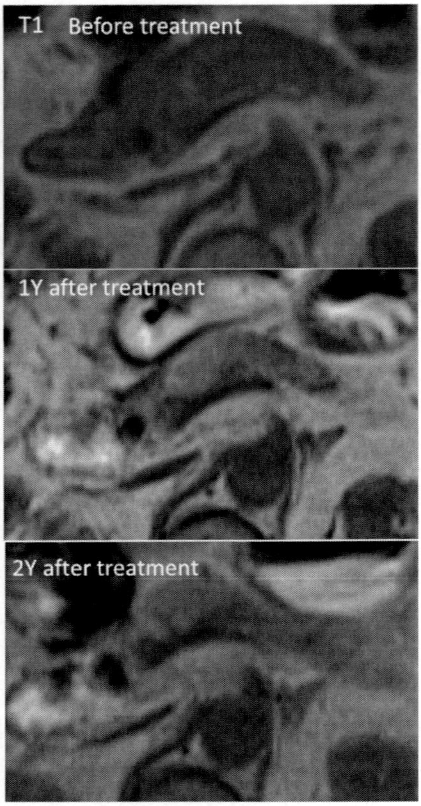

Figure 11. IgG 4-related pancreatitis in a 74-year-old woman. Follow-up axial T1-wighted MR images obtained before corticosteroid treatment (upper panel) and 1-year (middle panel) and 2 years after treatment (lower panel) show shrinkage of the enlarged pancreas.

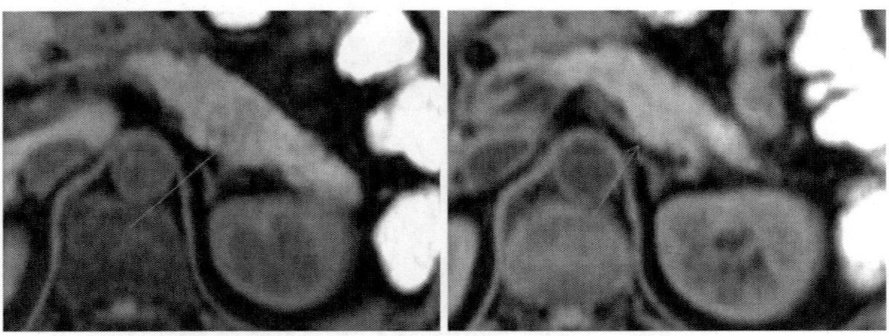

Figure 12. IgG4-related focal pancreatitis in a 63-year-old man. Axial T1-wighted fat saturated (FS) MR images show focal hypointense mass-like lesion (arrows).

Gadolinium Enhanced T1-Weighted MRI

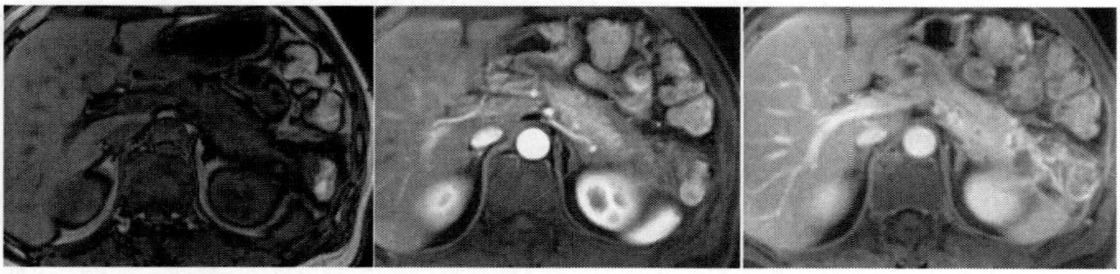

Figure 13. Autoimmune pancreatitis in a 63-year-old man. Axial gadolinium enhanced T1 MR image (arterial phase) (middle panel) shows reduced enhancement of the peri-pancreatic tissue compared to the pancreas (arrows). Axial T1 post-contrast equilibrium phase shows delayed enhancement of the peri-pancreatic tissue (right panel).

T2-Weighted MRI

On T2-weighted MR images, autoimmune pancreatitis shows mild low signal when fibrosis is strong but may show mild high signal in cases with mild fibrosis. The signal intensity of the lesion in the T2-weighted image varies depending on the degree of fibrosis.

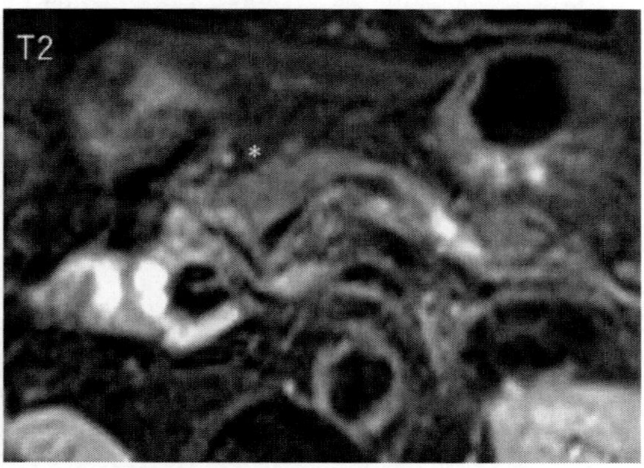

Figure 14. Autoimmune pancreatitis in a 75-year-old woman. Axial T2-weighted fat saturated (FS) image shows hyperintense T2 signal within the pancreas, but low T2 signal peri-pancreatic tissue (*).

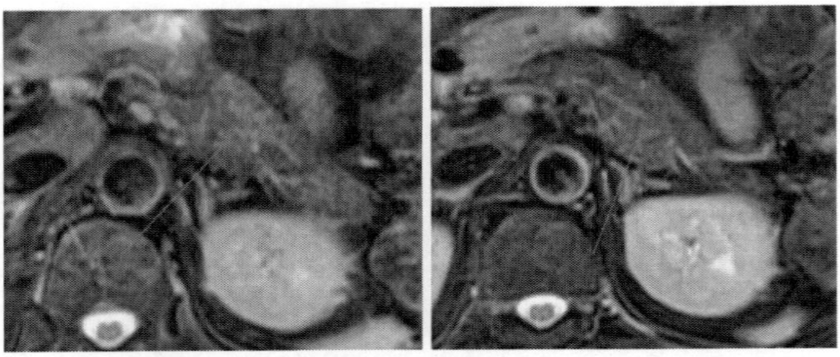

Figure 15. Focal autoimmune pancreatitis in a 63-year-old man. Axial T2-weighted fat saturated (FS) images show isointensity and slight hyperintensity signal of the nodule in the pancreas.

Diffusion-Weighted Imaging (DWI)

Diffusion-weighted imaging (DWI) can be useful in evaluating autoimmune pancreatitis (AIP).

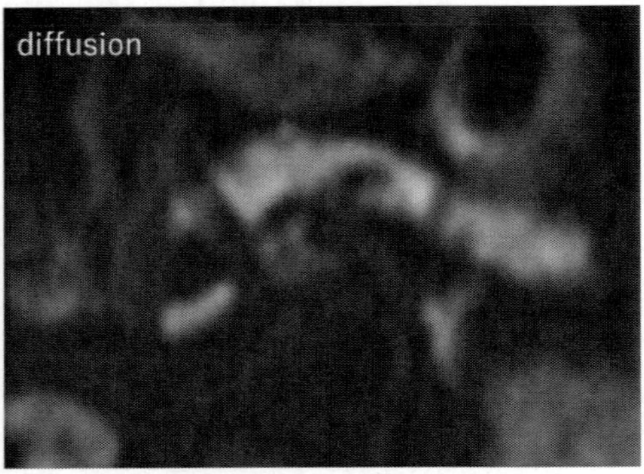

Figure 16. Autoimmune pancreatitis in a 75-year-old woman. Axial diffusion-weighted MR image shows the lesion with hyperintense relative to the pancreatic parenchyma because of inflammation.

Figure 17. Focal autoimmune pancreatitis in a 63-year-old man. On axial diffusion-weighted MR images, the lesion (arrow) is slightly hyperintense relative to the pancreatic parenchyma because of inflammation.

Dynamic MRI

Dynamic MRI is a method in which a contrast agent is administered while continuously acquiring MR images and the transferability of the contrast agent into the tissue is determined from the change in the obtained image intensity.

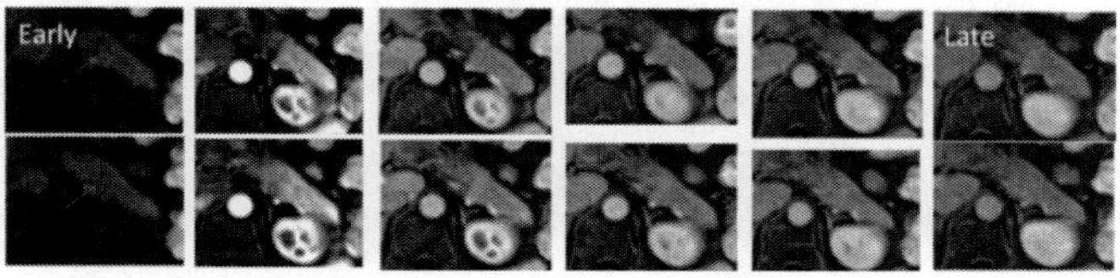

Figure 18. On dynamic MRI, focal autoimmune pancreatitis lesions show mild delayed staining.

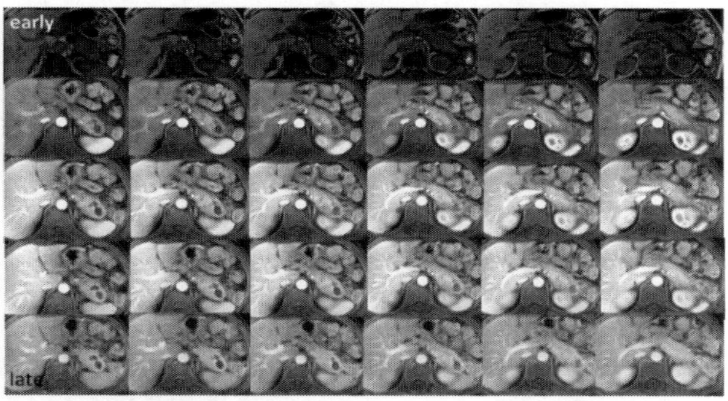

Figure 19. On dynamic MRI, focal autoimmune pancreatitis lesions show delayed staining of the peri-pancreatic tissue.

MR Cholangiopancreatography (MRCP)

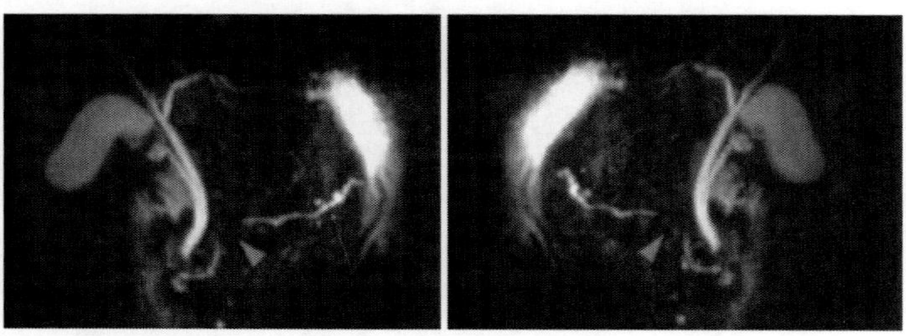

Figure 20. Autoimmune pancreatitis in a 74-year-old man. Coronal MR cholangiopancreatographic (MRCP) images show stenosis or defect in the affected segment of the main pancreatic duct (arrowheads), with upstream dilatation (arrows). Narrowing of the upstream pancreatic duct is smooth and tapered (ice pick sign).

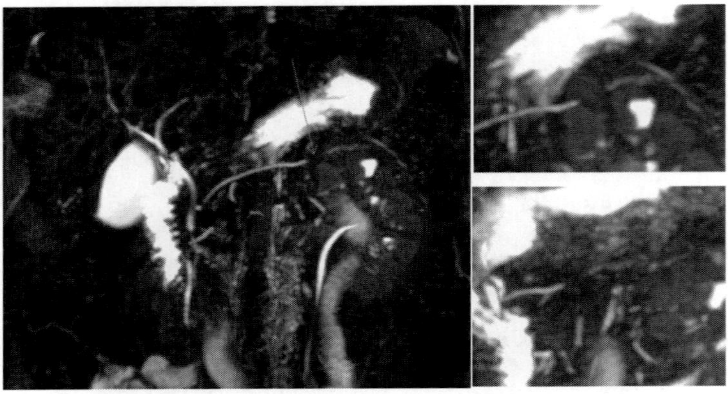

Figure 21. Focal autoimmune pancreatitis in a 63-year-old man. MR cholangiopancreatographic (MRCP) images show narrowing in the main pancreatic duct at the junction of the pancreatic body and tail. There is little dilation in the upstream pancreatic duct.

Gallium Scan

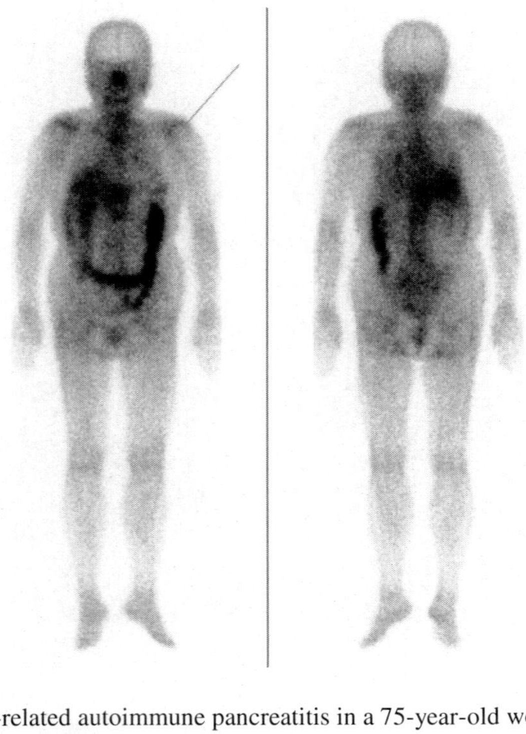

Figure 22. IgG4-related autoimmune pancreatitis in a 75-year-old woman. Gallium scan shows uptake in the pancreatic head (arrow).

Abdominal Ultrasonography

In a typical case, it generally exhibits a diffuse or focal enlargement with hypoechoic parenchyma and takes a form described as "sausage-like appearance." The swollen part shows a low-echo image, and high-echo spots may be scattered. In the case of focal enlargement of the pancreas, autoimmune pancreatitis requires a differential diagnosis from pancreatic cancer or mass-forming pancreatitis.

Differential Diagnosis

Pancreatic Cancer

Autoimmune pancreatitis results in obstructive jaundice and swelling of the pancreas, which can mimic pancreatic cancer (Kawa S 2019). The differentiation between pancreatic cancer and autoimmune pancreatitis is clinically difficult in some cases. However, the presence of the peri-pancreatic capsule in autoimmune pancreatitis is useful for differentiation (Zaheer A 2014). Another characteristic of autoimmune pancreatitis is that even if there is narrowing in the pancreatic duct, there is no or little upstream duct dilation (Sun GF 2013).

Pancreatitis

Autoimmune pancreatitis is not associated with pancreatic pseudocysts, peri-pancreatic fluid collections and retroperitoneal fluid. Lack of these findings differs from acute and chronic pancreatitis.

IgG4-Related Sclerosing Cholangitis

IgG4-associated sclerosing cholangitis (IgG4-SC) is cholangitis characterized by elevated serum IgG4 levels, dense infiltration in the bile duct walls by IgG4-positive plasma cells and lymphocytes, fibrosis, and occlusive phlebitis (Nakazawa 2012). IgG4-related sclerosing cholangitis is frequently associated with autoimmune pancreatitis and is the bile duct lesion of IgG4-related disease that is a systemic disease (Kamisawa T.. 2015). Becaise IgG4-sclerosing cholangitis is closely related to autoimmune pancreatitis, their co-existence helps diagnose both diseases (Nakazawa T. 2016).

Classification

Classification, based on bile duct images and the presence or absence of autoimmune inflammation, is used (Nakazawa T 2006).

Type 1 IgG4-SC presents with stenosis in the lower bile duct (intrapancreatic bile duct), and it is necessary to differentiate between lower bile duct cancer and pancreatic cancer.

Type 2 IgG4-SC has multiple stenoses in the bile ducts inside and outside the liver, and it is important to distinguish it from primary sclerosing cholangitis. Further, type 2 IgG4-SC is classified into type 2a IgG4-SC in which the intrahepatic bile ducts with prestenotic dilatation and type 2b IgG4-SC in which stricture of the intrahepatic bile ducts is without prestenotic dilation. Type 2 IgG4-SC has multiple stenoses in the bile ducts inside and outside the liver, so it is important to distinguish it from the "pruned-tree" appearance in primary sclerosing cholangitis (PSC).

Type 3 IgG4-SC presents stenosis in the lower bile duct and hilar hepatic bile duct lesions. Type 4-SC presents only with strictures of the hilar bile ducts. Types 3 and 4 IgG4-SC need to be differentiated from cholangiocarcinoma.

Differential Diagnosis

Because IgG4-related sclerosing cholangitis is widely distributed throughout the biliary system, it is important to differentiation lower bile duct lesions of IgG4-rellated sclerosing cholangitis from pancreatic cancer and intrahepatic or hilar lesions of primary sclerosing cholangitis and bile duct malignancies.

CT

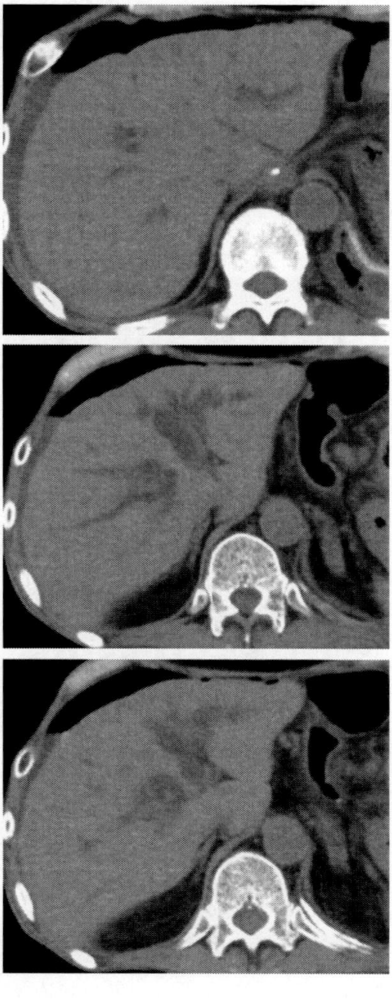

Figure 23. IgG4-related disease in a 56-year-old man. Axial non-contrast enhanced abdominal CT images show remarked intrahepatic biliary tract dilatation.

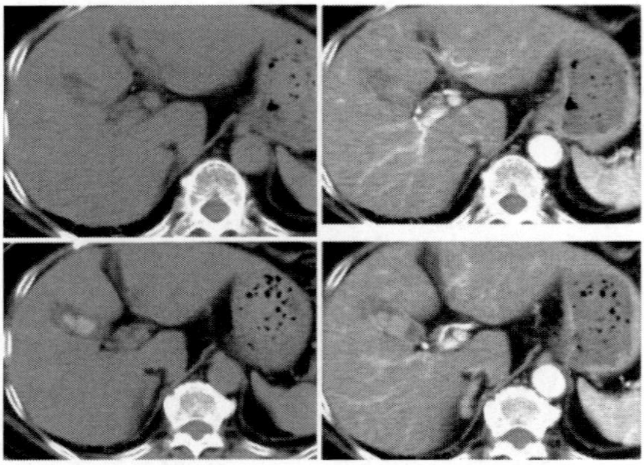

Figure 24. IgG4-related disease in a 75-year-old woman. Axial non-contrast enhanced and contrast enhanced abdominal CT images show thickened and irregular bile duct walls, with surrounding inflammation.

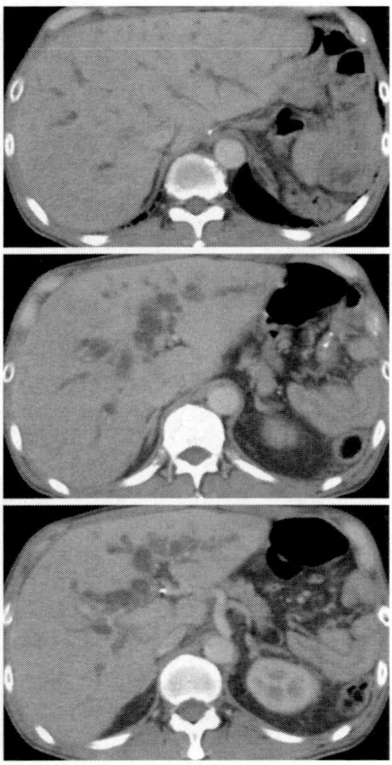

Figure 25. IgG4-related disease in a 54-year-old man. Axial contrast enhanced abdominal CT images show moderate intrahepatic biliary tract dilatation.

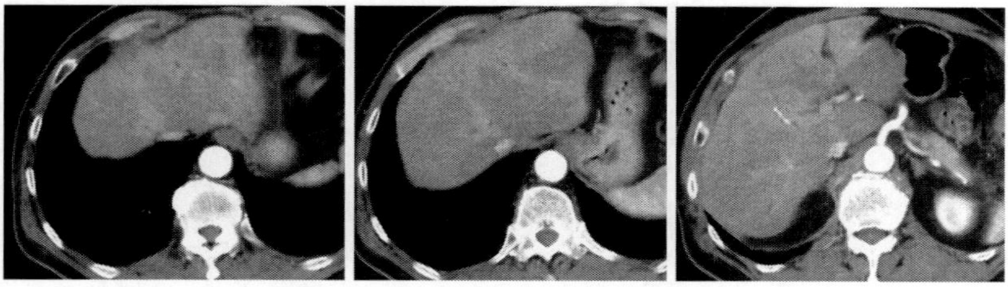

Figure 26. IgG4-related disease in a 65-year-old man. Coronal contrast enhanced abdominal CT images show multiple early and strong contrast-enhanced lesions with segments in both liver lobes, and the boundaries are relatively clear. In addition, intrahepatic bile duct dilation is conspicuous.

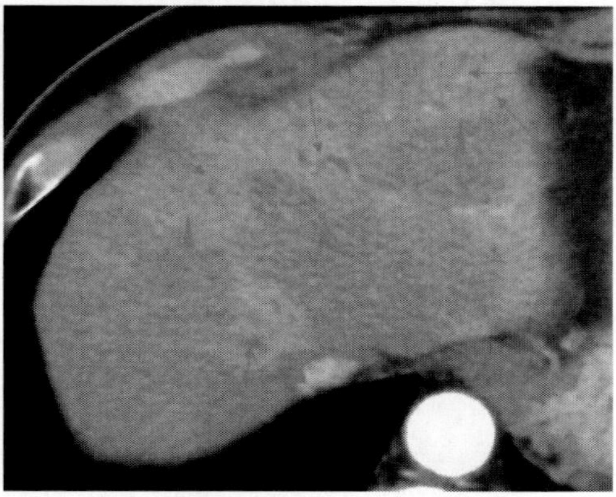

Figure 27. IgG4-related disease in a 65-year-old man. Coronal contrast enhanced abdominal CT images show multiple early contrast-enhanced lesions in both liver lobes with intrahepatic bile duct dilation.

MRI

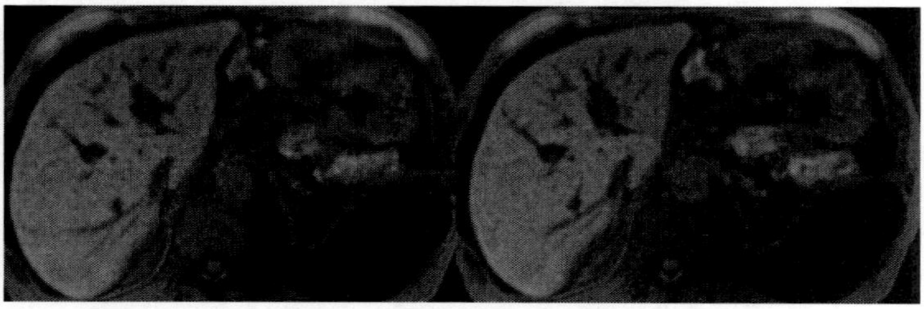

Figure 28. IgG4-related disease in a 56-year-old man. Axial T1-weighted abdominal MR images show remarked intrahepatic biliary tract dilatation.

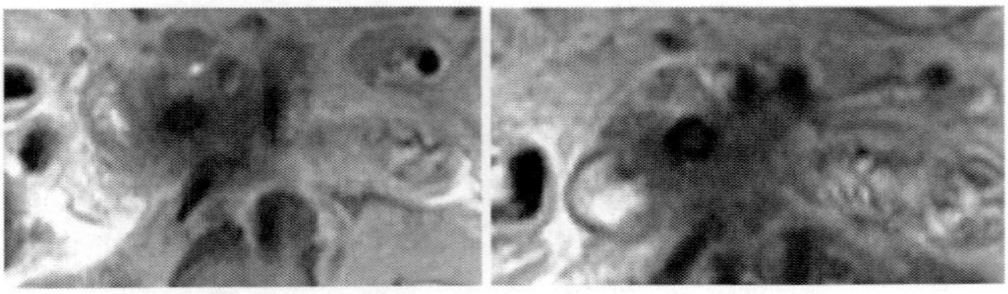

Figure 29. IgG4-related disease in a 56-year-old man. Axial T2-weighted MR images show hyperintense T2 signal of mass lesion in the common bile duct.

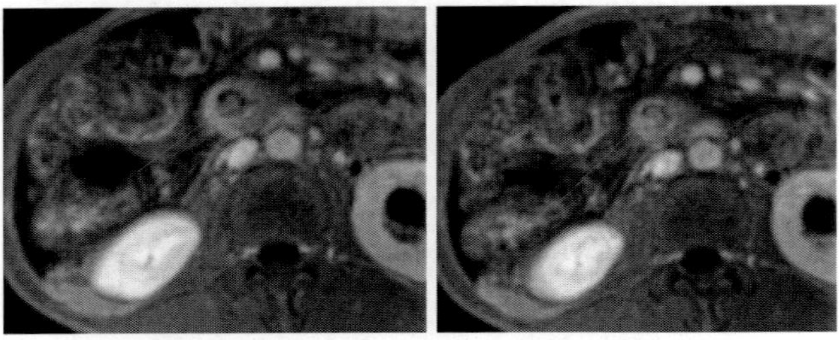

Figure 30. On dynamic MRI, mass lesion of the common bile duct shows mild delayed staining.

ERCP Images

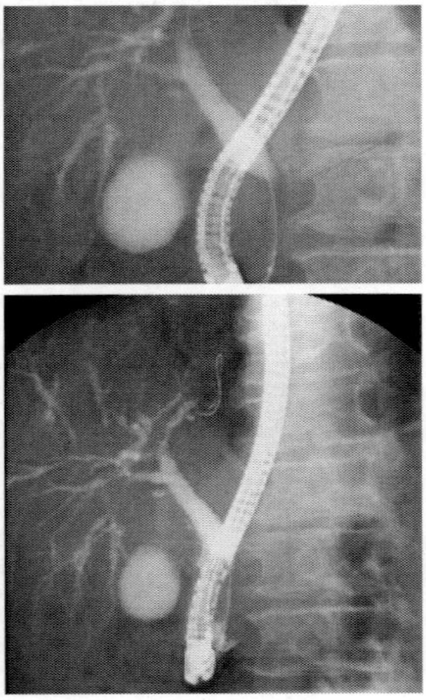

Figure 31. ERCP(ERC) images of a 63-year-old patient with autoimmune pancreatitis involving pancreatic head show narrowing of the distal common duct (arrow). Mild dilation and stenosis of the common hepatic duct to intrahepatic bile ducts appear.

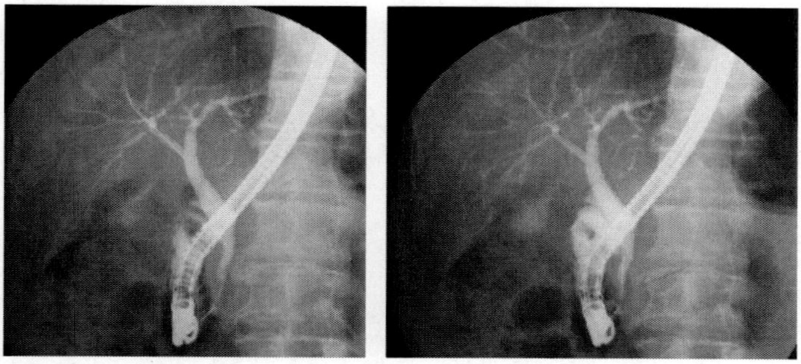

Figure 32. ERCP(ERC) images of a 64-year-old patient with autoimmune pancreatitis involving pancreatic head show narrowing of the distal common duct (arrows).

PET-CT Images

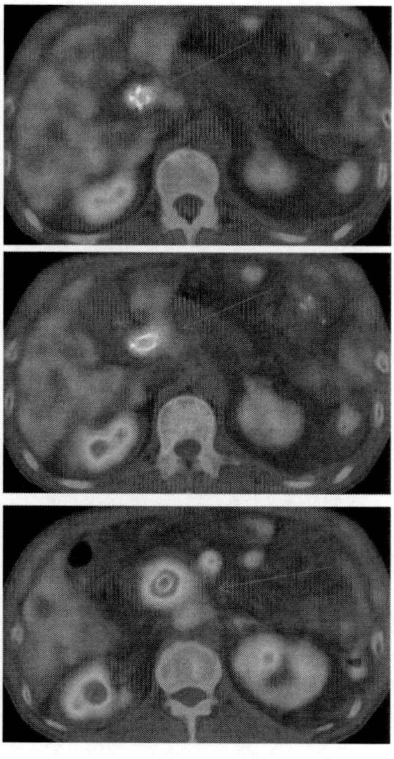

Figure 33. IgG4-related disease in a 56-year-old man. Axial FDG-PET/CT images show uptake in the common bile duct.

IgG4-Related Ascites

Ultrasound

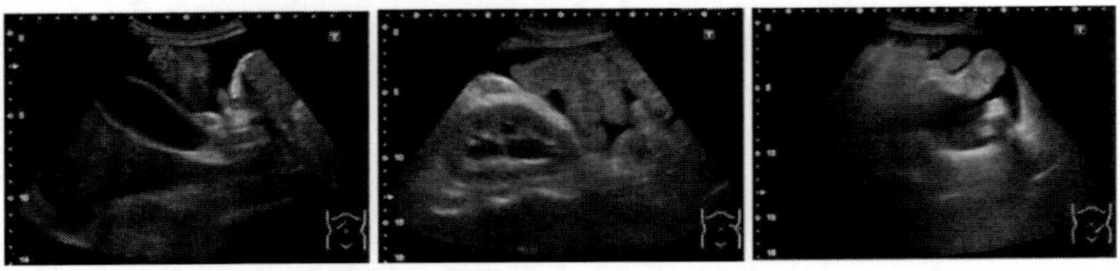

Figure 34. IgG4-related disease in a 75-year-old man. Abdominal ultrasound images show a massive amount of ascites.

CT

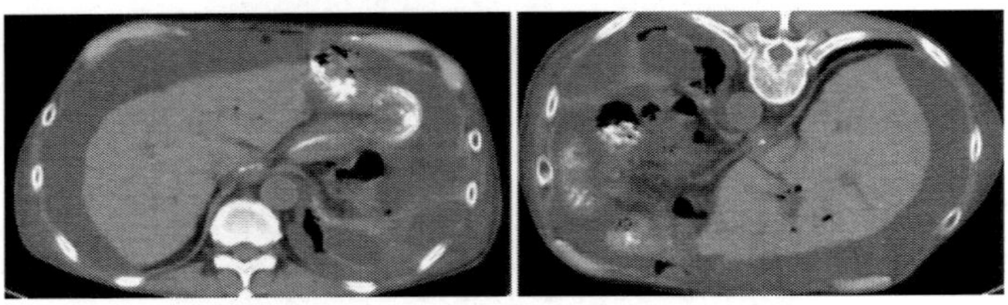

Figure 35. IgG4-related disease in a 56-year-old man. Abdominal non-contrast enhanced CT images show a massive amount of ascites.

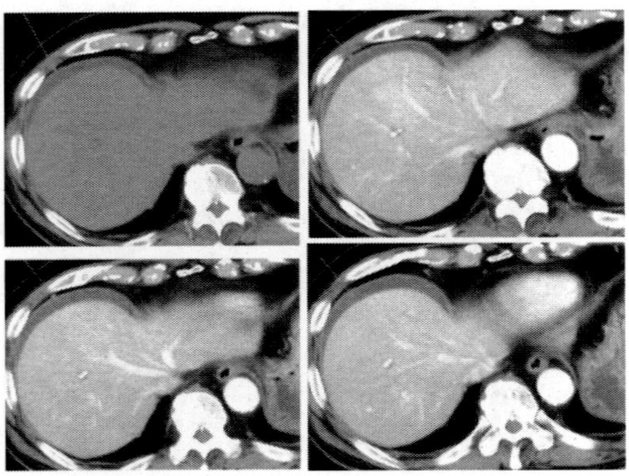

Figure 36. IgG4-related disease in a 75-year-old woman. Axial non-contrast and contrast enhanced abdominal CT images show a small amount of ascites.

MRI

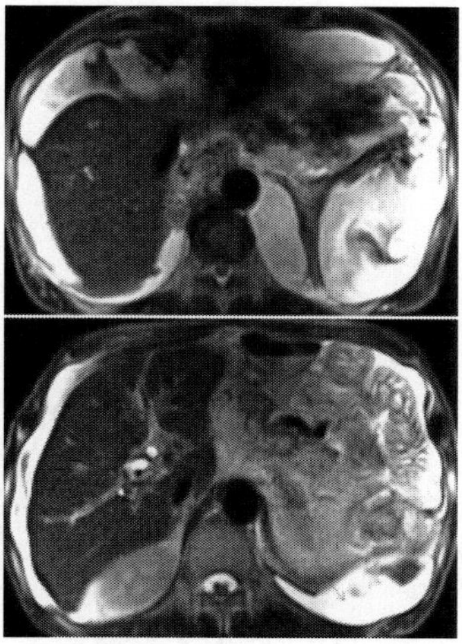

Figure 37. IgG4-related disease in a 56-year-old woman. Axial T2-weighted abdominal MR images show ascites.

IgG4-Related Gastrointestinal Tract Lesions

Rare cases of gastrointestinal tract due to IgG4-related disease have been reported (Kim JH. 2013).

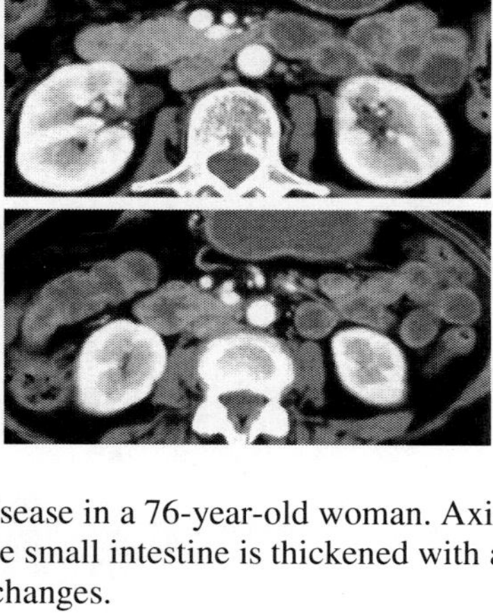

Figure 38. IgG4-related disease in a 76-year-old woman. Axial contrast enhanced chest CT images. The wall of the small intestine is thickened with a contrast effect, suggesting inflammatory changes.

Mucosa-Associated Lymphoid Tissue (MALT) Lymphoma

Lymphomas can develop in patients with IgG4-related disease. If lymphadenopathy or extranodal masses persists despite proper treatment of IgG4-related disease, strong suspicion must be given. Co-occurrence of IgG4-related disease and lymphoma suggests a possible etiological association (Bledsoe JR 2018).

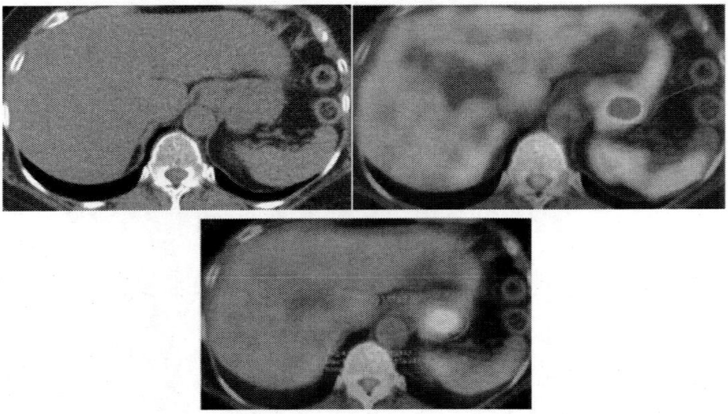

Figure 39. IgG4-related disease in a 75-year-old woman. FDG-PET/CT images show intense uptake in the stomach (arrows) and multiple lymph nodes. Mucosa-associated lymphoid tissue (MALT) lymphoma was diagnosed by stomach biopsy. It is not easy to detect the lesion using plain abdominal CT.

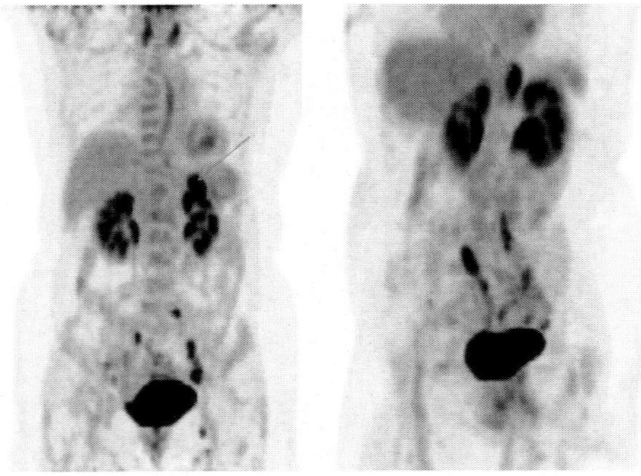

Figure 40. IgG4-related disease in a 75-year-old woman. FDG-PET/CT images show uptake in the stomach (arrows) and multiple lymph nodes. Mucosa-associated lymphoid tissue (MALT) lymphoma was diagnosed by stomach biopsy.

ABDOMINAL LYMPHADENOPATHY

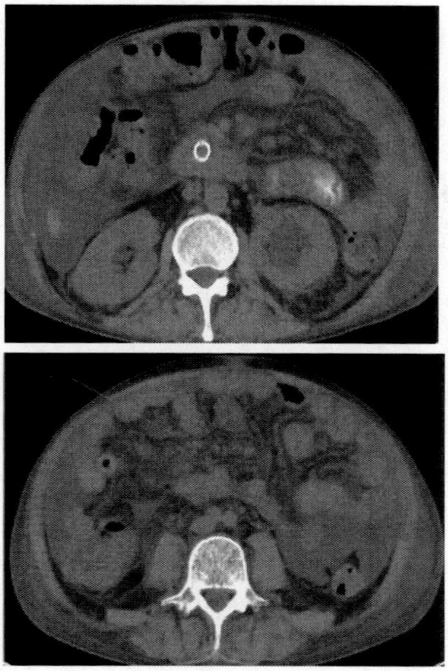

Figure 41. IgG4-related disease in a 56-year-old man. Axial non-contrast enhanced abdominal CT images show swelling of the mesenteric and para-aortic lymph nodes.

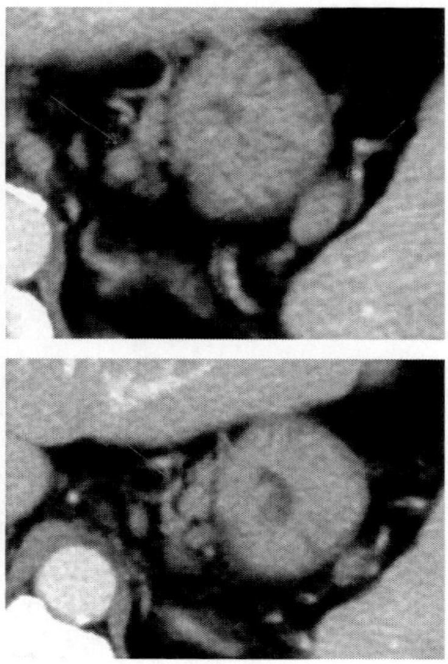

Figure 42. IgG4-related disease in a 67-year-old man. Axial contrast enhanced abdominal CT images show swelling of the gastric lymph nodes.

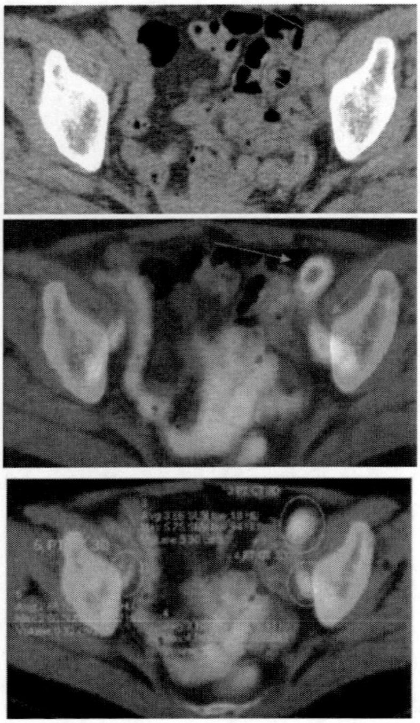

Figure 43. IgG4-related disease in a 75-year-old woman. Axial FDG-PET/CT images through the pelvic cavity show the left internal iliac lymphadenopathy (arrows).

MALT Lymphoma

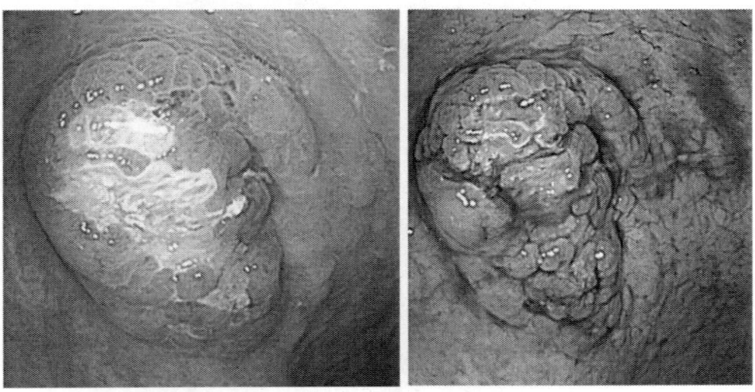

Figure 44. Upper gastrointestinal endoscopy of a patient with IgG4-related disease shows an irregular mass lesion with a large ulcer on the greater curvature of the stomach. The lesion is a MALT lymphoma.

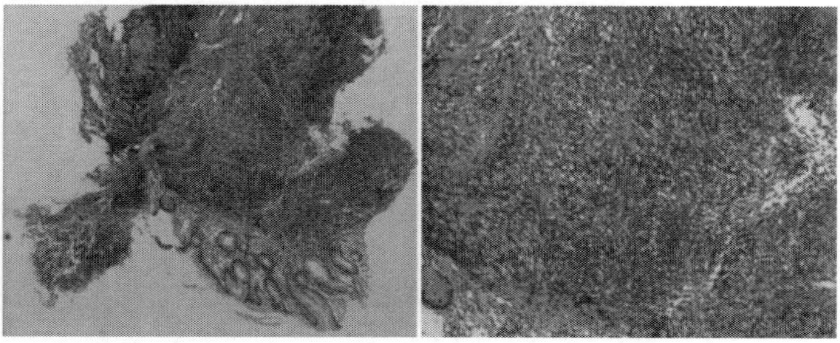

Figure 45. Mucosa-associated lymphoid tissue (MALT) lymphoma, stomach, biopsy from a patient with IgG4-related disease. In the lamina propria, medium-sized atypical lymphocytes proliferate. The main component are centrocyte-like cells with constricted nucleuses.

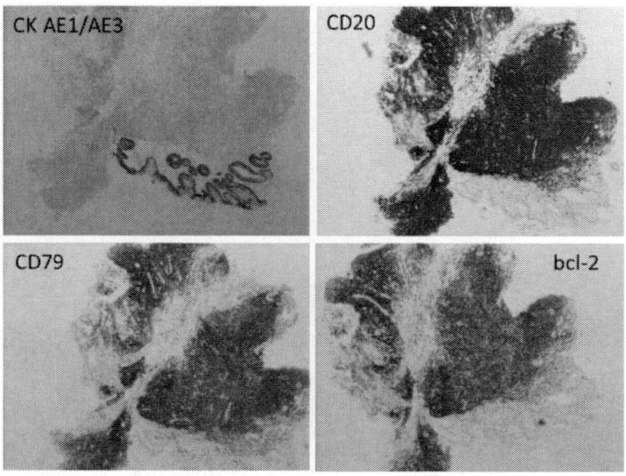

Figure 46. Mucosa-associated lymphoid tissue (MALT) lymphoma, stomach, biopsy from a patient with IgG4-related disease. Immunohistologically atypical lymphocytes are CD20, CD79a, and bcl-2 positive.

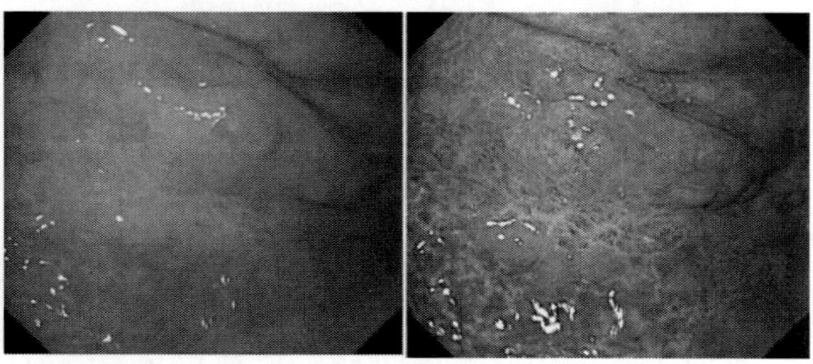

Figure 47. Upper gastrointestinal endoscopy after eradication therapy for Helicobacter pylori. MALT lymphoma of the upper gastric body curvature is scarred, flattened, and shrunk.

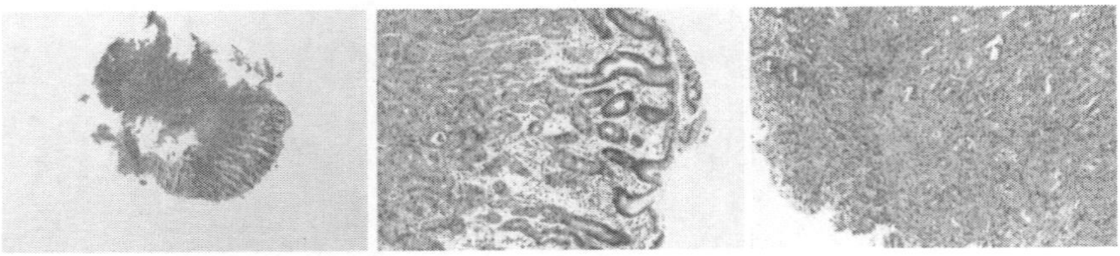

Figure 48. Histology of gastric mucosa after eradication treatment of Helicobacter pylori in a patient with MALT lymphoma and IgG4-related disease. Gastric mucosa with chronic inflammation, erosions and fibrosis are seen. It is chronic gastritis. No findings suggestive of MALT lymphoma.

IgG4-Related Liver Disease (IgG4 Hepatopathy), (IgG4-Related Autoimmune Hepatitis, IgG4-AIH)

IgG4-related disease can cause liver disease and may take on a condition like autoimmune hepatitis (AIH) (Umemura T 2007) (Nakanuma Y 2016).

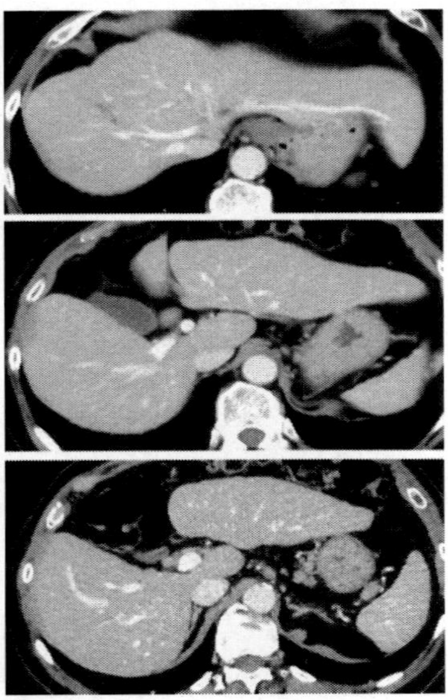

Figure 49. IgG4-related disease in a 67-year-old man. Axial contrast enhanced abdominal CT images show swelling of the left and caudate lobes of the liver and irregularities on the surface of the liver. These findings are consistent with the pattern of chronic liver injury.

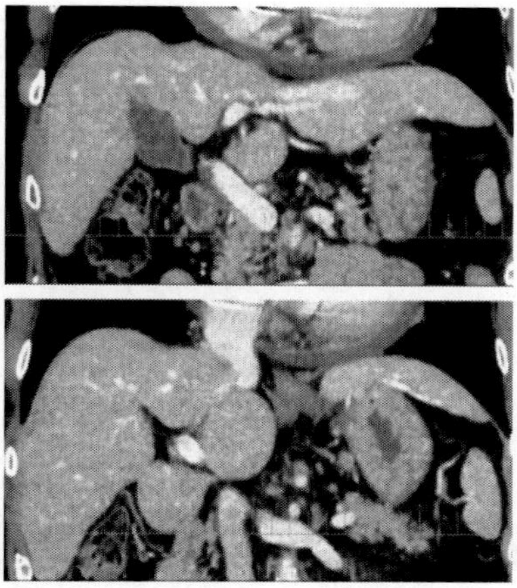

Figure 50. IgG4-related disease in a 67-year-old man. Coronal contrast enhanced abdominal CT images show swelling of the left and caudate lobes of the liver and irregularities on the surface of the liver.

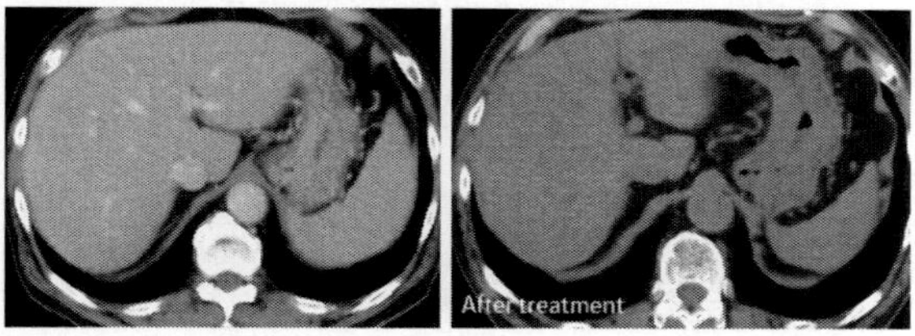

Figure 51. IgG4-related disease in a 72-year-old man. Axial CT images (left panel; before treatment, right panel; after treatment) show hepatomegaly. Hepatomegaly was resolved after glucocorticoid treatment.

SPLEEN

CT

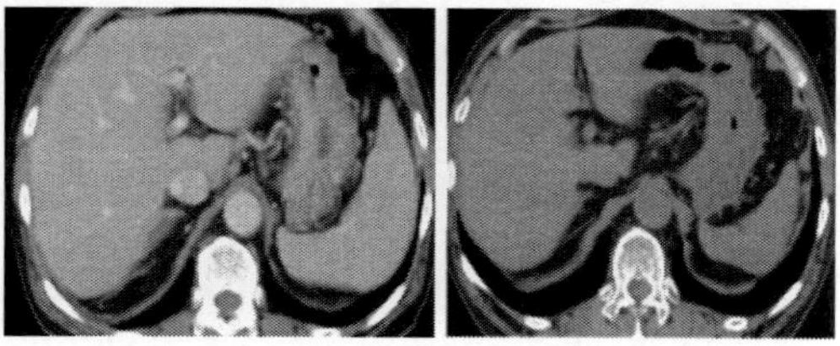

Figure 52. IgG4-related disease in a 72-year-old man. Axial CT images (left panel; before treatment, right panel; after treatment) show swelling of spleen (splenomegaly). Splenomegaly was improved after glucocorticoid treatment.

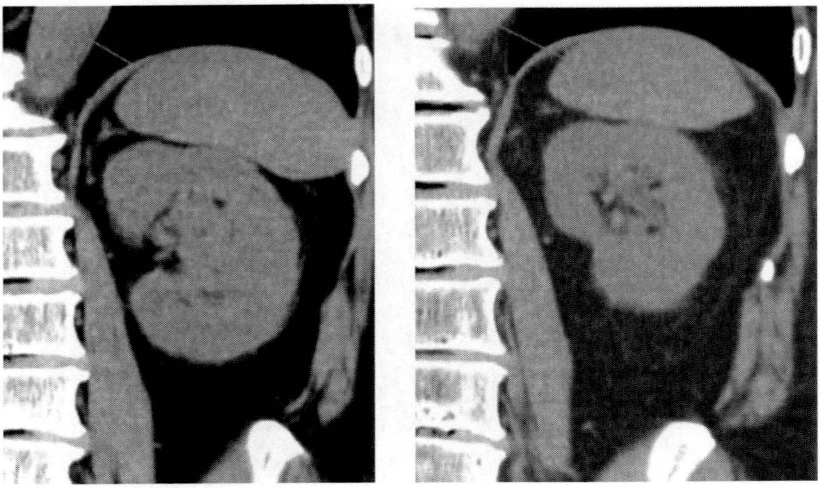

Figure 53. IgG4-related disease in a 72-year-old man. Coronal non-contrast enhanced abdominal CT images (left panel; before treatment, right panel; after treatment) show swelling of the spleen (splenomegaly). Splenomegaly was improved after glucocorticoid treatment.

Ultrasound Imaging

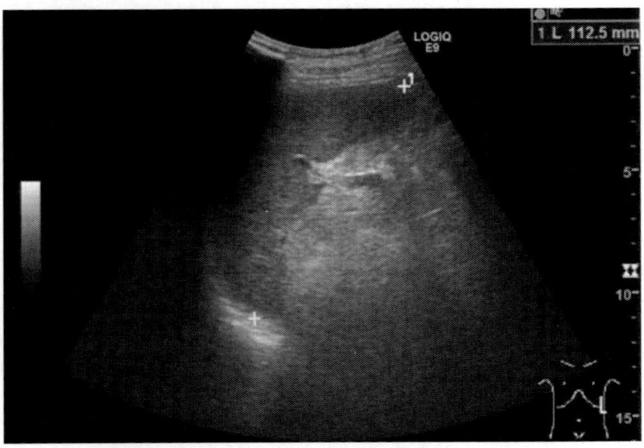

Figure 54. IgG4-related disease in a 72-year-old man. Longitudinal ultrasound image shows swelling of spleen (splenomegaly).

INGUINAL LYMPHADENOPATHY

Right Inguinal Lymph Nodes

Lymphadenopathy is common in patients with IgG4-related disease. Inguinal lymph nodes are those in the groin. They are in the femoral triangle of the inguinal region.

Lymphadenopathy in IgG4-related disease tends to be small (less than 2 cm), and patients with IgG4-reated disease usually have no fever or weight loss. Lymphadenopathy may appear as the first symptom, but imaging often finds it in asymptomatic situations.

Contrast Enhanced Abdominal CT

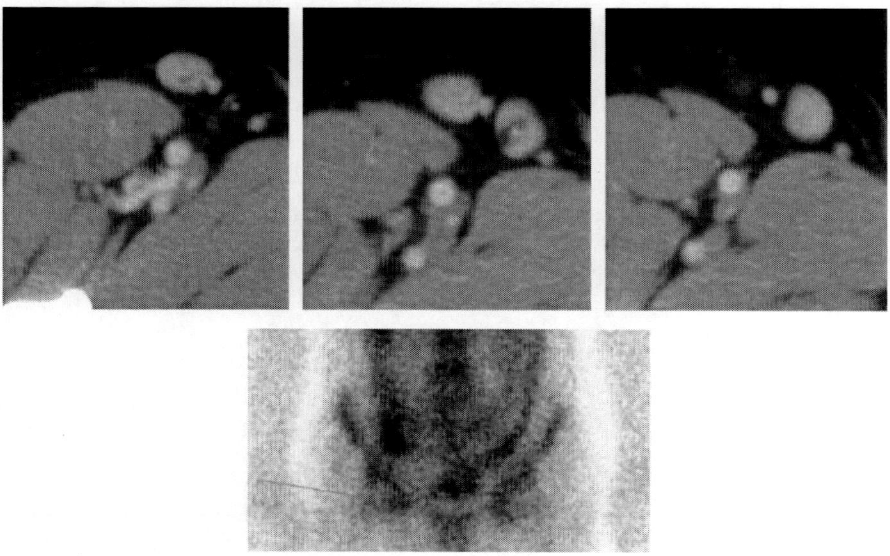

Figure 55. IgG4-related inguinal lymphadenopathy in a 38-year-old man. Axial contrast enhanced CT images of the abdomen reveal multiple enlarged right inguinal lymph nodes. Gallium scan shows uptake in the right inguinal lymph nodes (arrow).

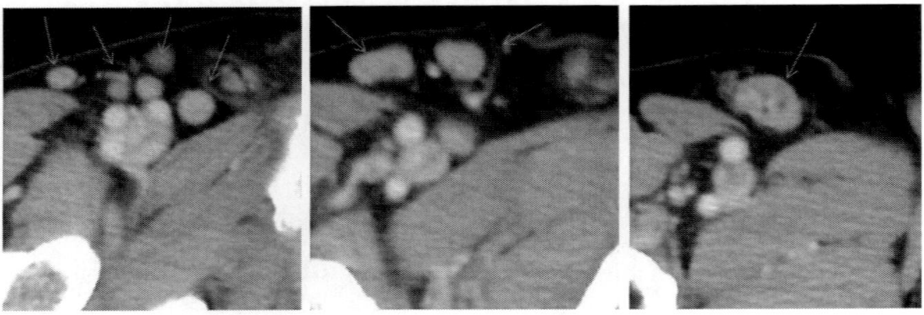

Figure 56. IgG4-related inguinal lymphadenopathy in a 72-year-old man.
Axial contrast enhanced CT images of the abdomen show multiple enlarged right inguinal lymph nodes (arrows).

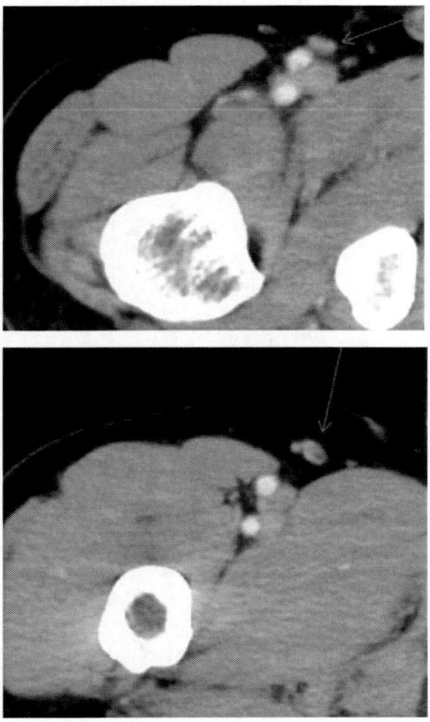

Figure 57. IgG4-related inguinal lymphadenopathy in a 67-year-old man.
Axial contrast enhanced CT images of the abdomen show the right small inguinal lymph nodes (arrows).

Left Inguinal Lymph Nodes

Contrast Enhanced Abdominal CT

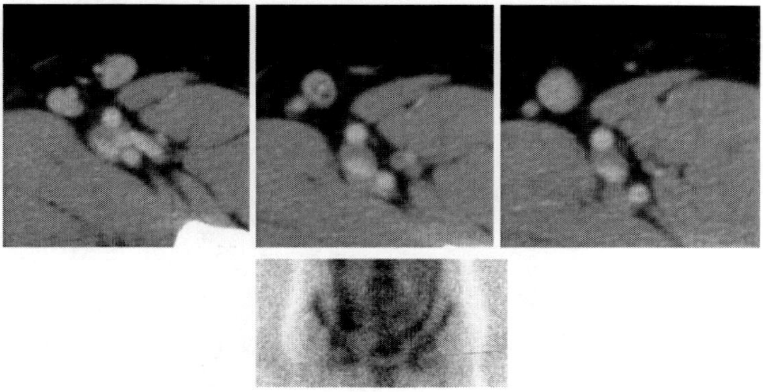

Figure 58. IgG4-related inguinal lymphadenopathy in a 38-year-old man. Axial contrast enhanced CT images of the abdomen reveal multiple enlarged left inguinal lymph nodes. Gallium scan shows uptake in left inguinal lymph nodes (arrow).

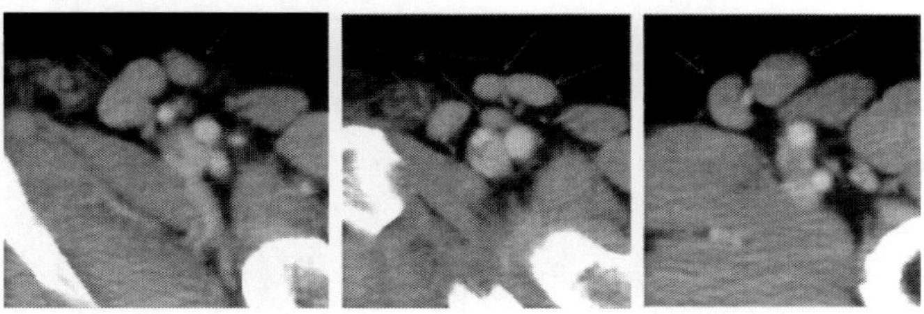

Figure 59. IgG4-related inguinal lymphadenopathy in a 72-year-old man. Axial contrast enhanced CT images of the abdomen show multiple enlarged left inguinal lymph nodes (arrows).

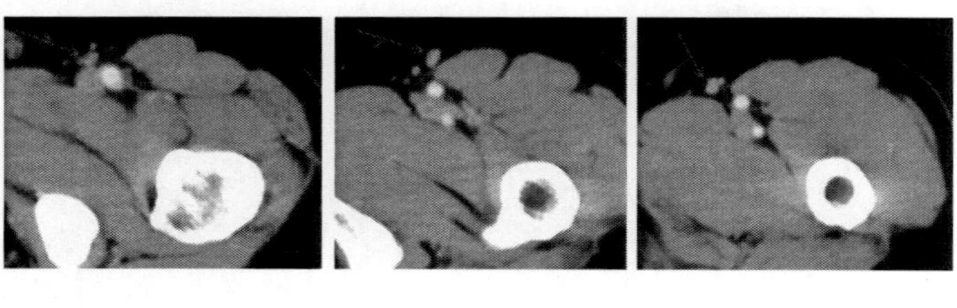

Figure 60. IgG4-related inguinal lymphadenopathy in a 67-year-old man. Axial contrast enhanced CT images of the abdomen show the left small inguinal lymph nodes (arrows).

PET/CT

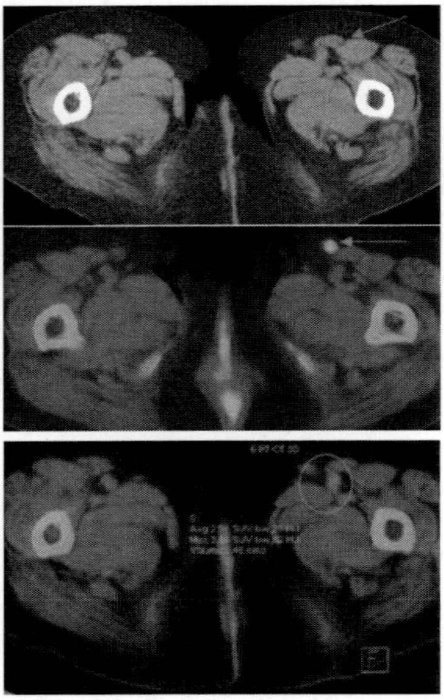

Figure 61. IgG4-related disease in a 75-year-old woman. FDG-PET/CT images show uptake in the left inguinal lymph node (arrows).

Histological Finding

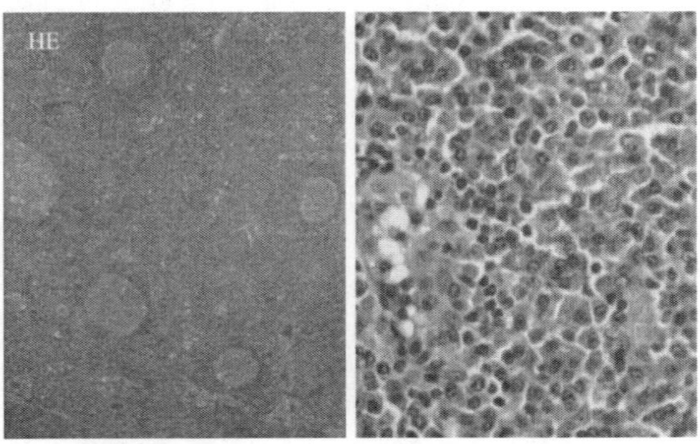

Figure 62. Histological finding of inguinal lymph nodes in a patient with IgG4-related lymphadenopathy reveals follicular hyperplasia with germinal center formation and infiltration of plasma cells. Storiform fibrosis and obliterative phlebitis are absent (Koarada S. 2013).

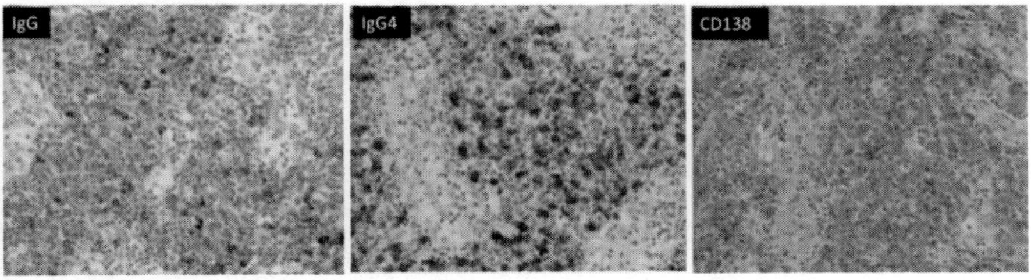

Figure 63. Immunohistochemistry of specimen for IgG (left panel) and IgG4 (middle panel) shows markedly increased IgG secreting plasma cells (right panel), a majority of which are positive for IgG4. (Koarada S. 2013).

REFERENCES

Abraham SC, Wilentz RE, Yeo CJ et al. "Pancreaticoduodenectomy (Whipple resections) in patients without malignancy: are they all 'chronic pancreatitis'?" *Am J Surg Pathol* 27 (2003): 110-120.

Bledsoe JR, Wallace ZS, Stone JH, Deshpande V, Ferry JA. "Lymphomas in IgG4-related disease: clinicopathologic features in a Western population." *Virchows Arch* 472 (2018): 839-852.

Cheuk W., Chan JK. "IgG4-related sclerosing disease: a critical appraisal of an evolving clinicopathologic entity." *Adv Anat Pathol 2010;17(5):303–332.* 17 (2010): 303-332.

Hamano H., Kawa S, Horiuchi A, et al. "High serum IgG4 concentrations in patients with sclerosing pancreatitis." *N Engl J Med.* 344 (2001): 732-738.

Ishigami K, Tajima T, Nishie A, et al. "MRI findings of pancreatic lymphoma and autoimmune pancreatitis: a comparative study." *Eur J Radiol* 74 (2010): e22-e28.

JPS, 2012 Members of the Criteria Committee for Autoimmune Pancreatitis. "Diagnostic criteria for autoimmune pancreatitis." *Suizo* 27 (2011): 17-25.

Kamisawa T., Okamoto A. "Autoimmune pancreatitis: proposal of IgG4-related sclerosing disease." *J Gastroenterol.* 41 (2006): 613-625.

Kamisawa T.., Zen Y, Pillai S, et al. "IgG4-related disease." *Lancet* 385 (2015): 1460-1471.

Kawa S. "Immunoglobulin G4-related Disease: An Overview." *JMAJ* 2 (2019): 11-27.

Kawa, S. "Current Concepts and Diagnosis of IgG4-Related Pancreatitis (Type 1 AIP)." *Semin Liver Dis. 2016;36(3):257-73.* 36 (2016): 257-73.

Kim HJ, Kim YK, Jeong WK, Lee WJ, Choi D. "Pancreatic duct "icicle sign" on MRI for distinguishing autoimmune pancreatitis from pancreatic ductal adenocarcinoma in the proximal pancreas." *Eur Radiol* 25 (2015): 1551–1560.

Kim JH., Byun JH, Lee SS, Kim HJ, Lee MG. "Atypical manifestations of IgG4-related sclerosing disease in the abdomen: imaging findings and pathologic correlations." *AJR Am J Roentgenol* 200 (2013): 102-112.

Koarada S., Tashiro S, Nagao N, Suematsu R, Ohta A, Tada Y. "Increased RP105-Negative B Cells in IgG4-Related Disease." *Open Rheumatol J* 7 (2013): 55-57.

Matsubayashi H, Kakushima N, Takizawa K, Tanaka M, Imai K, Hotta K, Ono H. "Diagnosis of autoimmune pancreatitis." *World J Gastroenterol* 20 (2014): 16559-69.

Muhi A, Ichikawa T, Motosugi U et al. "Mass-forming autoimmune pancreatitis and pancreatic carcinoma: differential diagnosis on the basis of computed tomography and magnetic resonance cholangiopancreatography, and diffusion-weighted imaging findings." *J Magn Reson Imaging* 35 (2012): 827-836.

Nakanuma Y, Ishizu Y, Zen Y, et al. "Histopathology of IgG4-Related Autoimmune Hepatitis and IgG4-Related Hepatopathy in IgG4-Related Disease." *Semin Liver Dis* 36 (2016): 229-41.

Nakazawa T, Ohara H, Sano H, et al. "Schematic classification of sclerosing cholangitis with autoimmune pancreatitis by cholangiography." *Pancreas* 32 (2006): 229.

Nakazawa T., Shimizu S, Naitoh I. "IgG4-Related Sclerosing Cholangitis." *Semin Liver Dis* 36 (2016): 216-28.

Nakazawa, Naitoh I, Hayashi K, et al. "Diagnostic criteria for IgG4-related sclerosing cholangitis based on cholangiographic classification." *J Gastroenterol* 47 (2012): 79—87.

Nishimori I, Tamakoshi A, Otsuki M, Research Committee on Intractable Diseases of the Pancreas, Ministry of Health, Labour, and Welfare of Japan. "Prevalence of autoimmune pancreatitis in Japan from a nationwide survey in 2002. J Gastroenterol 2007; 42 Sup." *J Gastroenterol.* 42 Suppl 18 (2007): 6.

Okazaki K., Uchida K, Koyabu M, Miyoshi H, Takaoka M. "Recent advances in the concept and diagnosis of autoimmune pancreatitis and IgG4-related disease." *J Gastroenterol* 46 (2011): 277–288.

Sah RP, Chari ST, Pannala R, et al. "Differences in clinical profile and relapse rate of type 1 versus type 2 autoimmune pancreatitis." *Gastroenterology* 139 (2010): 140.

Sahani DV, Kalva SP, Farrell J et al. "Autoimmune pancreatitis: imaging features." *Radiology* 233 (2004): 345–352.

Sangha Brar JS, Gupta S, Haja Mohideen SM, Liauw L, Lath N. "The pancreatic and extrapancreatic manifestations of IgG4-related diseas." *Diagn Interv Radiol* 24 (2018): 83-88.

Shimosegawa T, Kanno A. "Autoimmune pancreatitis in Japan: overview and perspective." *J Gastroenterol.* 44 (2009): 503.

Shimosegawa T., Chari ST, Frulloni L, Kamisawa T, Kawa S, Mino-Kenudson M, Kim MH, Klöppel G, Lerch MM, Löhr M, Notohara K, Okazaki K, Schneider A, Zhang L. "International consensus diagnostic criteria for autoimmune pancreatitis: guidelines of the International Association of Pancreatology." *Pancreas* 40 (2011): 352-358.

Sun GF, Zuo CJ, Shao CW, Wang JH, Zhang J. "Focal autoimmune pancreatitis: radiological characteristics help to distinguish from pancreatic cancer." *World J Gastroenterol* 19 (2013): 3634–3641.

Suzuki K, Itoh S, Nagasaka T, Ogawa H, Ota T, Naganawa S. "CT findings in autoimmune pancreatitis: assessment using multiphase contrast-enhanced multisection CT." *Clin Radiol* 65 (2010): 735–743.

Tang CSW, Sivarasan N, Griffin N. "Abdominal manifestations of IgG4-related disease: a pictorial review." *Insights Imaging* 9 (2018): 437–448.

Umemura T, Zen Y, Hamano H, et al. "Immunoglobin G4-hepatopathy: association of immunoglobin G4-bearing plasma cells in liver with autoimmune pancreatitis." *Hepatology* 46 (2007): 463-71.

Yang DH, Kim KW, Kim TK et al. "Autoimmune pancreatitis: radiologic findings in 20 patients." *Abdom Imaging* 31 (1996): 94-102.

Zaheer A, Singh VK, Akshintala VS et al. "Differentiating autoimmune pancreatitis from pancreatic adenocarcinoma using dual-phase computed tomography." *J Comput Assist Tomogr* 38 (2014): 146-152.

In: IgG4 Related Disease
Editor: Syuichi Koarada

ISBN: 978-1-53618-050-3

Chapter 8

Other Involved Organs and Tissues, Candidate Members of IgG4-RD and Uncommon Manifestations of Each IgG4-RD

Syuichi Koarada* and Mariko Sakai
Division of Rheumatology, Faculty of Medicine,
Saga University, Nabeshima, Saga, Japan

Abstract

IgG4-related disease has various lesions in various organs. The main pathological conditions have been described in the previous chapters, but here, bone marrow lesions and skin lesions are described as other rare lesions. There is no characteristic finding for these disorders, and it is necessary to make the diagnosis based on histopathological findings, coexistence with other organ lesions, and clinical course.

---

* Corresponding Author's Email: koarada@cc.saga-u.ac.jp.

BONE MARROW

Histopathology

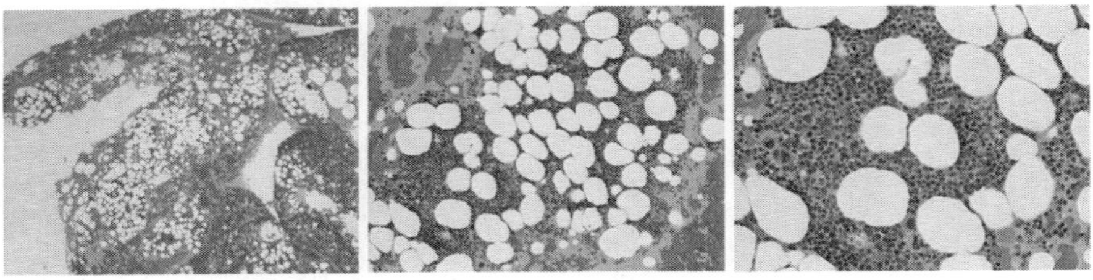

Figure 1. Histologically, nucleated cells are about 30% and normocellular marrow. Hematopoietic cells have been confirmed to exist in all three lines, and there is no apparent differentiation disorder. The M/E (myeloid cells to erythroblastic cells) ratio is about 3.

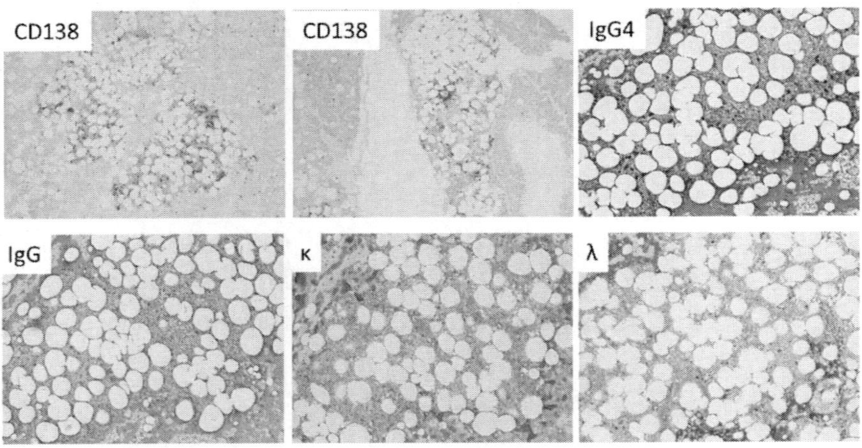

Figure 2. About 10% of CD138-positive plasma cells are present, but there are no atypical plasma cells. There is no large bias in the distribution of κ and λ, and there is no monoclonal growth or aggregation. The IgG4/IgG ratio is over 40%, and the number of IgG4 positive cells is 24/HPF. Bone marrow lesions are consistent with an IgG4-related disease.

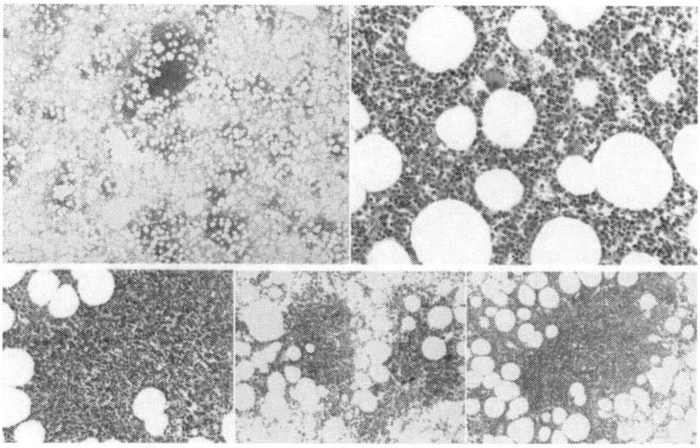

Figure 3. Hematopoietic cell components account for approximately 40% of the specimen. Normocellular marrow and all three lines are maintained. M/E ratio is about 3-4. Hematopoietic cell maturation and differentiation are normal, but some lymphocyte aggregations are seen.

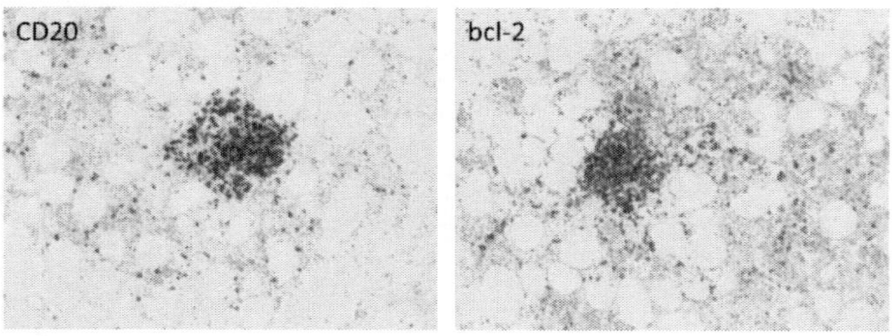

Figure 4. Bone marrow biopsy specimens are positive for CD20 and bcl-2 by immunostaining. Bone marrow infiltration of MALT lymphoma is suspected.

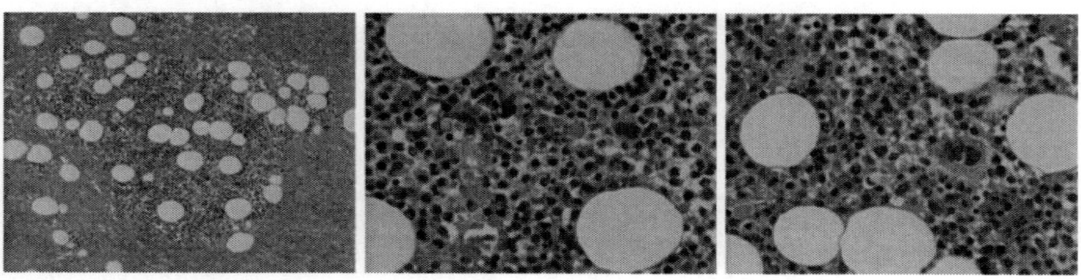

Figure 5. Normocellular bone marrow with about 40-50% of hematopoietic cell components is seen. The megakaryocytes are 1-2/HPF. Mature granulocytes are observed and no clear maturation disorder is observed. The erythroblasts have a G/E ratio of 4. No atypical lymphocyte proliferation is found.

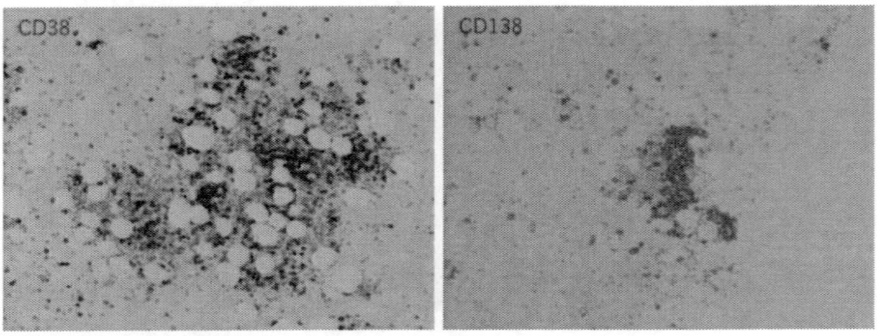

Figure 6. CD38 or CD138 positive cells account for about 30-50% of bone marrow by immunohistochemistry.

IgG4-Related Skin Disease

IgG4-related skin disease is the recommended disease name for skin symptoms of IgG4-related disease (Stone J. H., 2012).

Although a clear understanding of the various skin lesions in IgG4-related diseases is not yet sufficient, at present skin lesions are categorized into the following subtypes based on the case: (Tokura Y., 2014)

- Angiolymphoid hyperplasia with eosinophilia
- Cutaneous pseudolymphoma
- Cutaneous plasmacytosis
- Eyelid swelling (as part of Mikulicz's disease)
- Psoriasis-like eruptions
- Unspecified maculopapular or erythematous eruptions
- Unspecified purpura
- Hypergammaglobulinemic purpura and urticarial vasculitis
- Impaired blood supply to fingers or toes, leading to Raynaud's phenomenon or gangrene
- Wells syndrome (Karashima T., 2014)
- Leg edema

Eyelid Swelling (As Part of Mikulicz's Disease)

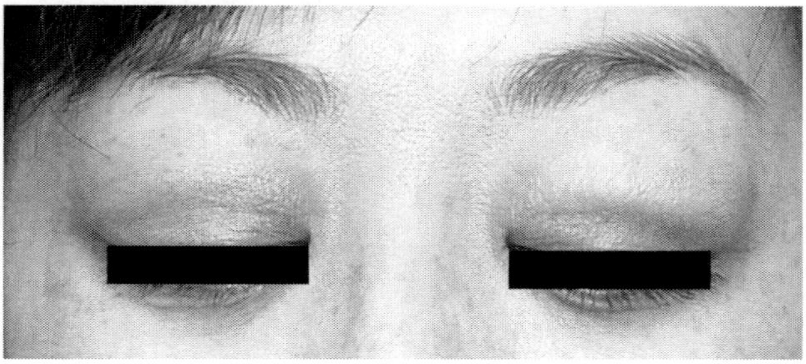

Figure 7. IgG4-related skin disease in a 43-year-old woman. Bilateral eyelid swelling as part of Mikulicz's disease is observed.

Unspecific Purpura

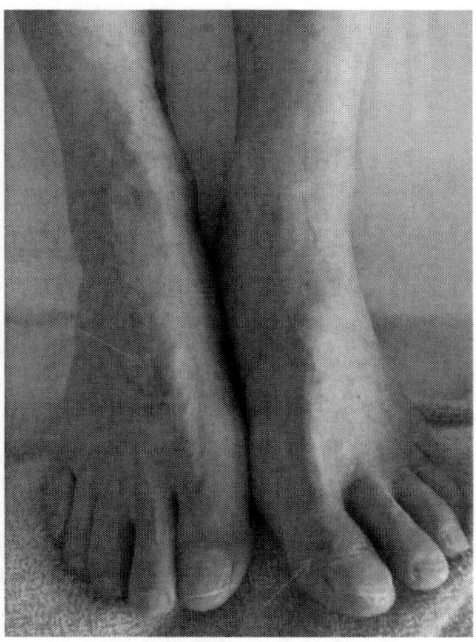

Figure 8. IgG4-related skin disease in a 72-year-old man. Unspecific purpura of the feet is observed.

Figure 9. IgG4-related skin disease in a 72-year-old man. Unspecific purpura of the feet is observed.

Edematous Change of Lower Limb

Plain Radiography

Edematous change of lower limbs may be caused by IgG4-related inflammation and obstruction of veins and lymphatic vessels.

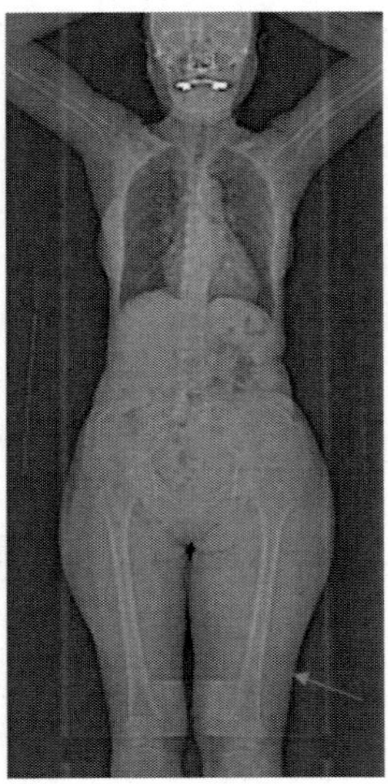

Figure 10. IgG4-related disease in a 56-year-old woman. Conventional X-ray image shows swelling and edematous change in the left lower limb.

CT

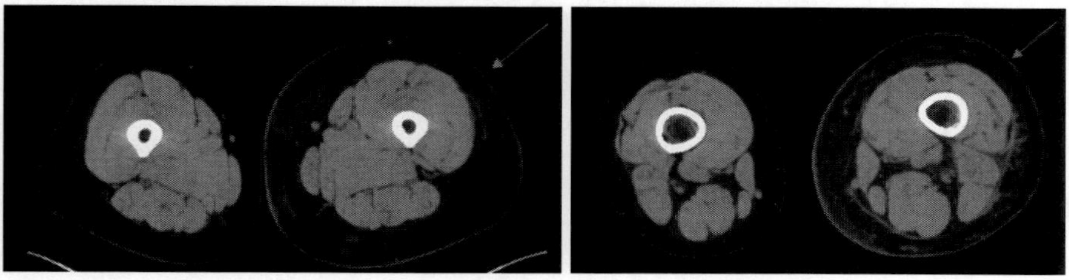

Figure 11. IgG4-related disease in a 56-year-old woman. Coronal non-contrast enhanced CT images show swelling and edematous change in the left lower limb (arrows).

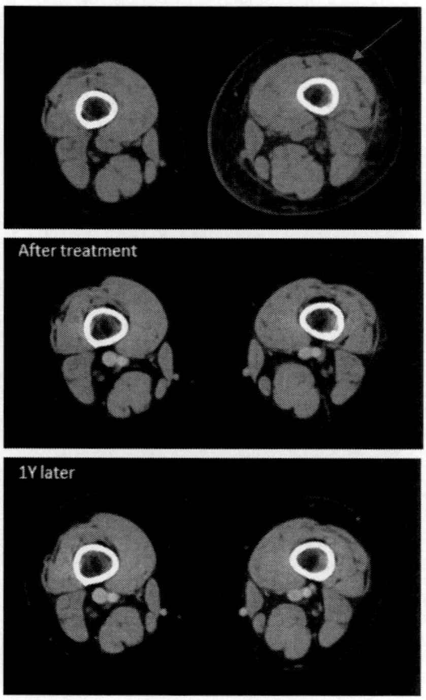

Figure 12. IgG4-related disease in a 56-year-old woman. Coronal non-contrast enhanced CT images show swelling in the left lower limb (arrow). This lesion was resolved after glucocorticoid treatment.

Photography

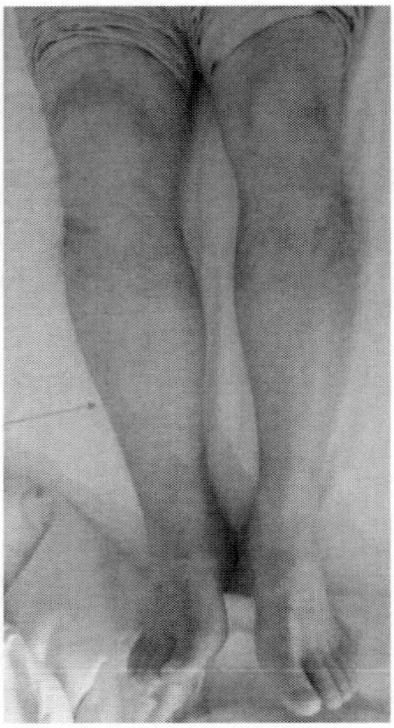

Figure 13. IgG4-related disease in a 71-year-old man. Clinical photograph shows swelling and edema of the right lower limb.

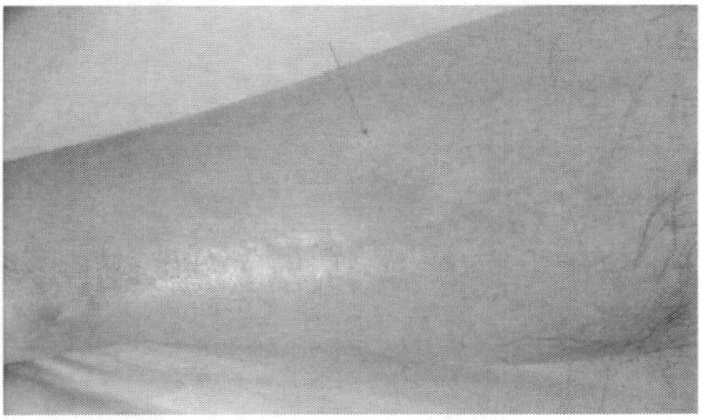

Figure 14. IgG4-related disease in a 71-year-old man. Clinical photograph shows unilateral pretibial pitting edema of the right lower limb.

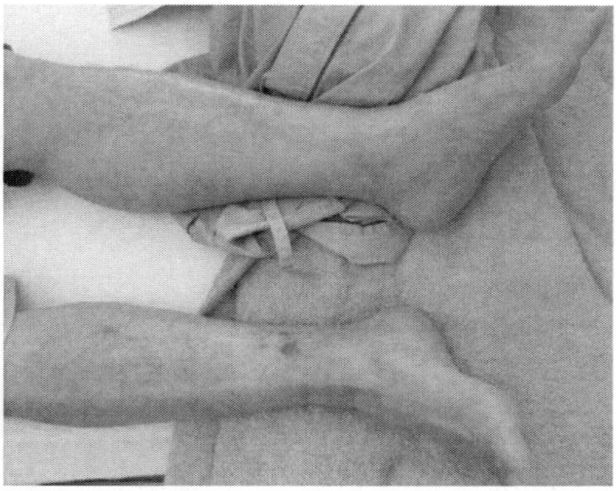

Figure 15. IgG4-related disease in a 73-year-old man. The photographic image shows swelling and edema of the left lower limb.

Development of Malignancies

The activity of IgG4-related disease is a strong risk factor for the development of malignancies (Asano J., 2015). In particular, a close link between IgG4-related disease and malignancy in the elderly has been reported, possibly associated with persistent inflammatory tissue damage and/or impaired immunological surveillance (Yamamoto M., 2012) (Shiokawa M., 2013).

References

Asano J., Watanabe T., Oguchi T., et al., "Association between immunoglobulin G4-related disease and malignancy within 12 years after diagnosis: an analysis after longterm followup." *J Rheumatol* 42 (2015): 2135-42.

Karashima T., Taniguchi Y., Shimamoto T., et al., *"IgG4-related disease of the paratestis in a patient with Wells syndrome: a case report."* 9 (2014): 225.

Shiokawa M., Kodama Y., Yoshimura K., et al., "Risk of cancer in patients with autoimmune pancreatitis." *Am J Gastroenterol* 108 (2013): 610-7.

Stone J. H., Khosroshahi A., Deshpande V., et al., "Recommendations for the nomenclature of IgG4-related disease and its individual organ system manifestations." *Arthritis & Rheumatism* 64 (2012): 3061-3067.

Tokura Y., Yagi H., Yanaguchi H., Majima Y., Kasuya A., Ito T., Maekawa M., Hashizume H. "IgG4-related skin disease." *British Journal of Dermatology* 171 (2014): 959-967.

Yamamoto M., Takahashi H., Tabeya T., et al., "Risk of malignancies in IgG4-related disease." *Mod Rheumatol* 22 (2012): 414-8.

In: IgG4 Related Disease
Editor: Syuichi Koarada
ISBN: 978-1-53618-050-3

Chapter 9

OVERVIEW OF IGG4-RELATED DISEASES BY PICTORIAL CLINICAL IMMUNOLOGY

Syuichi Koarada*[*] *and Yoshinobu Nakao
Division of Rheumatology, Faculty of Medicine,
Saga University, Nabeshima, Saga, Japan

ABSTRACT

IgG4-related disease has various lesions in multiple organs and is comprehensively diagnosed according to diagnostic criteria based on high serum IgG4 levels, various images and histopathological findings. For diagnosis, differential diagnosis from various similar diseases is very important. However, diagnosis can be difficult in some cases, such as when serum IgG4 levels are normal, like malignant tumors, or when no histopathological findings are available. Regarding treatment, corticosteroids are responsive, and the prognosis of the disease is good, but refractory or relapsed cases may require treatment with rituximab or immunosuppressants.

[*] Corresponding Author's Email: koarada@cc.saga-u.ac.jp.

The position of IgG4-related diseases among autoimmune diseases has not yet been established. We make a three-dimensional interpretation of the concept of autoimmune diseases. The acquired immunity and innate immunity are arranged on the X axis, the degree of B cell differentiation is arranged on the Y axis, and immune cells, autoantibodies, cytokines, chemokines, and target tissues are layered on the Z axis. By considering diseases in this three-dimensional distribution, it has become possible to make immunological interpretations and treatment strategies for IgG4-related disease.

INTRODUCTION

Despite the great attention, the pathophysiology of IgG4-related diseases is not yet known.

The immune response can be broadly divided into two components, innate immunity and acquired immunity. Innate immunity functions immediately after exposure to pathogens, inducing clonal expansion and acquired immunity. IgG4-related immunological abnormalities are associated with both innate and adaptive immune systems.

Because of the variety of immunological changes in autoimmune diseases, it is often difficult to understand the pathophysiology of autoimmune diseases for medical students. However, it becomes easier to understand if one recognizes that an immune disease basically has a three-dimensional and four-layer immune structure.

The description in this chapter is the content of my lectures on clinical immunology to students and residents at Saga University. This lecture is designed to attract students' interest, and is highly evaluated by students and residents.

TWO-DIMENSIONAL PATHOLOGY

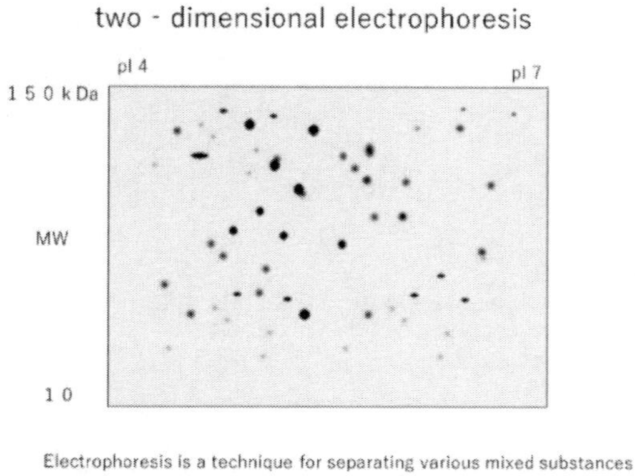

Figure 1. Electrophoresis is a technique for separating various mixed substances. Among them, two-dimensional electrophoresis is a separation method in which various proteins are electrophoresed (developed) twice in two dimensions, that is, in the X and Y directions. Currently, by combining different separation conditions (sample and electrophoresis conditions) for the first and second rounds, the resolution is better than one-dimensional (one round) electrophoresis. This figure shows a method for precisely dividing molecules into spots based on molecular weight and isoelectric point.

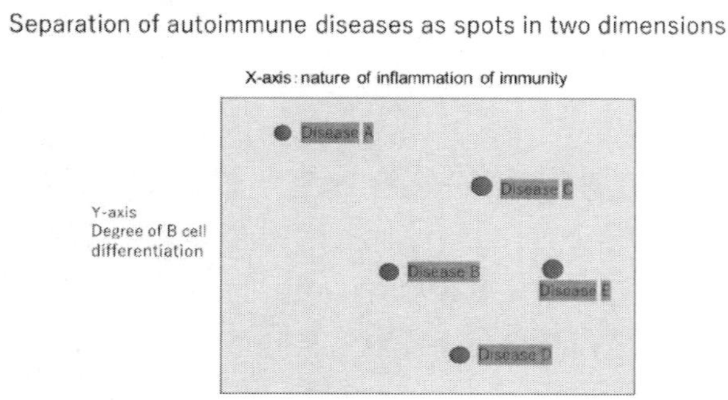

Figure 2. The pathology of autoimmune diseases is extremely complex and cannot be separated in one indicator, one dimension. What we are thinking is to understand autoimmune diseases in three dimensions. Therefore, first, the X-axis is developed based on the nature of inflammation of immunity, whether innate immunity or acquired immunity. And it develops according to the degree of B cell differentiation which is one of the clearest immunological markers on the Y-axis. In this way, the idea is to separate autoimmune diseases as spots in two dimensions. Based on this distribution map, the location of the disease, its relation to a group of closely related diseases, cytokines, chemokines, adhesion molecules, and treatment and prognosis can be considered.

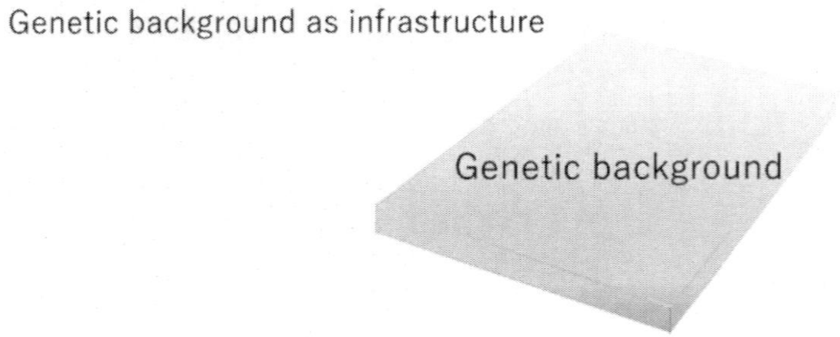

Figure 3. The beginning of an autoimmune disease is that in a patient, some genetic background exists in its infrastructure.

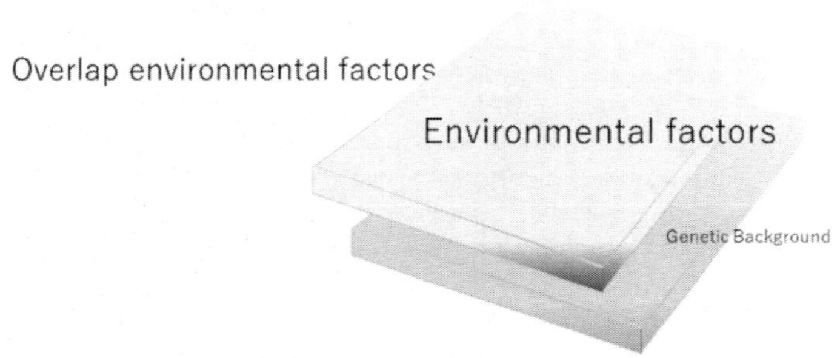

Figure 4. In the patient with the autoimmune disease, there is a genetic background and further environmental factors overlap.

THREE-DIMENSIONAL PATHOLOGY

First, consider the first layer of cells. Given the two-dimensional distribution of EGPA, the X-axis has a high degree of acquired immune system abnormalities and eosinophils play a central role in pathophysiology. Then, regarding the degree of B cell differentiation, the ratio of RP105-negative B cells that are autoantibody-producing B cells is extremely large, and the degree of B cell differentiation is high. However, some patients do not have an increase in RP105-negative B cells, and their two-dimensional distribution is quite diverse, with a wide range of B cell differentiation, from high to moderate or low.

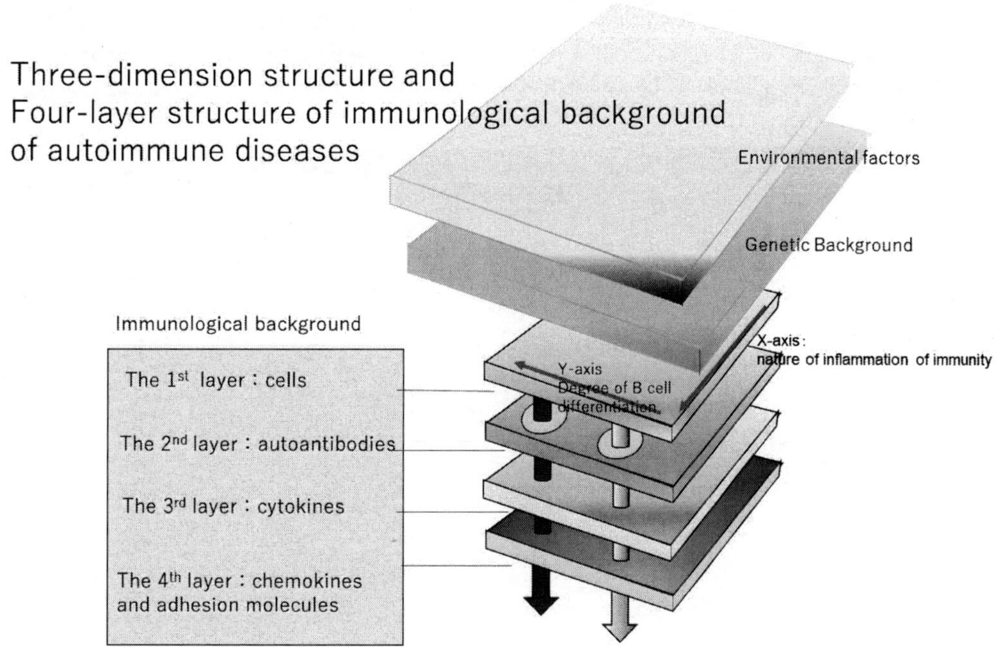

Figure 5. Further layering the immunological background results in a three-layer structure. However, the immunological background has a four-layer structure further below. The first layer is the cells, for immunological cells. Here, considering the nature of immunity on the X-axis, cells that function as the center in autoimmune pathophysiology are identified. Further, in order to identify the degree of B cell differentiation, the ratio of autoantibody producing cells is considered on the Y-axis. (Here, the autoantibody-producing cells are RP105-negative B cells in our system). The second layer is autoantibodies. The third layer is cytokines. The fourth layer, chemokines and adhesion molecules, defines the target tissue for the autoimmune phenomenon. The pathophysiology of each autoimmune disease will be considered based on the immunological four-layer structure.

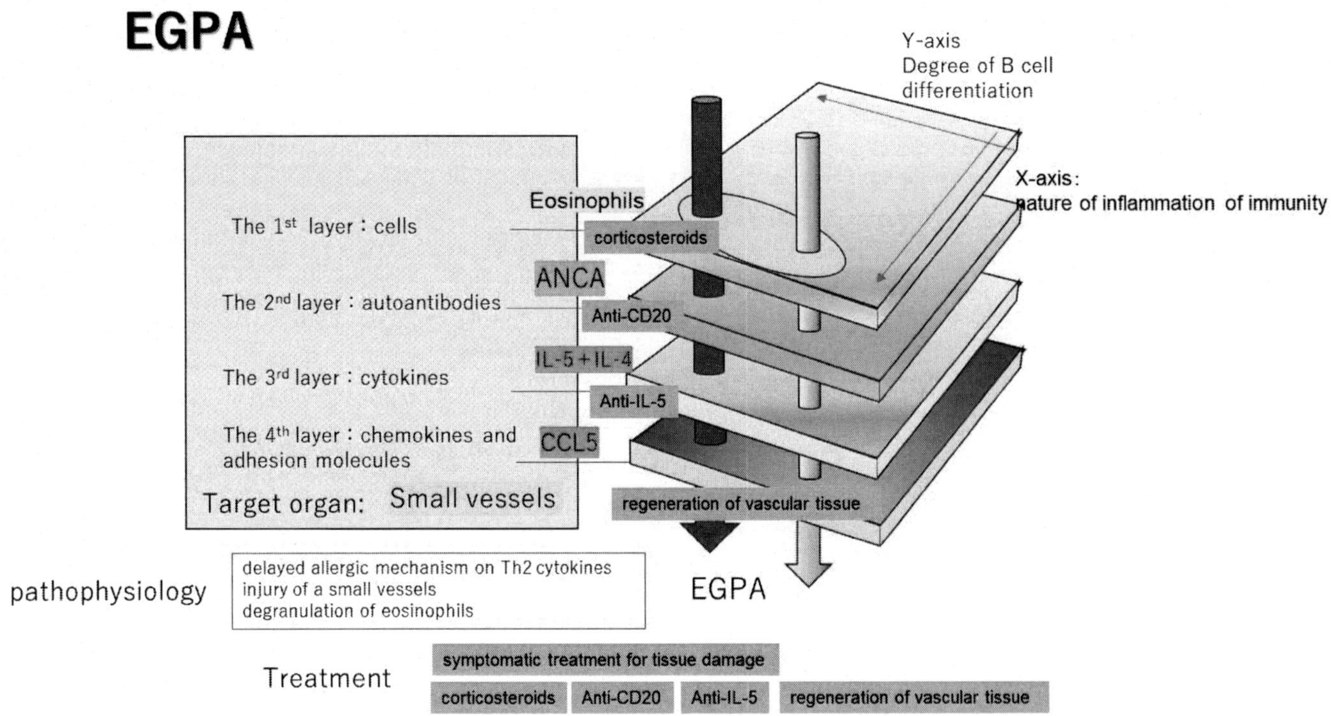

Figure 6. The composite image of the four-layer perspective view, that is, the three-dimensional structure is the essential feature of autoimmune diseases. As an example, consider the pathophysiology of EGPA (eosinophilic granulomatous polyangiitis) from this perspective view.

Next, regarding the second-layer autoantibodies, it is a well-known fact that EGPA patients produce ANCA (anti-neutrophil cytoplasmic antibody), and ANCA will be additionally described.

Furthermore, it is a cytokine of the third layer. In EGPA, IL-5 and IL-4 are deeply involved.

Finally, the fourth layer of chemokines has been reported to involve CCL5, CCL17 (chemokine（C-C motif）ligand 17）（TARC: thymus and activation regulated chemokine）, CCL26 (eotaxin-3) which may define a target tissue for autoimmunity.

In the case of EGPA, the target tissue is small vessels of the whole body.

From the above, the pathophysiology is considered based on this perspective view. In summary, a delayed allergic mechanism centered on Th2 cytokines is a background, and a mechanism of injury of small vessels, which is a target organ, by degranulation of eosinophils is a basic condition.

Next, based on this pathophysiology, a treatment strategy will be considered.

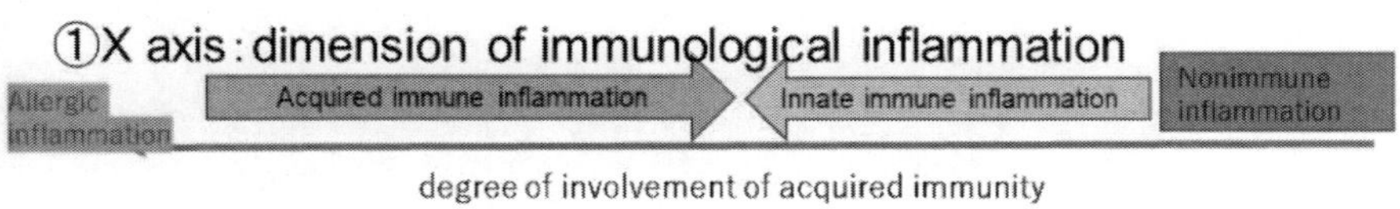

Figure 7. The X-axis is based on the nature of the immune inflammation. The dimension of immunological inflammation is defined by the degree of involvement of acquired immunity. The immune response in which acquired immunity is most involved is allergic inflammation, which is advanced, followed by acquired immune (autoimmune) inflammation, innate immune inflammation, and nonimmune inflammation.

First, corticosteroids are very effective for eosinophils in the first layer. Next, an anti-CD20 antibody that suppresses the production of ANCA, which is an autoantibody of the second layer, is used. As for the third layer cytokine, there is an anti-IL-5 antibody. For the fourth-layer chemokine CCL5, an anti-CCL5 antibody might be a candidate.

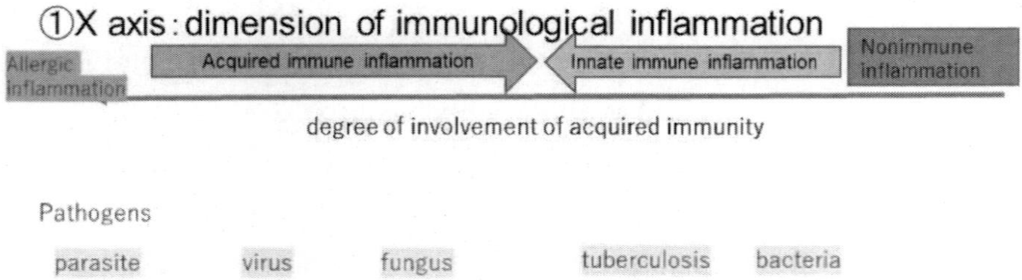

Figure 8. Each of these immunological inflammations is responsible for protection against pathogens. Allergic inflammation is responsible for parasites, acquired immune inflammation is for viruses and fungi, and innate immunity is responsible for protection against tuberculosis and bacteria. Nonimmune inflammation is responsible for protection against mechanical damages.

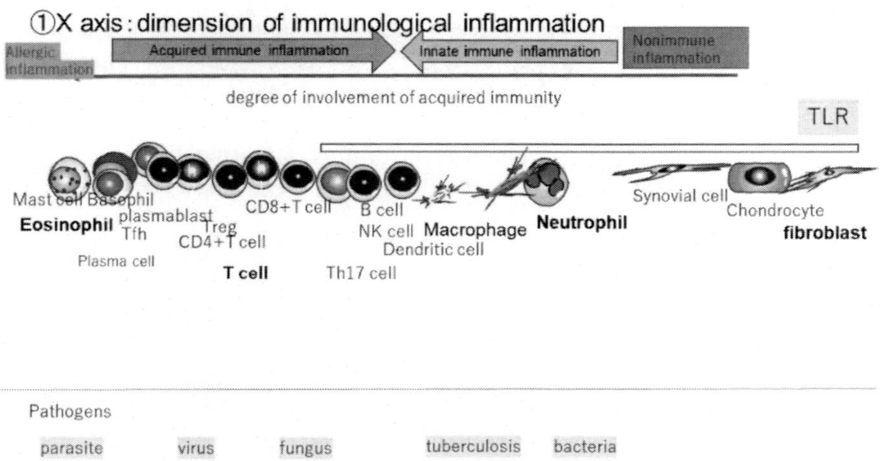

Figure 9. On the created X-axis, various immune and non-immune system cells are arranged depending on their inflammatory nature and the corresponding pathogens. Allergic immune system cells include mast cells and basophils, mainly eosinophils. In the acquired immune system cells, a cell group centered on T cells and plasma cells and plasmablasts that have been finally differentiated among B cell lines are arranged. The T cell line cell group is further divided into T follicular helper cells (Tfh), CD4 + T cells, CD8 + T cells, and Th17 cells, and arranged in that order. B cells could present antigens and are located at a position slightly closer to the innate immune system. Innate immune system cells are dendritic cells, macrophages, and neutrophils. Dendritic cells are closely related to acquired immunity and are therefore placed close to acquired immunity. Neutrophils are a highly differentiated cell population as innate immunity and are in innate immunity. Non-immune cells include synovial cells, chondrocytes, and fibroblasts.

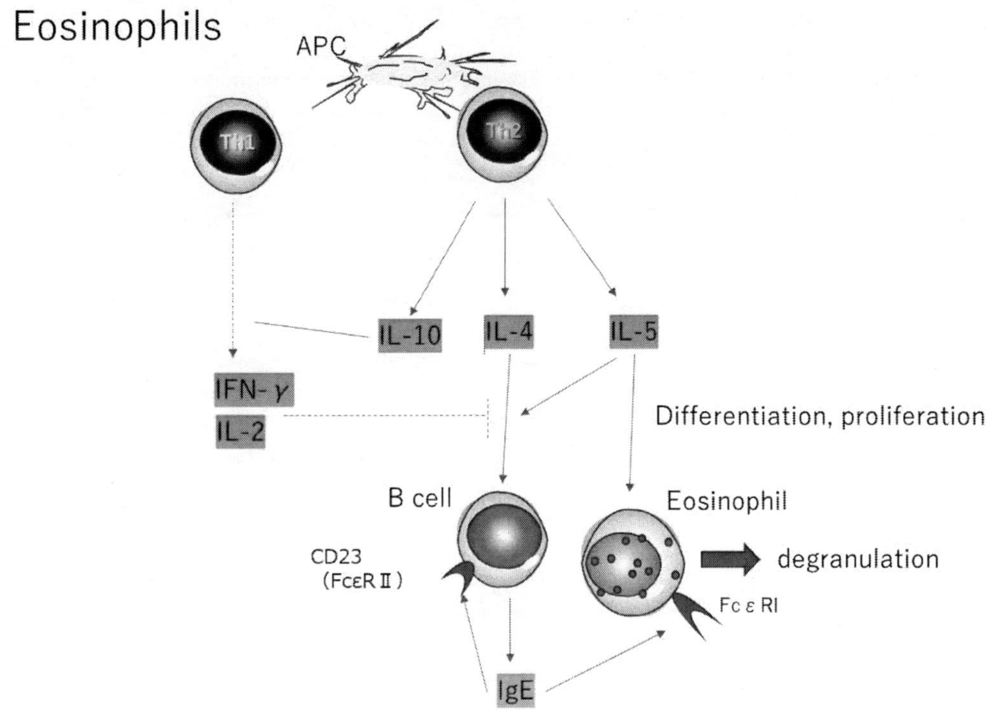

Figure 10. Eosinophils are considered cells belonging to the innate immune system but are not cells of the simple innate immune system. Eosinophils are very highly regulated by acquired immunity. IgE is only present in evolved mammals reflects the expertise of highly acquired immunity.

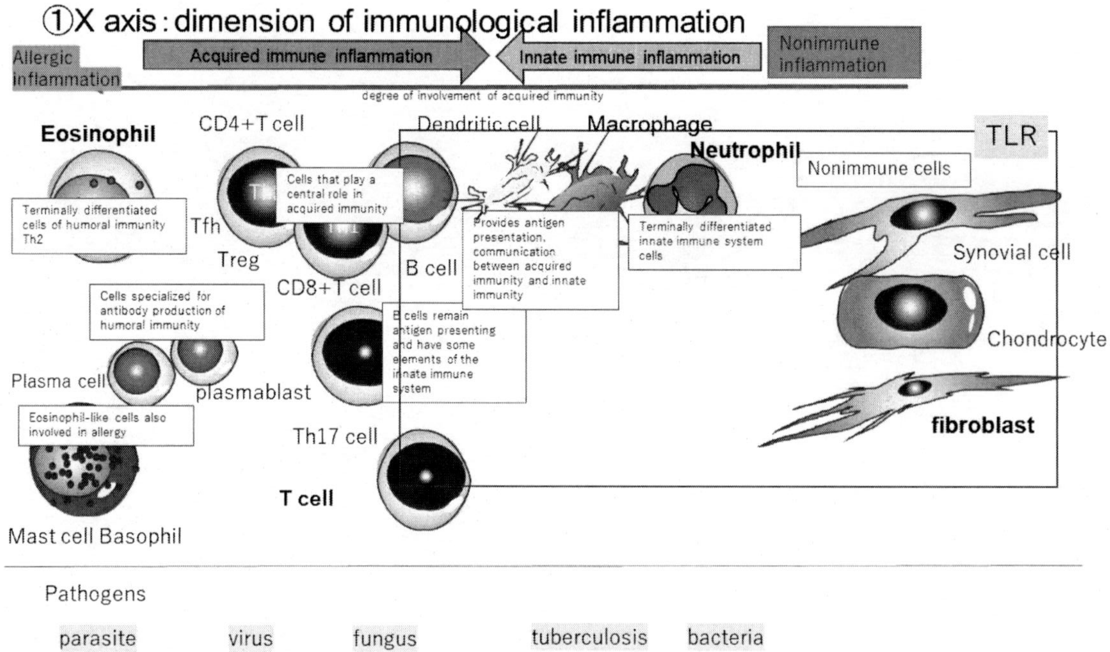

Figure 11. According to the above description, the cells are arranged in an easy-to-understand manner in this figure. Eosinophil: Terminally differentiated cells of humoral immunity Th2. Plasma cells and plasmablasts: Cells specialized for antibody production of humoral immunity. Mast cell and Basophil: Eosinophil-like cells also involved in allergy. T cells: Cells that play central roles in acquired immunity. B cells: Cells remain antigen presenting ability and have some elements of the innate immune system. Dendritic cell: Cells provide antigen presentation, communication between acquired immunity and innate immunity. Neutrophil: Terminally differentiated innate immune system cells. Nonimmune cells: synovial cells, chondrocytes and fibroblasts.

At present, there is only a symptomatic treatment for tissue damage, but the regeneration of vascular tissue will be an issue in the future.

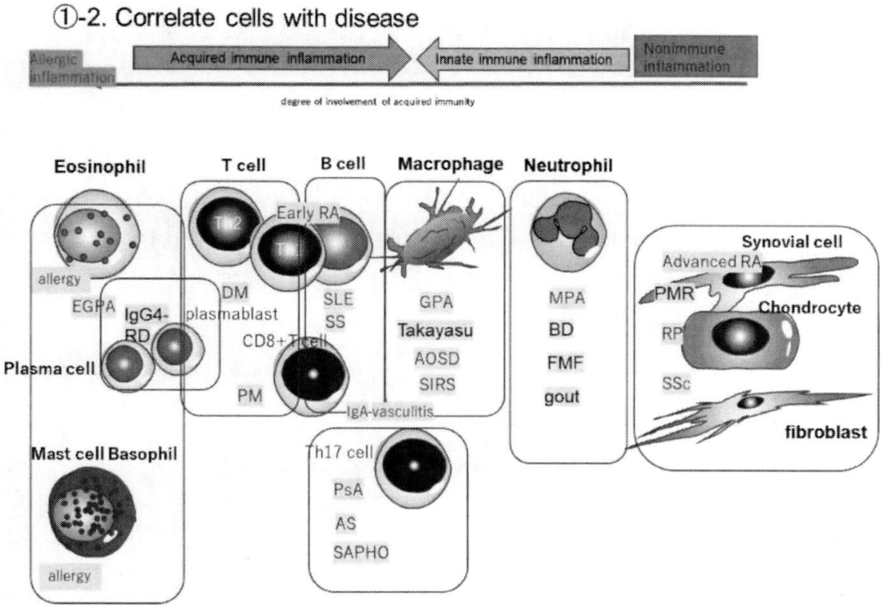

Figure 12. Correlate cells with disease.

Although various autoimmune diseases have complicated pathophysiology, one or two immune cells or non-immune cells play central roles in each disease. Based on the cells, the immune diseases are plotted on the X-axis. Eosinophil-related diseases include allergy and EGPA. Plasma cells and plasmablasts correspond to IgG4-related disease. In the T cell line, Th2, Th1, CD8 + T cells and Th17 are the main cells. These correspond to dermatomyositis (DM), early rheumatoid arthritis (RA), PM (polymyositis) and spondyloarthritis such as psoriatic arthritis, ankylosing spondylitis, SAPHO syndrome, respectively. B cell lines correspond to systemic lupus erythematosus (SLE), Sjögren's syndrome (SS), and IgA vasculitis. On the other hand, early rheumatoid arthritis straddles both Th1 and B cell lines. Macrophages correspond to granulomatous polyangiitis (GPA), Takayasu disease, adult-onset Still's disease (AOSD), and Systemic

Inflammatory Response Syndrome (SIRS). Neutrophil-related diseases include microscopic polyangiitis (MPA), Behçet's disease (BD), familial Mediterranean fever (FMF), and gout. In non-immune system inflammation, synovial cells correlate with late rheumatoid arthritis and polymyalgia rheumatica (PMR). Chondrocytes correspond to relapsing polychondritis (RP), and fibroblasts are correlated with scleroderma. However, only the distribution of cells on the X-axis cannot separate diseases because many diseases correspond to just one type of cells. Therefore, the pathophysiology of each disease cannot be clearly explained separately only by using indicators by the cells.

B CELL PATHOLOGY

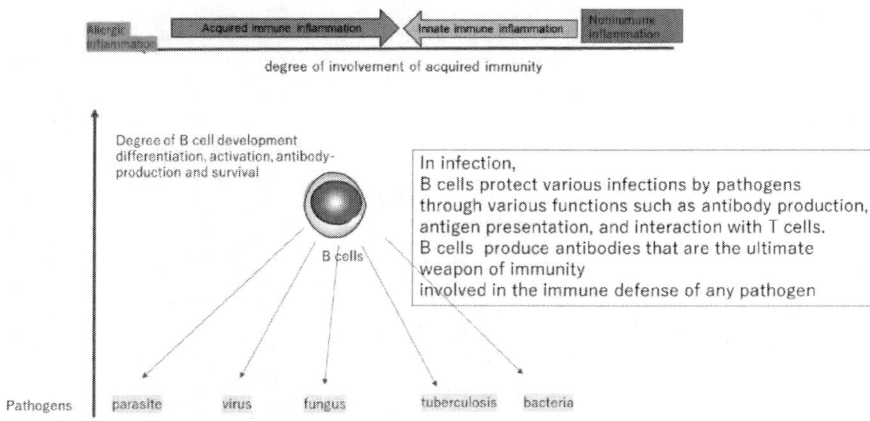

Figure 13. If only cells were used as indicators, multiple diseases correspond to one type of cells, and it is difficult to separate each disease. However, in each immune disease, the role and distribution of B cells are significantly different and have unique properties. This is because in infection immunology, B cells protect various infections by pathogens through various functions such as antibody production, antigen presentation, and interaction with T cells. In a sense, B cells are cells that produce antibodies that are the ultimate weapon of immunity and are involved in the immune defense of any pathogen. Therefore, even in autoimmune diseases, B cells have various disease-specific states. By using the B cells as an indicator on the Y-axis, it is possible to clearly separate a disease in two dimensions. Degree of B cell development includes differentiation, activation, antibody-production, survival and expression of various surface markers specific for the disease.

This is exactly the function corresponding to the degree of B cell development described above, and RP105 molecule can serve as an index on the Y-axis.

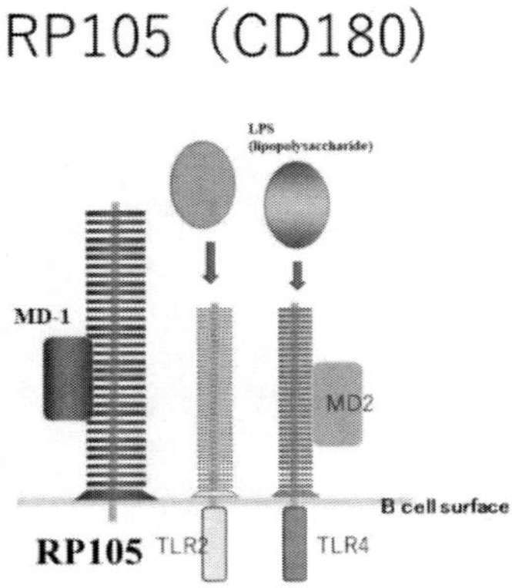

Figure 14. RP105 (CD180) molecule is an abbreviation for Radio-Protective MW105Kd. The RP105 molecule is a member of TLR-related molecules and is mainly expressed on the surface of B cells in association with MD-1. Its function is to assist the responsiveness of TLR2 and TLR4 to lipopolysaccharide (LPS), and regulates B cell activation, differentiation, antibody production, survival and expression of markers (Modified from Yamashita Y et al. J Exp Med. 1996).

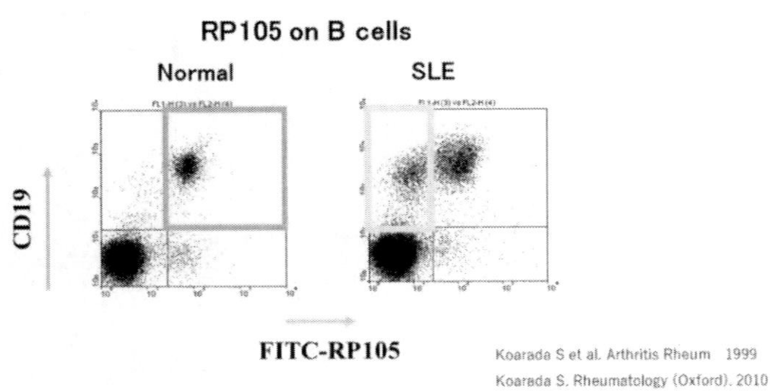

Figure 15. We analyzed expression of RP105 molecule on the surface of B cells from systemic lupus erythematosus (SLE) patients. Peripheral blood mononuclear cells (PBMCs) were isolated from fresh blood by specific gravity centrifugal method and analyzed by flow cytometry after double staining with RP105 and CD19. As a result, it became clear that many RP105-negative B cells, which are rarely found in normal, are present in SLE patients (Modified from Koarada S, et al. Arthritis Rheum, 1999) (Modified from Koarada S, et al. Rheumatology (Oxford), 2010).

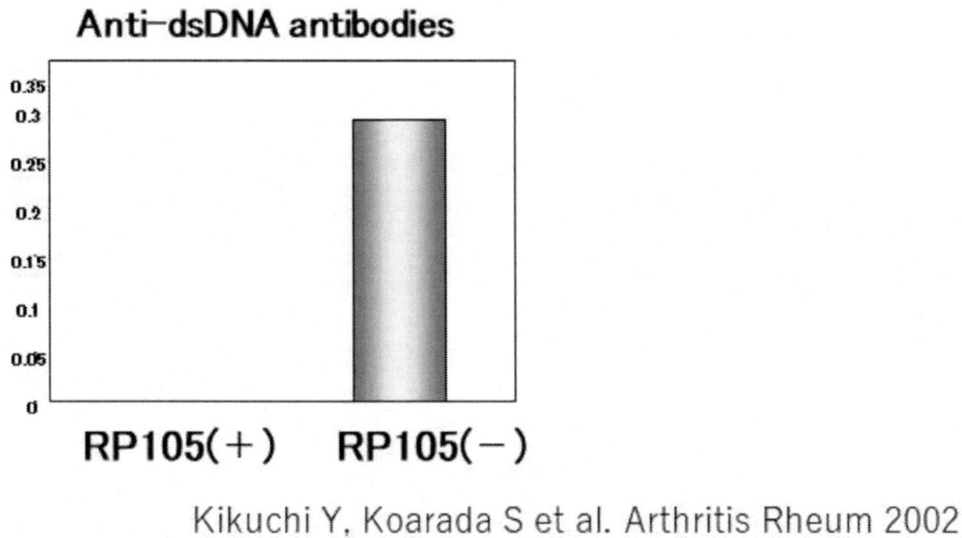

Figure 16. IgG class anti-dsDNA antibody production by RP105 negative B cells. After separating RP105 (-) and RP105 (+) B cells using cell sorter and stimulating and culturing them in vitro with activated T cells, ELISA analysis of IgG class anti-dsDNA antibody in the supernatant was performed. RP105-negative B cells produced anti-dsDNA antibodies, whereas RP105-positive B cells did not produce autoantibodies. This result indicates that RP105-negative B cells are autoantibody-producing B cells themselves. The cell ratio of RP105-negative B cells can be used as an indicator to suggest a breakdown of B cell tolerance (Modified from Kikuchi Y, Koarada S et al. Arthritis Rheum 2002).

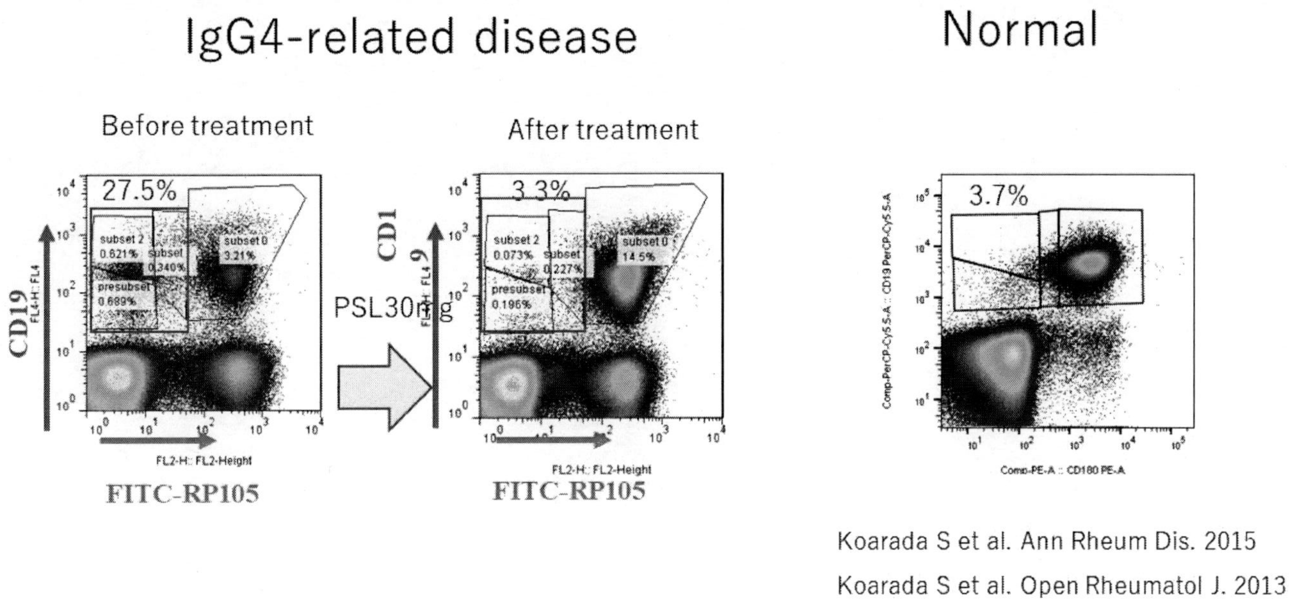

Figure 17. In IgG4-related disease, increase in the numbers of RP105-negative B cells has been observed before treatment. Corticosteroid treatment rapidly reduces RP105-negative B cells and returns to near normal levels. Thus, RP105-negative B cells are correlated with disease activity in IgG4-related disease (Modified from Koarada S et al. Ann Rheum Dis. 2015) (Modified from Koarada S et al. *Open Rheumatol J.* 2013).

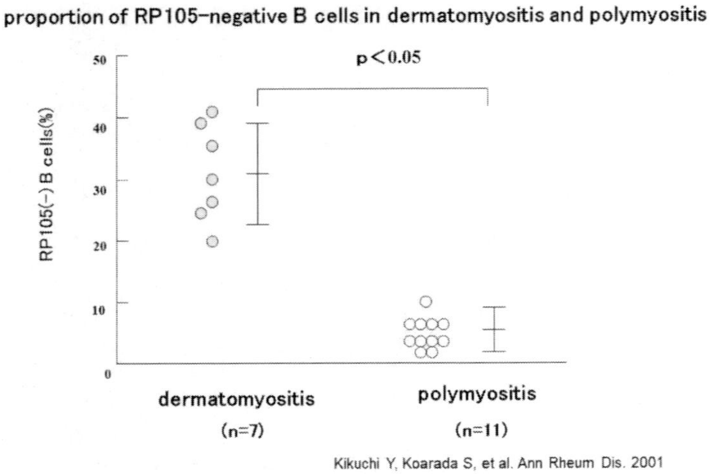

Figure 18. RP105 negative B cells in other autoimmune diseases are described. The proportion of RP105-negative B cells in dermatomyositis and polymyositis has been studied. Patients with dermatomyositis had an increase in RP105-negative B cells in all cases, whereas patients with polymyositis had little increase. The ratio of RP105 negative B cells is significantly different in both diseases ($p < 0.05$). B cell involvement may be different in the pathophysiology of dermatomyositis and polymyositis (Modified from Kikuchi Y, Koarada S, et al. *Ann Rheum Dis*. 2001).

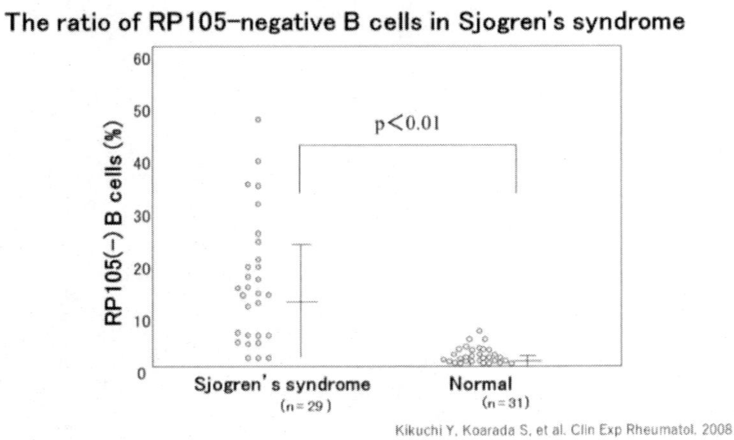

Figure 19. The ratio of RP105-negative B cells in Sjögren's syndrome has been studied. In Sjögren's syndrome, there was an increase in RP105-negative B cells, though to a varying degree in each patient. Since patients with Sjögren's syndrome have B cell activation and autoantibody production, an increase in RP105-negative B cells also suggests that B cell line immune abnormalities are present in the background (Modified from Kikuchi Y, Koarada S, et al. *Clin Exp Rheumatol*. 2008).

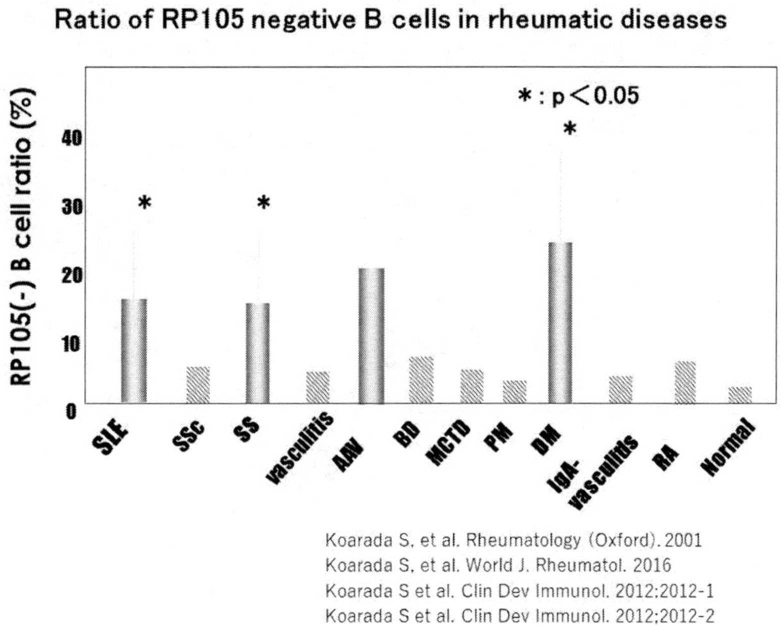

Figure 20. This figure shows the ratio of RP105-negative B cells in rheumatic diseases. Thus, it has been found that the ratio of RP105-negative B cells greatly differs depending on the underlying disease. SLE: systemic lupus erythematosus, SSc: systemic sclerosis, SS: Sjögren's syndrome, AAV: ANCA associated vasculitis, BD: Behçet's disease, MCTD: mixed connective tissue disease, PM: polymyositis, DM: dermatomyositis, RA: rheumatoid arthritis (Modified from Koarada S, et al. Rheumatology (Oxford). 2001) (Modified from Koarada S, et al. *World J. Rheumatol*. 2016) (Modified from Koarada S et al. Clin Dev Immunol. 2012;2012-1) (Modified from Koarada S et al. *Clin Dev Immunol*. 2012;2012-2).

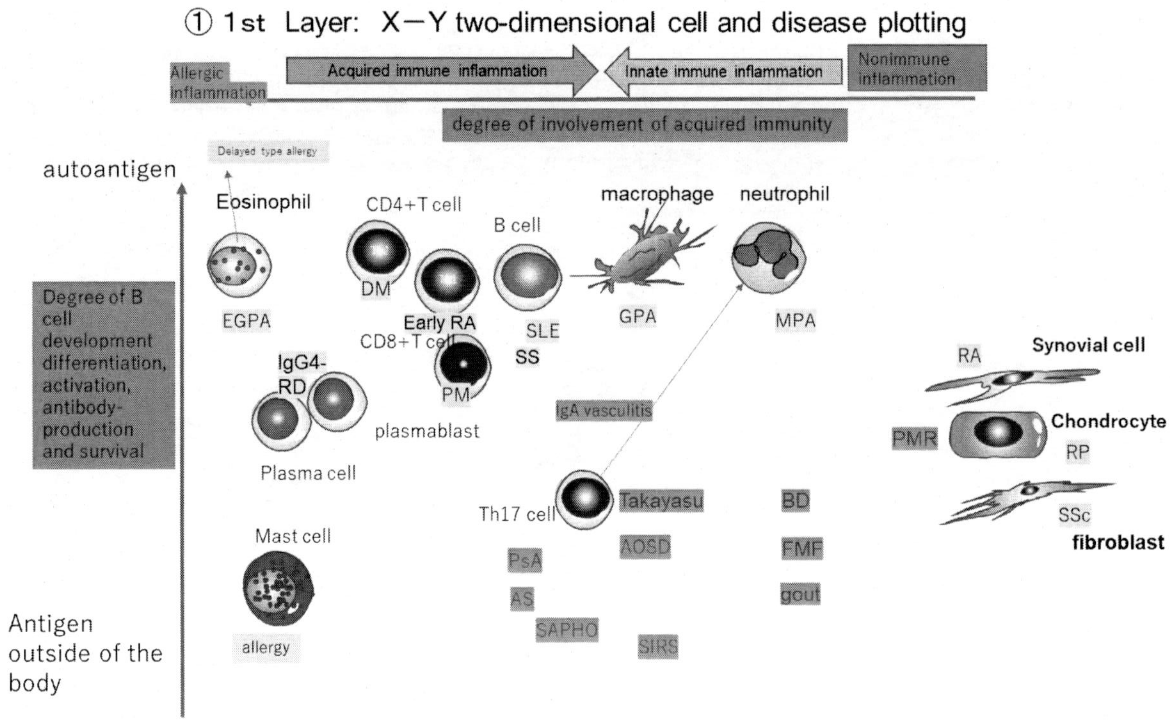

Figure 21. ① First layer, Separation of individual diseases by two-dimensional development based on the degree of immunological inflammatory response on the X-axis and the degree of B cell differentiation on the Y-axis. In this way, by developing in two dimensions, it is possible to plot each disease independently. For allergies, there will be axes outside and inside the body.

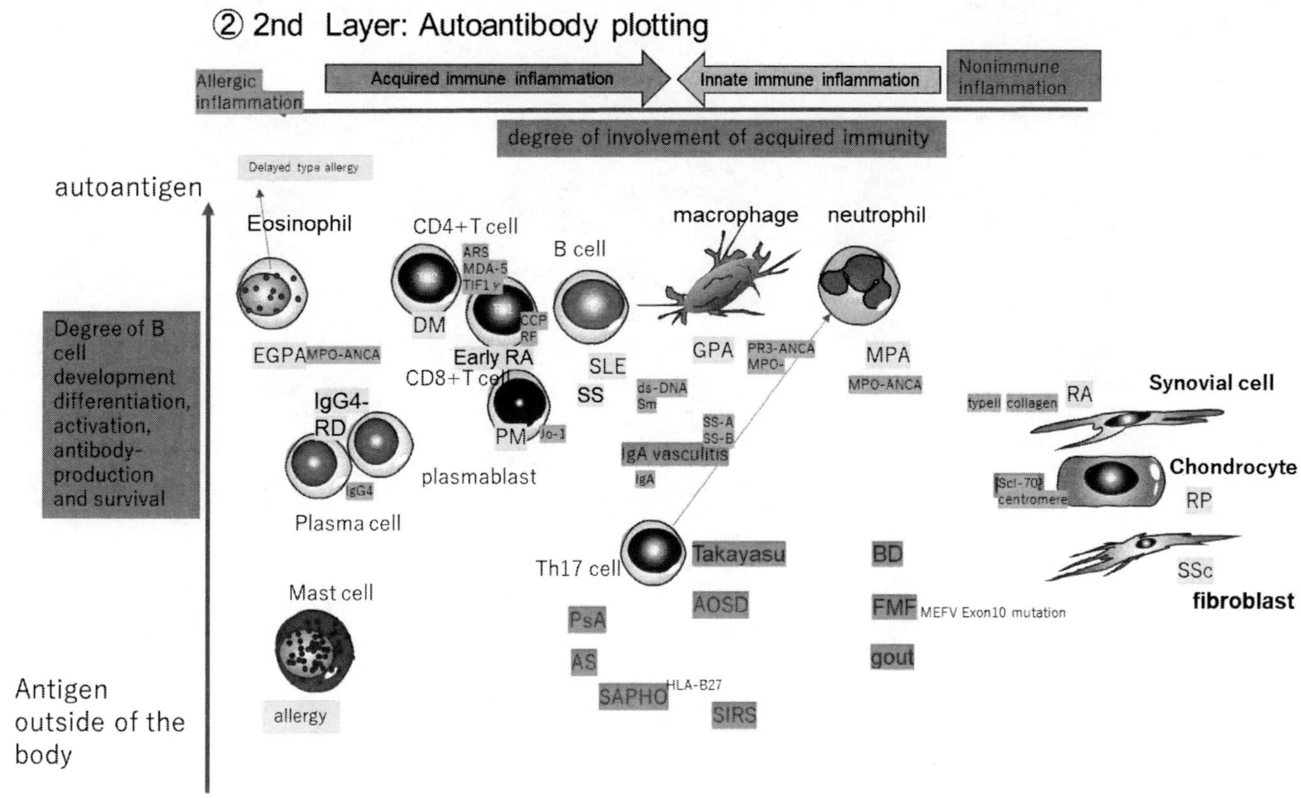

Figure 22. ②The second layer is autoantibody-production. Here, autoantibodies specific to each autoimmune disease are plotted.

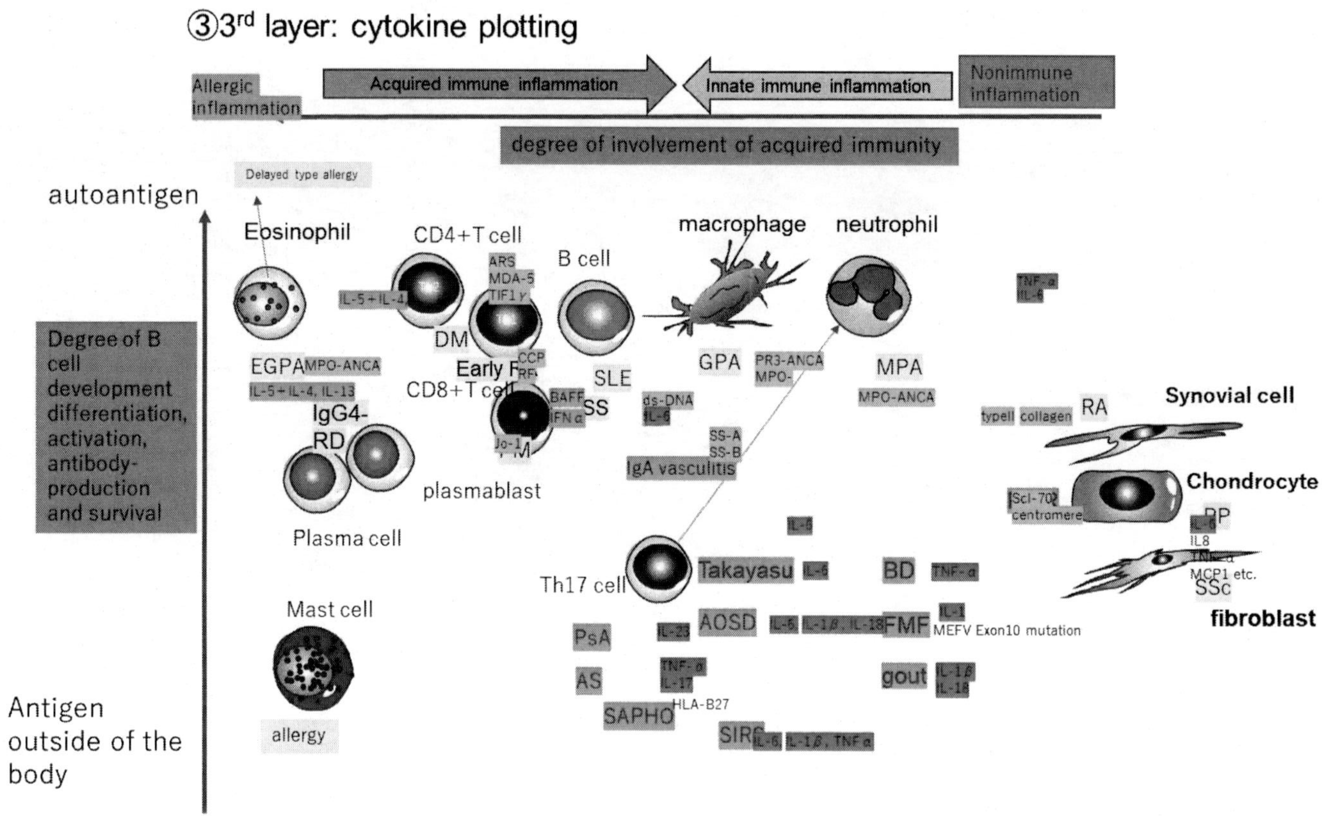

Figure 23. ③The third layer is a plot of cytokines. Various cytokines are plotted corresponding to disease and cells.

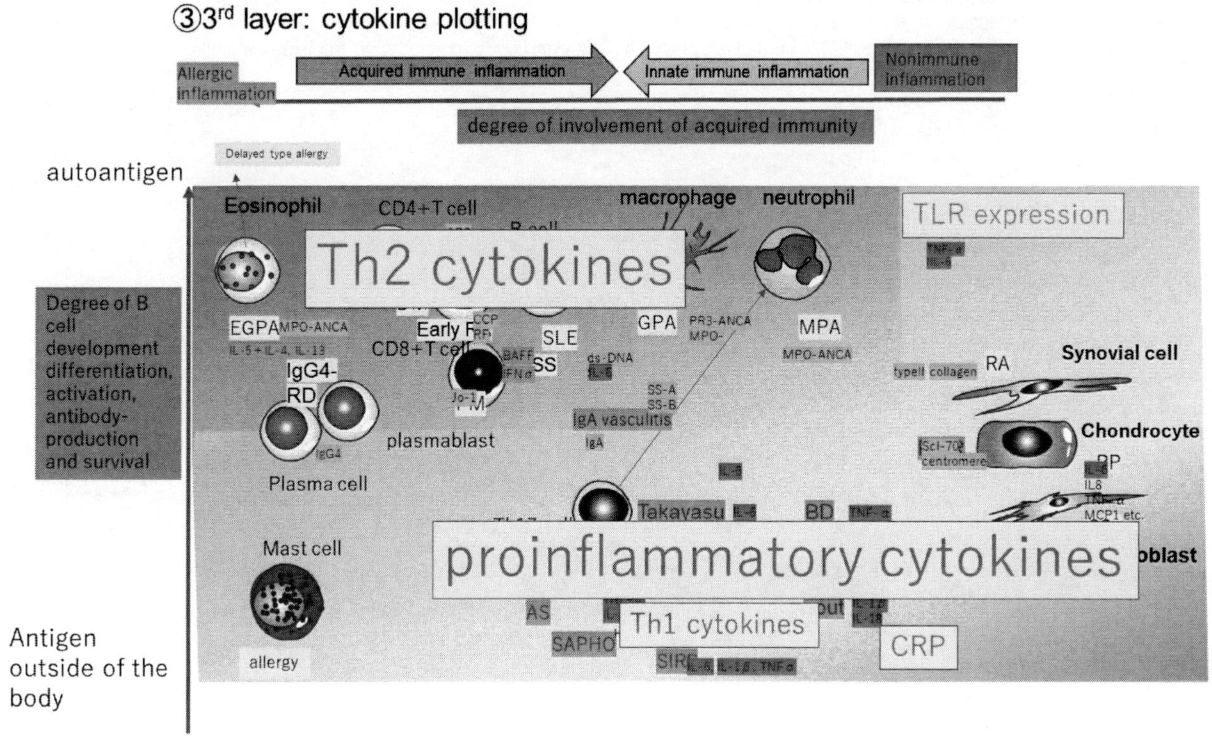

Figure 24. When plotting is performed in this manner, the Th2 cytokine is automatically arranged at the upper left, and the Th1 and inflammatory cytokine are arranged at the lower right. The upper left is a group of diseases involving Th2 cytokines with autoantibody-production, and the lower right is a group of diseases mainly involving inflammatory cytokines. The disease group located at the lower right tends to be positive for CRP, and the disease group at the upper right has pathophysiology in which TLR is deeply involved.

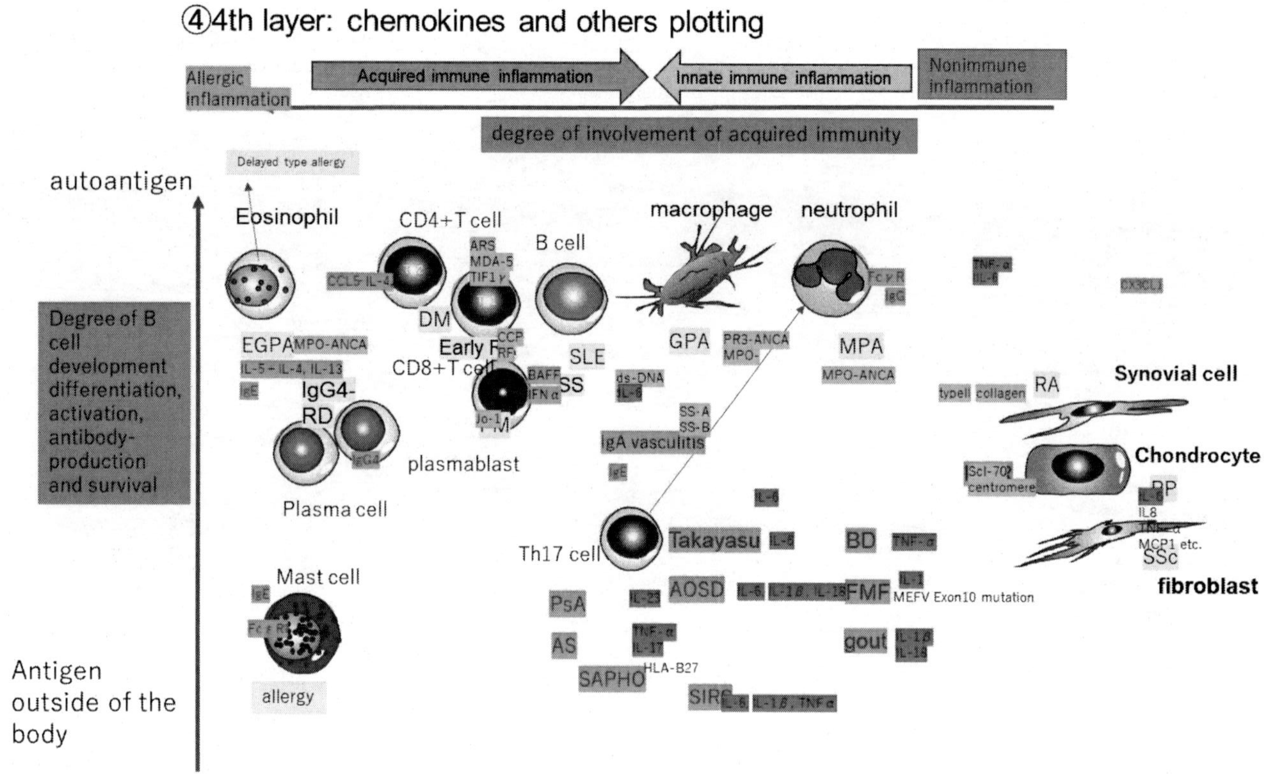

Figure 25. ④ Fourth layer: Tissue impairment factors such as chemokines (including adhesion molecules, fractalkine) and others are plotted in this figure. The condition is more complicated and not as simple as this. This plot could be an oversimplification. Any disease has both aspects of innate immunity and acquired immunity, and the center of disease and the specific gravity differ depending on the disease and the patient.

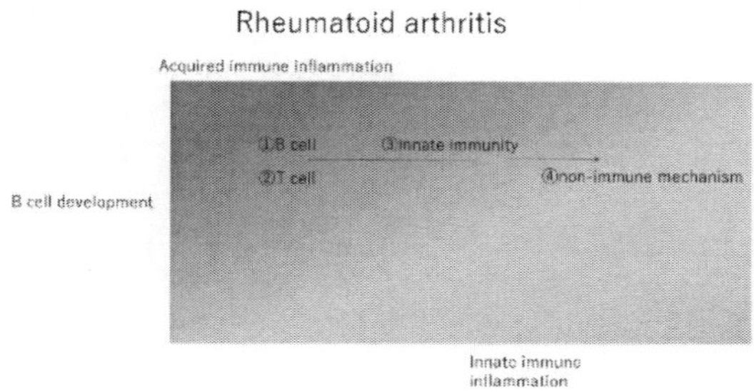

Figure 26. For example, in rheumatoid arthritis, B cells and T cells are the primary immunological abnormalities in the early stages. However, through the involvement of the innate immune system, it eventually shifts to non-immune inflammation, in which the synovial cells are at the center of pathophysiological reaction. The same disease does not always have the same immunological condition at different times.

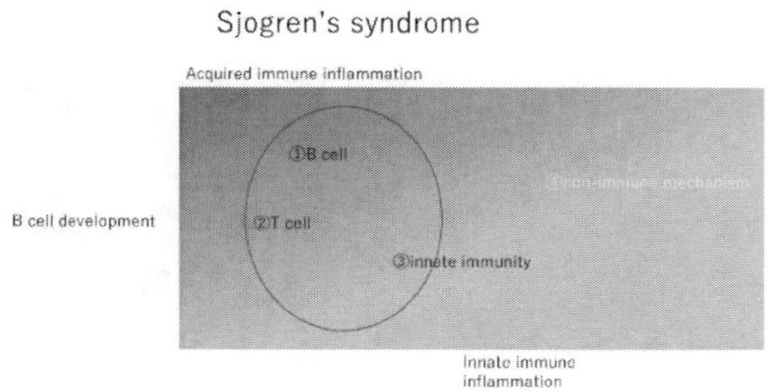

Figure 27. Further, even the same disease may include various disease states. For example, in Sjögren's syndrome, some patients focus on B cells, while others focus on T cells. In addition, there are various patients, such as those with a strong involvement of the innate immune system. In addition, one patient may have all these various conditions at the same time. However, it is usually considered that there is no patient with Sjögren's syndrome that has only non-immune system inflammation. No matter how diverse the pathology of Sjögren's syndrome is, it does not appear that the pathology does not involve immunity at all.

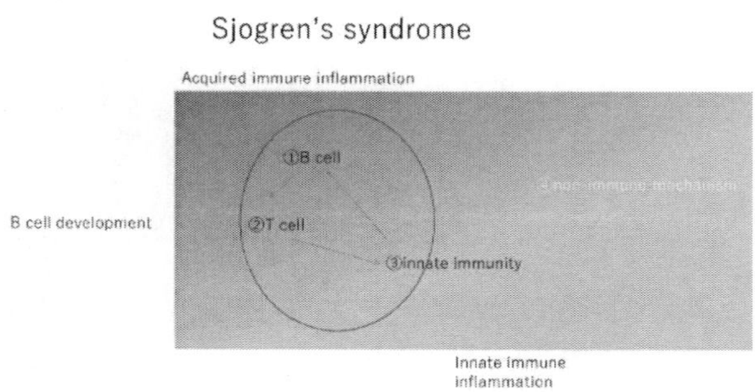

Figure 28. Even in the same Sjögren's syndrome patient, there is a possibility that there is a transition from a B cell-centered pathophysiology to a T cell-centered pathophysiology, or to a pathophysiology in which the involvement of innate immune system cytokines is strong.

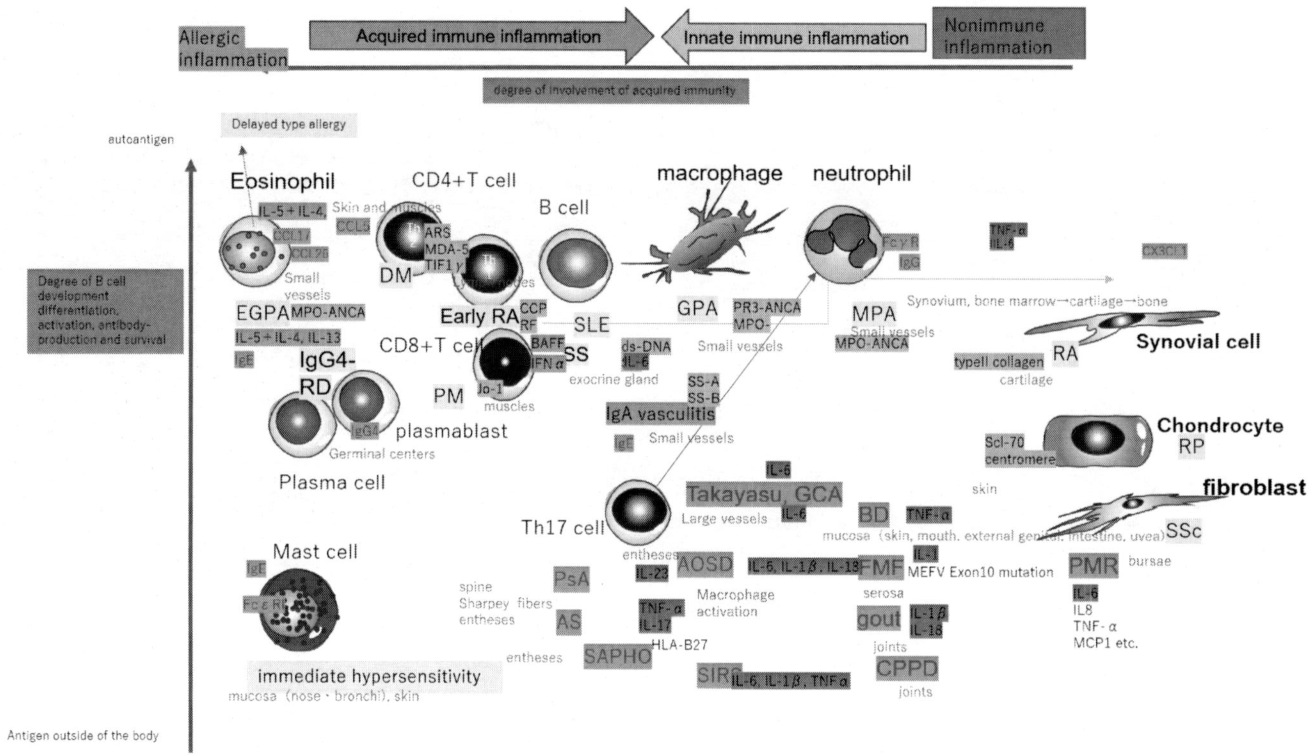

Figure 29. Target tissue. Finally, systemic autoimmune diseases target histologically common structural components such as muscle tissue, vascular tissue, skin tissue, cartilage tissue, synovial tissue, attachment tissue, exocrine glands, and mucosal tissue. These are plotted.

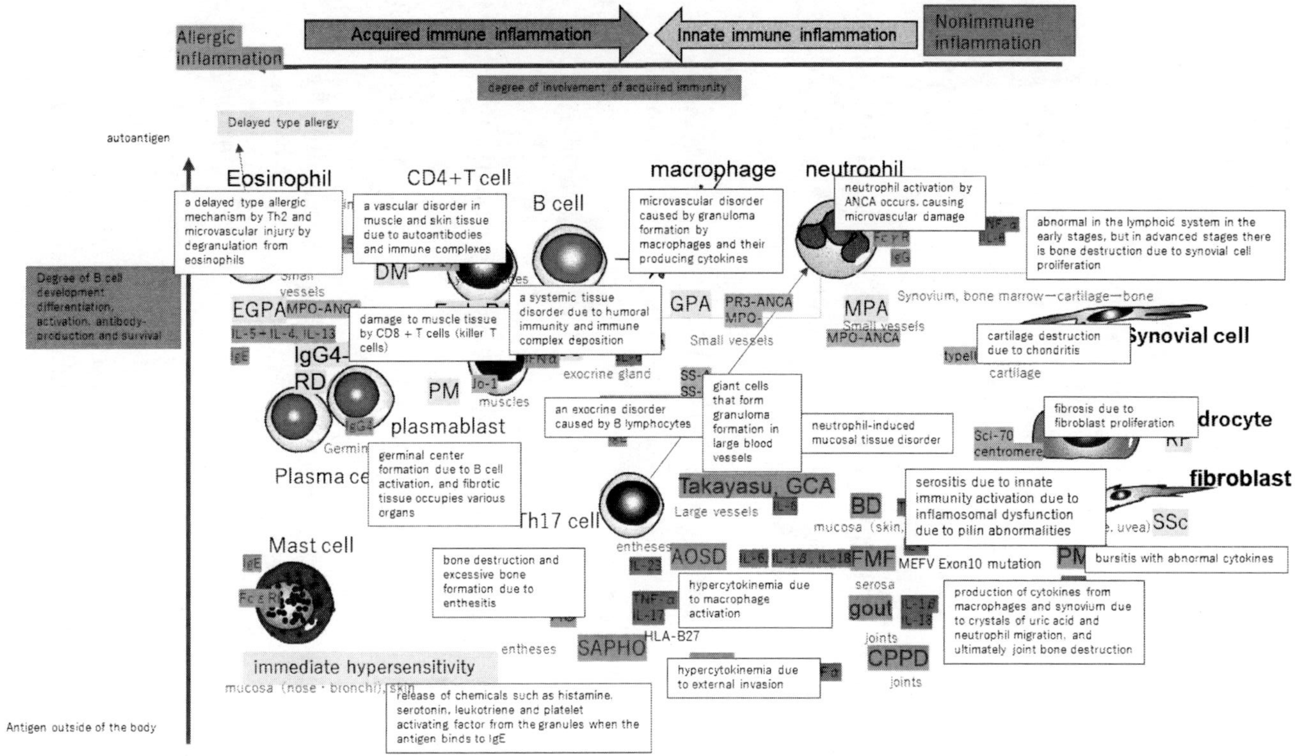

Figure 30. Pathophysiology of immune diseases.

The pathophysiology of eosinophilic granulomatosis with polyangiitis (EGPA) is a delayed type allergic mechanism by Th2 and microvascular injury by degranulation from eosinophils.

The basic pathophysiology of dermatomyositis is a vascular disorder in muscle and skin tissue due to autoantibodies and immune complexes.

Polymyositis is damage to muscle tissue by CD8 + T cells (killer T cells).

IgG4-related disease has germinal center formation due to B cell activation, and fibrotic tissue occupies in various organs.

Systemic lupus erythematosus (SLE) is a systemic tissue disorder due to humoral immunity and immune complex deposition.

Sjögren's syndrome (SS) is an exocrine disorder caused by B lymphocytes.

Spondyloarthropathies, such as psoriatic arthritis (PsA), ankylosing spondylitis (AS), and SAPHO syndrome, show bone destruction and excessive bone formation due to enthesitis.

Immediate type allergy (hypersensitivity) is due to the release of chemicals such as histamine, serotonin, leukotriene and platelet activating factor from the granules when the antigen binds to IgE.

Granulomatosis with polyangiitis (GPA) is a microvascular disorder caused by granuloma formation by macrophages and their producing cytokines.

In microscopic polyangiitis (MPA), neutrophil activation by ANCA occurs, causing microvascular damage.

Adult-onset Still's disease (AOSD) is hypercytokinemia due to macrophage activation.

Systemic inflammatory response syndrome (SIRS) is hypercytokinemia due to external invasion.

Takayasu's arteritis (TA) and giant cell arteritis (GCA) are giant cells that form granuloma in the large blood vessels.

Rheumatoid arthritis (RA) has abnormality of the lymphoid system in the early stages, but in advanced stages there is bone destruction due to synovial cell proliferation.

Relapsing polychondritis (RP) is cartilage destruction due to autoimmune chondritis.

Systemic sclerosis (SSc) is fibrosis due to fibroblast proliferation.

Behçet's disease (BD) is a neutrophil-induced mucosal tissue disorder.

Familial Mediterranean fever (FMF) is serositis by innate immunity activation and inflammasomal dysfunction due to pilin abnormalities.

Rheumatic polymyalgia (PMR) is bursitis with abnormal cytokines.

Gout causes the attack by the production of cytokines from macrophages and synovium due to crystals of uric acid and neutrophil migration, and ultimately joint destruction.

TREATMENT

Neutrophils are recruited into peripheral blood by corticosteroids, but do not alter cell numbers throughout the body. However, corticosteroids decrease the migration ability of neutrophils. Glucocorticoids reduce the numbers of monocytes and macrophages slightly. In addition, migratory ability, phagocytic ability, antigen presenting ability, and cytokine/eicosanoid producing ability also decrease due to glucocorticoids. For lymphocytes, corticosteroids reduce cell numbers. Proliferation ability, migration ability, activation, and cytokine production ability also decrease by glucocorticoids. In eosinophils, apoptosis is induced, and the cell number is significantly reduced by glucocorticoids.

Table 1. The reason for arranging the disease in this way is that it has relevance to treatment. The first is the therapeutic effect of corticosteroids. As a prerequisite for understanding treatment, it is necessary to describe the effects of corticosteroids on blood cells. Immune cells are more vulnerable to corticosteroids as their degree of differentiation and the nature of the acquired immunity increase

Relevance to treatment: Corticosteroids

	effects of corticosteroids on blood cells	Cell numbers
Neutrophils	Recruited into peripheral blood Migration ability decreases	→
Monocytes and macrophages	Migratory ability, phagocytic ability, antigen presenting ability, and cytokine / eicosanoid producing ability decrease	↘
Lymphocytes	Proliferation ability, migration ability, activation, and cytokine production ability decrease	↓
Eosinophils	Apoptosis	↓ ↓

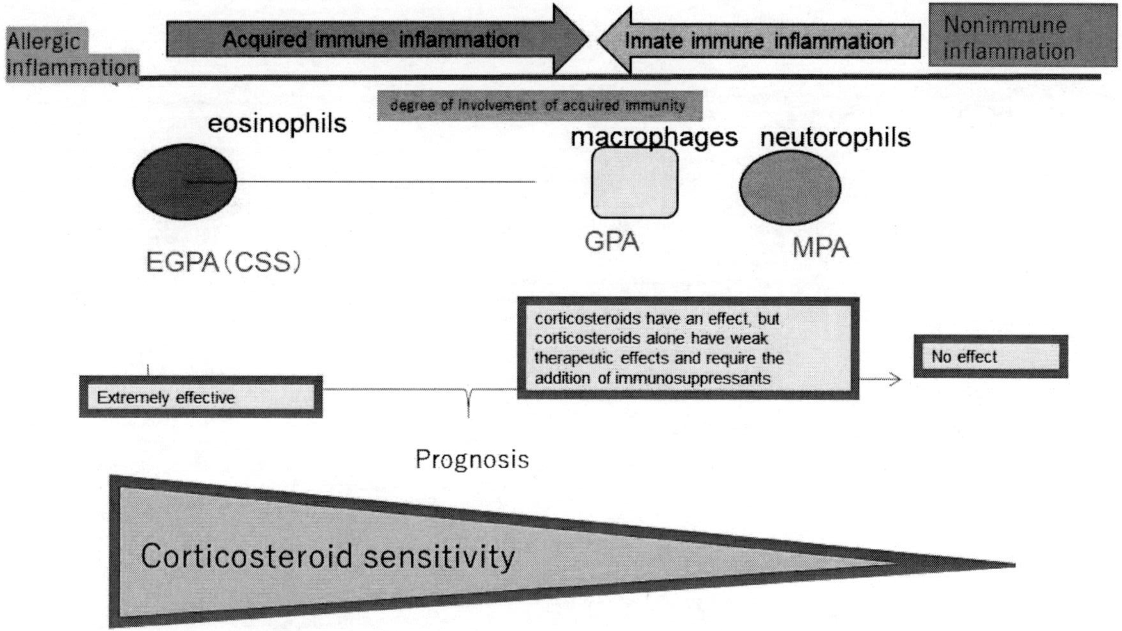

Figure 31. Treatment Implications: Corticosteroids. Consider the corticosteroid sensitivity of autoimmune diseases. Diseases located on the left side of the X-axis have enhanced adaptive immunity and enhanced corticosteroid effects. Therefore, even in the three diseases of ANCA-associated vasculitis (AAV) having similar pathophysiology, EGPA is located at the leftmost (GPA is located at the middle, and MPA is located at the right) and is extremely effective with corticosteroids. Since GPA and MPA are further on the right side than the middle, corticosteroids alone have weak therapeutic effects and require the addition of immunosuppressants. And the prognosis also tends to be as good as the left and not as good as the right. Therefore, the prognosis of vasculitis is also favorable for EGPA, followed by GPA and MPA.

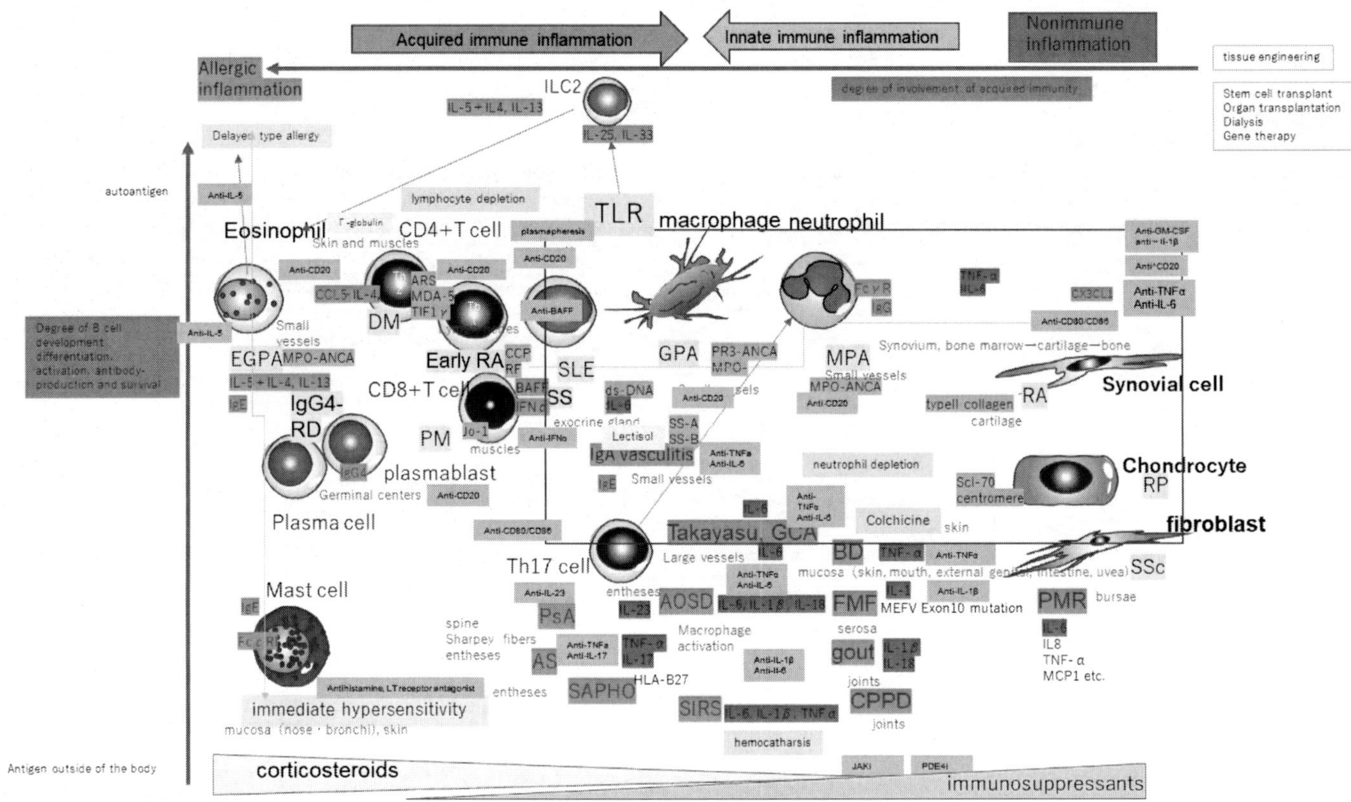

Figure 32. Interpretation of treatment. The treatment is naturally determined by the location of the disease in the chart of 3-D immunohysiology.

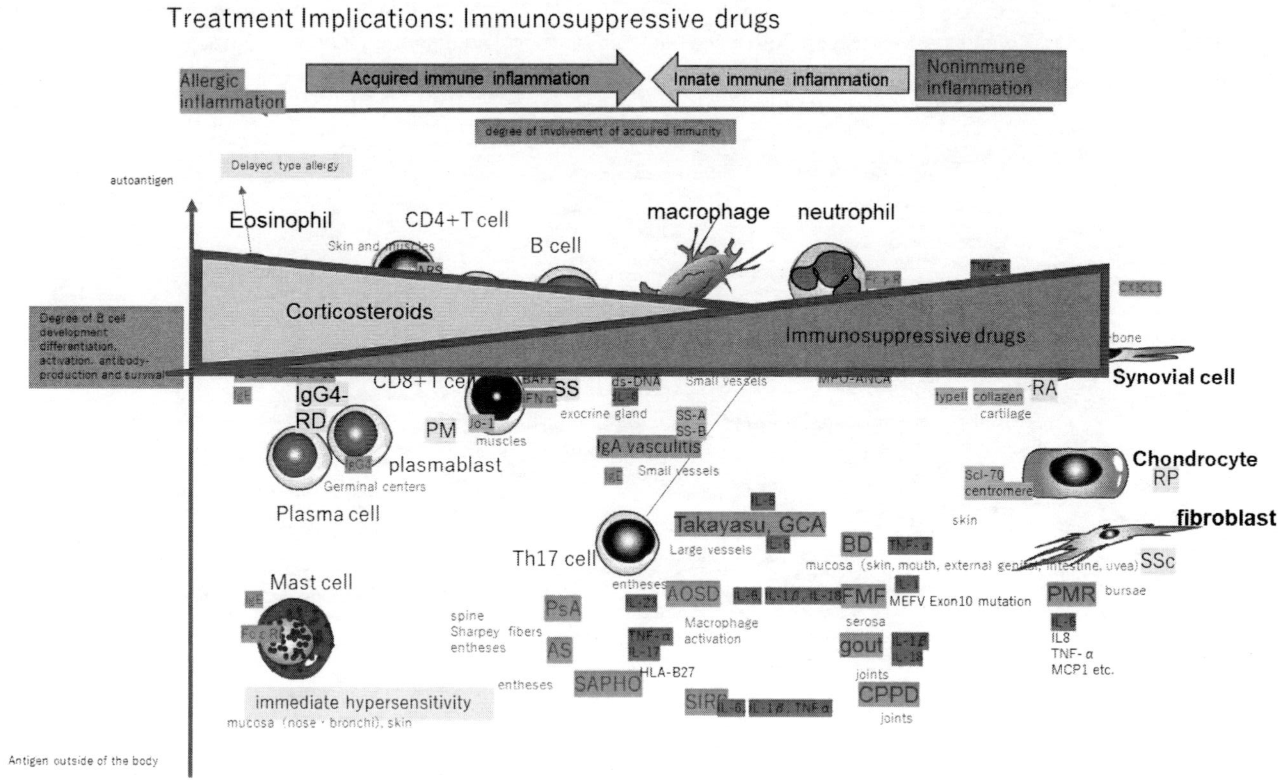

Figure 33. In this chart, the effects of corticosteroids and the treatment of immunosuppressive drugs that compensate for the lack of the effects are arranged.

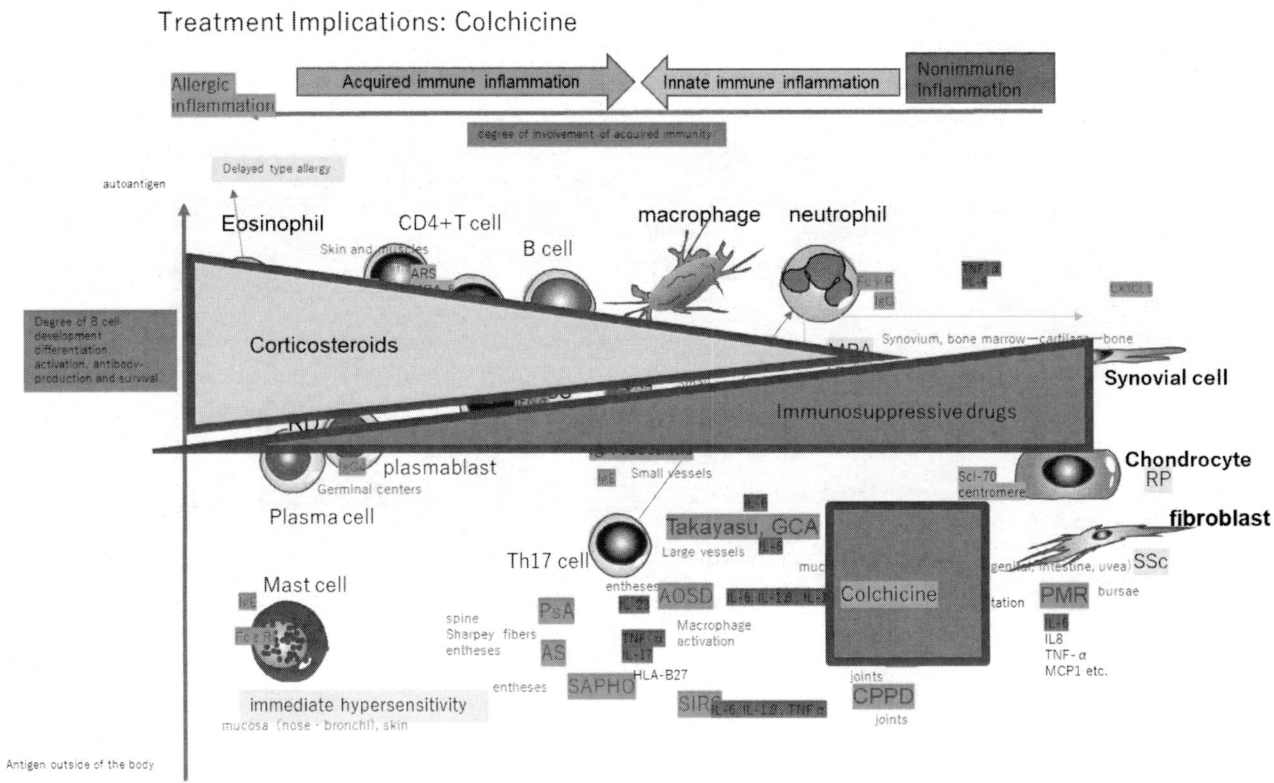

Figure 34. Next, consider the treatment of colchicine. Because colchicine is a drug that suppresses neutrophils, the position of colchicine is in parts of neutrophil-related diseases.

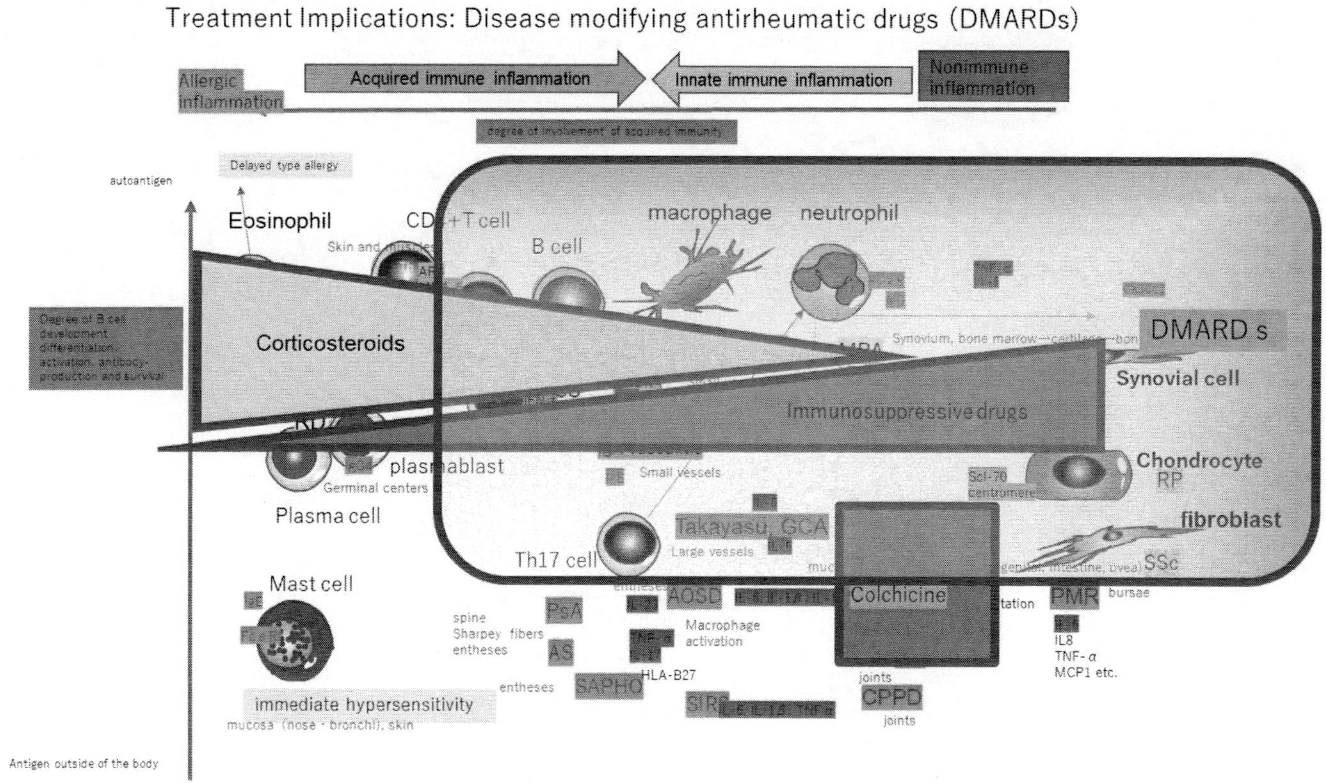

Figure 35. DMARDs are mainly used for rheumatoid arthritis, but their types and mechanisms are diverse, and they have been widely used for various diseases and their effects have been recognized.

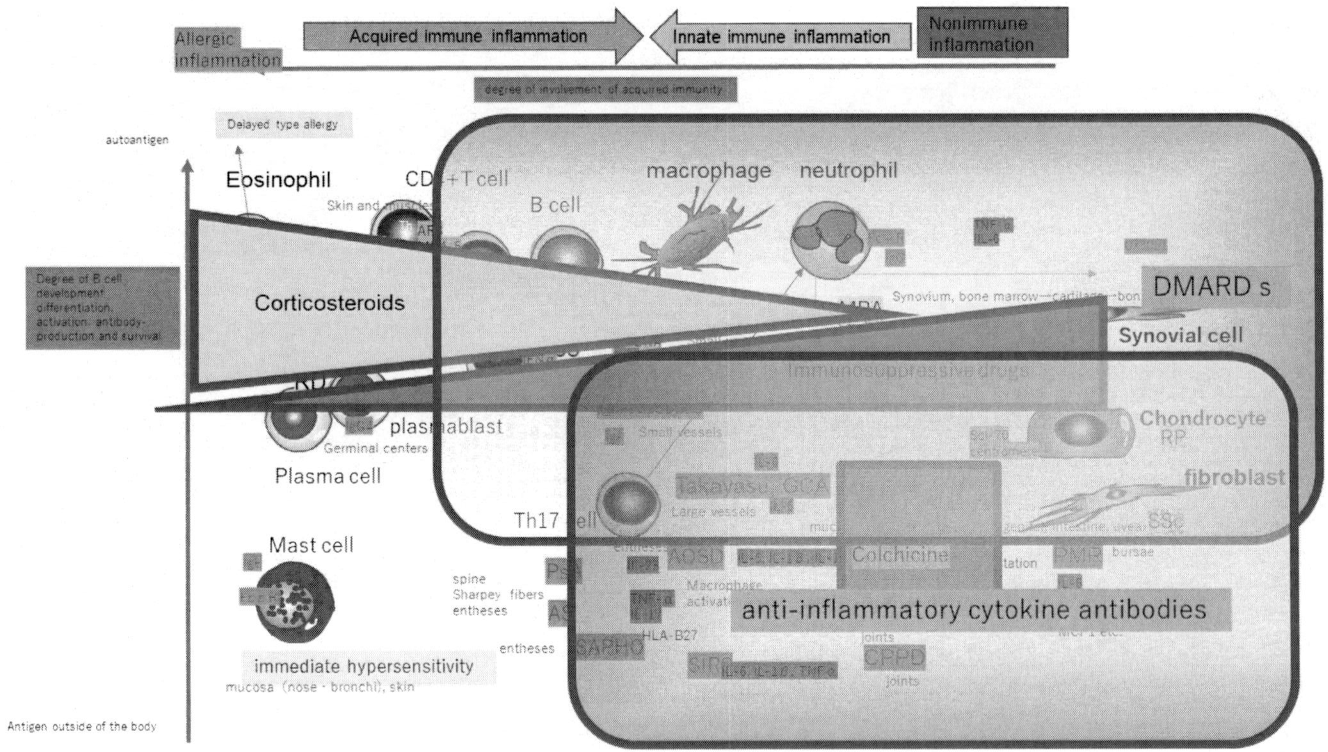

Figure 36. Therapeutic implications: Biologics: anti-inflammatory cytokine antibodies. It is often used mainly in the lower right group of diseases in which inflammatory cytokines are the main pathophysiological roles in the diseases.

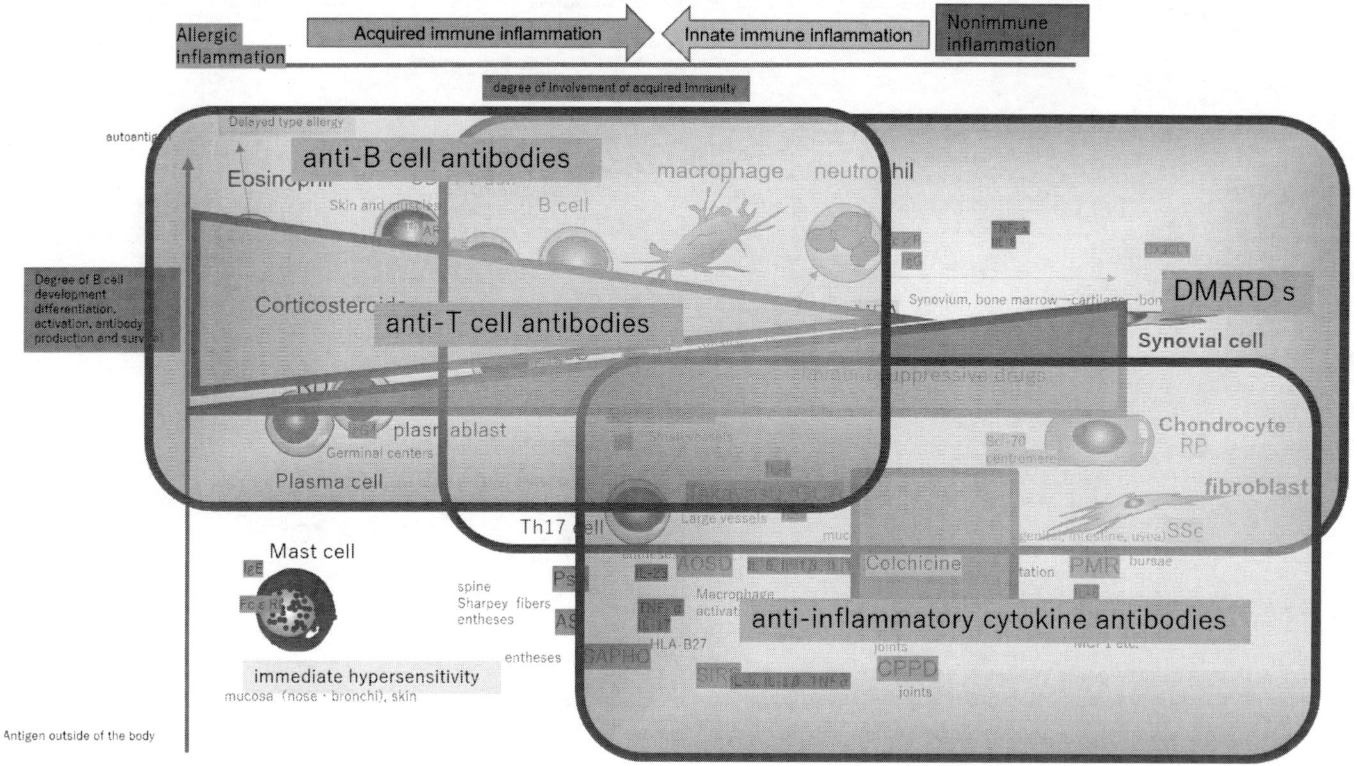

Figure 37. Therapeutic implications: Biologics: Anti-T and anti-B cell antibodies. Antibodies that suppress T cells or B cells are placed in T cell and B cell related disease groups. Anti-B cell antibodies are also useful for a group of diseases that produce autoantibodies.

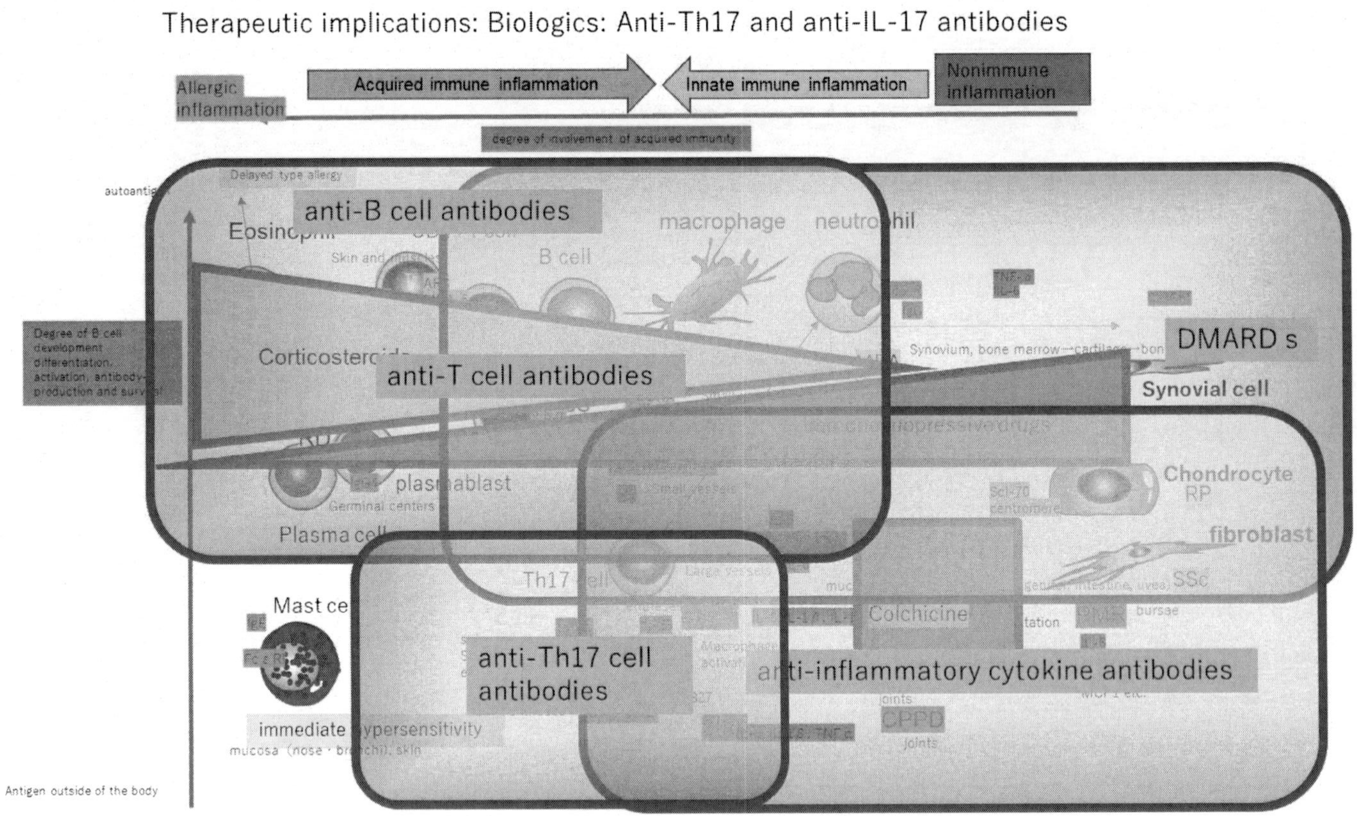

Figure 38. Therapeutic implications: Biologics: IL-17-suppressing biologics are useful in a group of diseases that produce Th17.

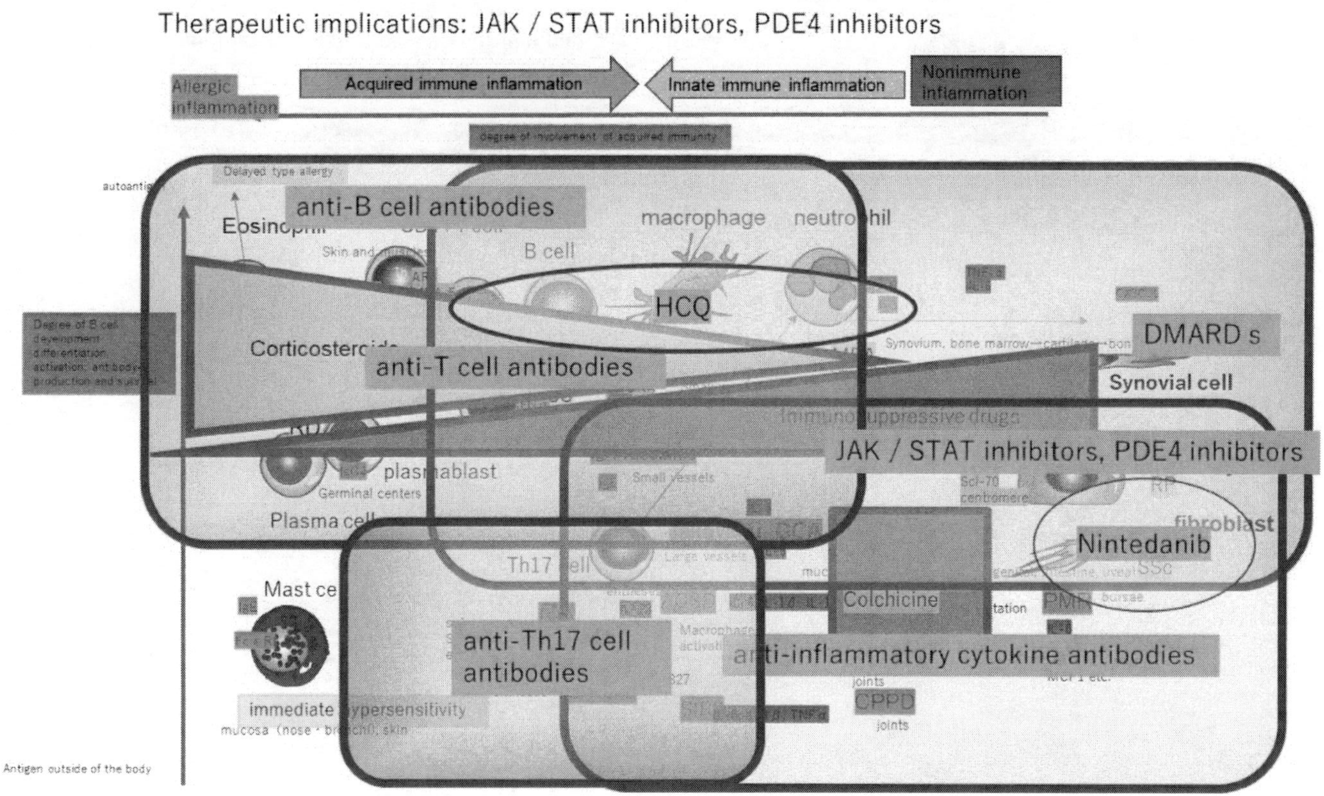

Figure 39. Relevance for treatment: JAK / STAT inhibitor, PDE4 inhibitor. The position of these new drugs is not yet clear but they are useful for groups of diseases associated with various cytokines.

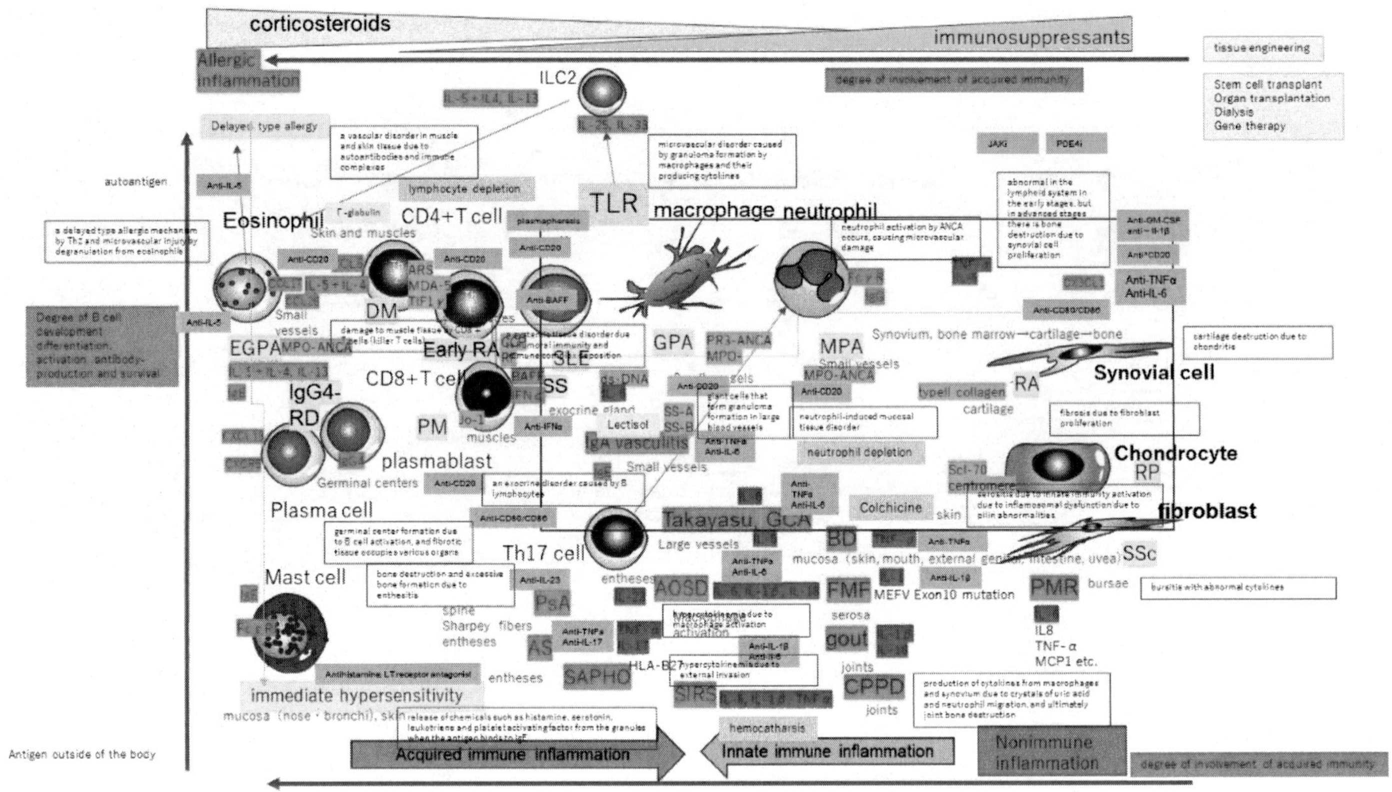

Figure 40. Final immunological perspective chart of immunological diseases.

SLE

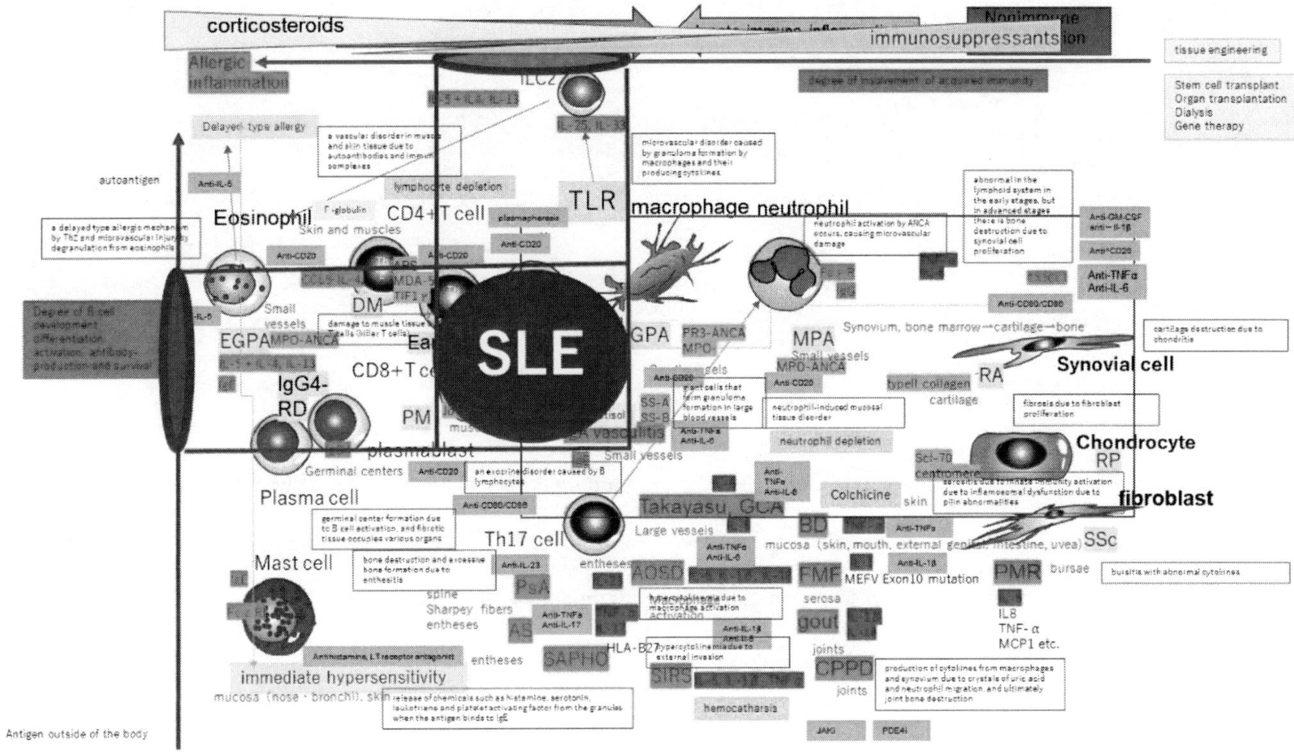

Figure 41. (Continued).

X-axis: B cell diseases of acquired immunity and autoimmune inflammation.
Y-axis: B cell differentiation (ratio of RP105-negative B cells) is very higher degree.
Layer 1: cells; B cells.
Layer 2: autoantibody; anti-dsDNA antibodies, anti-Sm antibodies.
Layer 3: cytokines; BAFF, IFNα.
Layer 4: Target tissue; immune complex deposited tissue → systemic tissue injury, mainly blood vessels.
Pathophysiology and Treatment.

Corticosteroids work to some extent, but usually treatment requires a combination of immunosuppressants. In the cases of conventional treatment resistance, CD20 antibody and BAFF antibody are considered. Plasma exchange may be performed in severe cases.

Figure 41. Position of systemic lupus erythematosus (SLE) in immunopathophysiological chart.

GPA

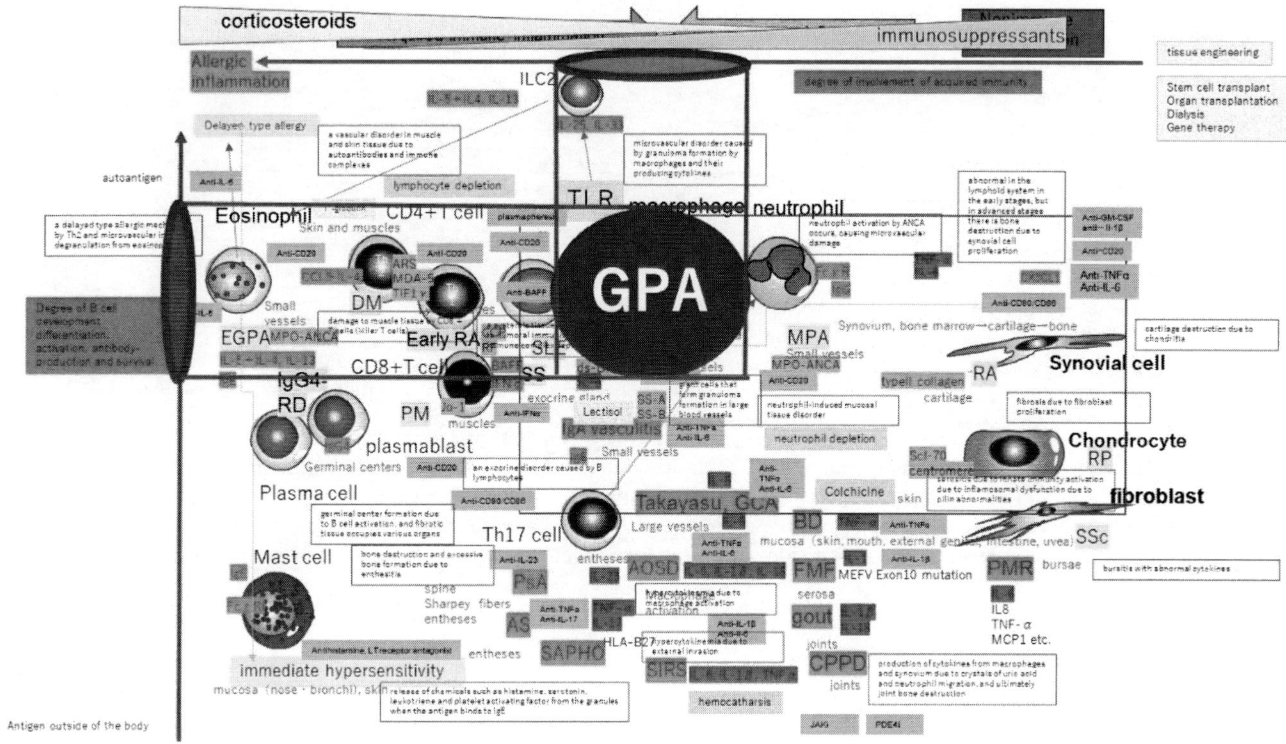

Figure 42. (Continued).

X-axis: An autoimmune disease at the position of macrophages that bridges innate and acquired immunity.
Y-axis: B cell differentiation (ratio of RP105negative B cells) is higher degree.
Layer 1: Cell; Macrophages (including nearby B cells and neutrophils).
Layer 2: Autoantibody; PR3-ANCA (or MPO-ANCA).
Layer 3: Cytokine; (TNFα).
Layer 4: Chemokines:
Target tissue: small blood vessels: ELK: ear and nose, lung, kidney.
Pathophysiology and treatment:

The main cause is microangiopathy caused by granuloma formation by macrophages and cytokines produced by the macrophages. Treatment is corticosteroids and immunosuppressants (cyclophosphamide: CY). Anti-CD20 antibody that suppresses autoantibody production is effective and is also selected for induction of remission. Although cytokine production is not the main pathophysiology, there have been reports of treatments of GPA patients with infliximab. In mild cases, it can be treated with corticosteroids and MMF or MTX. In severe cases, plasma exchange is also performed.

Figure 42. Position of GPA in immunopathophysiological chart.

PsA

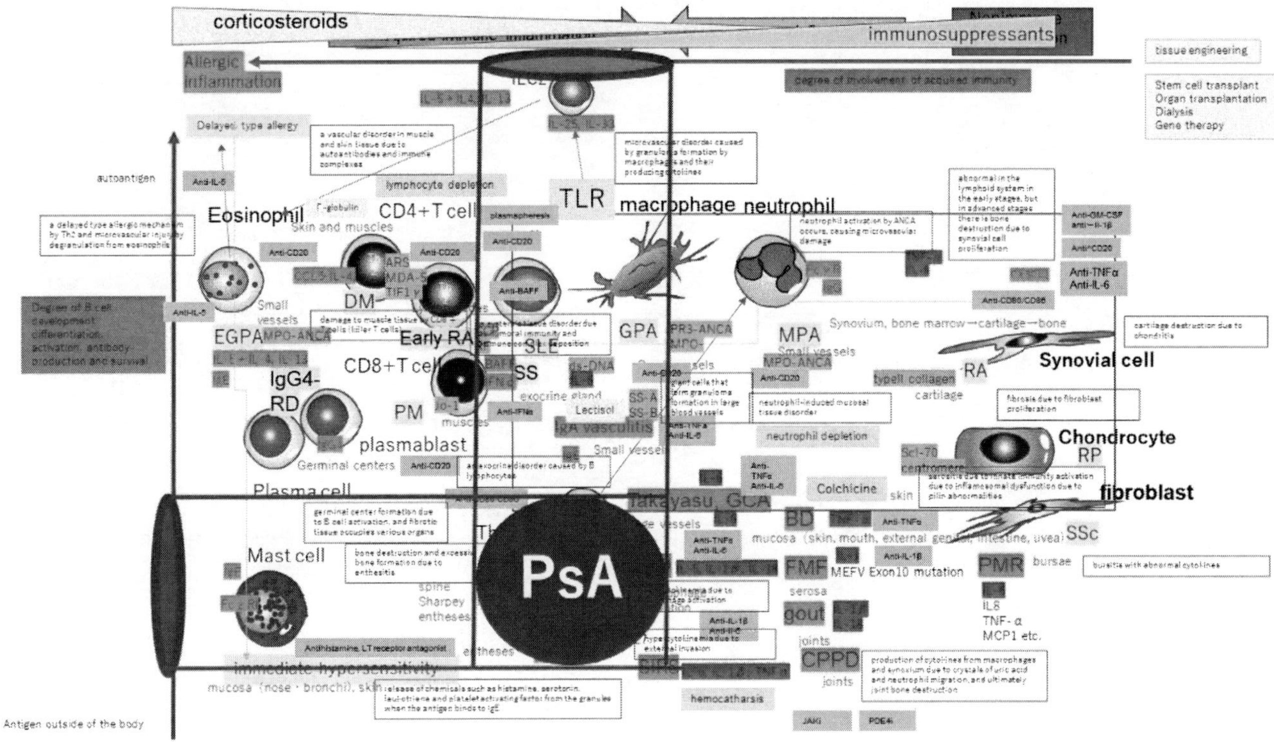

Figure 43. (Continued).

X-axis: Th17-related diseases that play central roles in autoimmune reactions.
Y-axis: low level of B cell differentiation (ratio of RP105negative B cells) is lower degree.
Layer 1: cells; Th17 cells.
Layer 2: autoantibody; none.
Layer 3: Cytokines; IL-23, TNF-alpha, IL-17, (GM-CSF).
Layer 4: Chemokines:
Target tissue: entheses
Pathophysiology and treatment:

Bone destruction and excessive bone formation due to enthesitis are the main features. Treatment with glucocorticoids is not effective. Anti-cytokine therapy involves anti-IL-23, anti-IL-17, and anti-TNFα antibodies. However, disease-modifying antirheumatic drugs (DMARDs) such as methotrexate (MTX) and salazosulfapyridine (SASP) may be used for peripheral arthritis, like rheumatoid arthritis.

Figure 43. Position of PsA in immunopathophysiological chart.

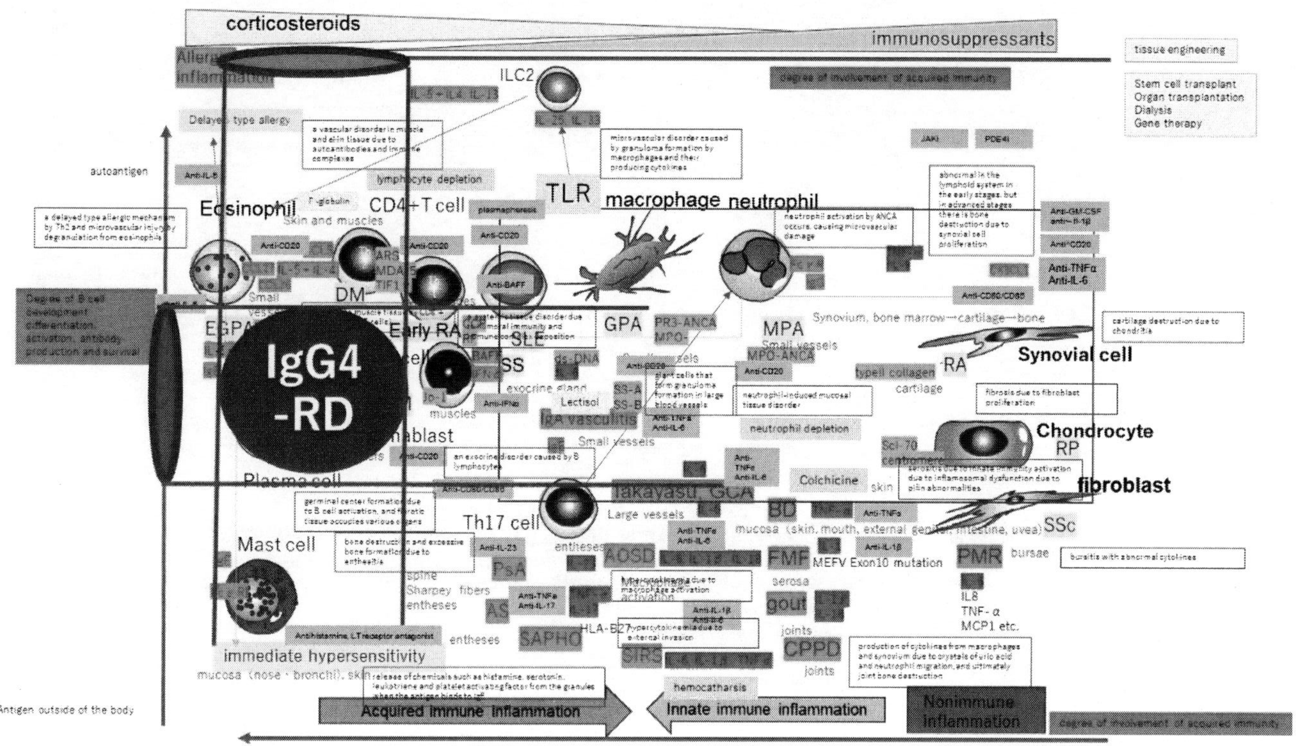

Figure 44. (Continued).

X-axis: Disease involving plasma cells and plasmablasts that are antibody-producing cells.
Y-axis: B cell differentiation (ratio of RP105-negative B cell s) is moderate and higher degree.
Layer 1: cells; plasma cells, plasmablasts (B cell line).
Layer 2: autoantibody; none.
Layer 3: Cytokine; BAFF?.
Layer 4: Chemokine: CXCR5, CXCR13.
Target tissue: systemic
Pathophysiology and treatment:

There is IgG4 production by plasma cells and organ damage associated with tissue occupation by and germinal center formation and fibrosis. It responds well to corticosteroids, but anti-CD20 antibody is considered for relapsed or refractory cases of IgG4-related disease.

Figure 44. Position of IgG4-related disease in immunopathophysiological chart.

Fundamental Policy of Diagnosis

Patients with IgG4-related disease usually respond to corticosteroid therapy, and timely diagnosis can avoid unnecessary invasive procedures or delays in treatment. Therefore, it is important for physicians to make a correct diagnosis based on the recognition that IgG4-related disease is the systemic disease.

Classification Criteria of IgG4-Related Disease

Although there are clinical and pathological differences in IgG4-related disease in organs, a consensus was reached in two ways for the definitive diagnosis of IgG4-related disease: (i) serum IgG4 levels > 135 mg/dl and (ii) more than 40% of IgG-positive plasma cells that are IgG4-positive, with more than 10 IgG4-positive cells per high-power field of biopsy sample.

Although clinical, serologic, radiological, and pathological features contribute to classification of IgG4-related disease, these approaches alone do not provide definitive evidence for accurate classification of patients. Proper classification of patients for both research and clinical purposes relies on the integration of data from all four areas of evidence (Wallace ZS., 2020).

The new classification criteria are the first one for IgG4-related disease and have been developed and tested using a data-driven approach and multi-criterion decision analysis.

Table 2. Exclusion criteria definitions (Wallace ZS., 2020)

Clinical
Fever: Documented, recurrent temperature>38°C, with fever being a prominent part of the patient's overall presentation with the underlying disease, in the absence of any clinical features of infection.
No objective response to glucocorticoids: If the patient has been treated with prednisone at a minimum of 40 mg/day (~0.6 mg/kg/day) for a period of 4 weeks, the patient has not demonstrated an objective clinical response. An objective response includes unequivocal improvement of the clinical lesions, biochemical abnormalities, or radiological findings. There are two two additional points to consider with regard to glucocorticoid response: Improvement only in the serum IgG4 concentration should not be regarded as a clinical response without improvement in other aspects of the disease. Some forms of IgG4-related disease (IgG4-RD) associated with advanced fibrosis, for example, some cases of retroperitoneal fibrosis or sclerosing mesenteritis, may not demonstrate obvious radiological responses to glucocorticoids.
Serological
Leucopenia and thrombocytopenia without alternative explanation: Reduction in the total white cell count and platelet count to levels below those normal for the reference laboratory, having no apparent explanation except for the underlying disease. Reductions in both the white cell count and platelet count are unusual in IgG4-RD but are typical of, for example, myelodysplastic syndromes, haematopoietic malignancies, and autoimmune conditions within the systemic lupus erythematosus spectrum.
Peripheral eosinophilia: To a concentration of>3000 mm^3.
Positive antineutrophil cytoplasmic antibody (ANCA): ELISA results positive for ANCA targeted against proteinase three or myeloperoxidase.
Positive antibodies: Ro, La, double-stranded DNA, RNP, or Sm antibodies positive in titrers greater than normal suggest an alternative diagnosis. Other autoantibody associated with high specificity for another immune-mediated condition is a reasonable explanation for the patient's presentation. Such specific autoantibodies include antisynthetase antibodies (e.g., anti-Jo-1), anti-topoisomerase III (Scl-70), and anti-phospholipase A2 receptor antibodies. This does not include autoantibodies of low specificity, such as rheumatoid factor, antinuclear antibodies, antimitochondrial antibodies, anti-smooth muscle antibodies, and antiphospholipid antibodies.
Cryoglobulinemia: Cryoglobulinemia (type I, II, or III) occurring in a clinical context that provides a reasonable explanation for the patient's presentation.

Radiological
Known radiological findings suspicious for malignancy or infection that have not been investigated sufficiently: Such radiological findings include mass lesions that have not been evaluated thoroughly, necrosis, cavitation, hypervascular or exophytic mass, bulky or matted lymphadenopathy, loculated abdominopelvic fluid collection, among others.
Rapid radiological progression: Defined as significant worsening within a 4–6 week interval.
Long bone abnormalities consistent with Erdheim-Chester disease: Multifocal osteosclerotic lesions of the long bones, usually associated with bilateral diaphyseal involvement.
Splenomegaly:>14 cm in the absence of alternative explanation (e.g., portal hypertension).
Pathological
Cellular infiltrates suspicious for malignancy that have not been investigated sufficiently: A high likelihood of malignancy may be suggested by cellular atypia, a monotypic nature of immunohistochemistry findings, or light chain restriction on in situ hybridizsation studies. If malignancy is suspected, this must be excluded by appropriate studies before inclusion.
Markers consistent with inflammatory myofibroblastic tumour: Known positivity for a marker suggestive of inflammatory myofibroblastic tumour, for example, anaplastic lymphoma kinase one or ROS, a receptor tyrosine kinase that is encoded by the gene *ROS1*
Prominent neutrophilic inflammation: Neutrophilic infiltrates are unusual in IgG4-RD, with the exception of occasional examples in the lung or near mucosal sites. Extensive neutrophilic infiltrates or neutrophilic abscesses strongly indicate the possibility of a non-IgG4-RD diagnosis.
Necrotising vasculitis: Although vascular injury (e.g., obliterative phlebitis or arteritis) is a hallmark of IgG4-RD, the presence of fibrinoid necrosis within blood vessel walls provides strong evidence against IgG4-RD.
Prominent necrosis: Small foci of necrosis may rarely be present around the luminal surface of ductal organs, but zonal necrosis with no alternative explanation (e.g., stenting) provides strong evidence against IgG4-RD.
Primary granulomatous inflammation: Inflammation rich in epithelioid histiocytes, including multinucleated giant cell formation and granuloma formation, is highly atypical of IgG4- RD
Pathological features of a macrophage/histiocytic disorder: For example: known S100-positive macrophages demonstrating emperipolesis, a pathological feature of Rosai-Dorfman disease.
Specific disease exclusions
Known diagnoses of the following diseases are exclusion criteria: Multicentric Castleman's disease, Crohn's disease (if pancreatobiliary disease is present), ulcerative colitis (if pancreatobiliary disease is present), Hashimoto thyroiditis (if the thyroid is the only proposed disease manifestation).: Patients with IgG4-RD can certainly have Hashimoto thyroiditis separately from IgG4-RD, but Hashimoto thyroiditis is part of the IgG4-RD spectrum.

Table 3. Inclusion criteria definitions (Wallace ZS., 2020)

Immunostaining
IgG+cells can be identified using either IgG staining or CD138 staining.
Head and neck gland involvement
A 'set' of glands refers to both lacrimal glands or both submandibular glands among others. If a gland has been surgically removed for the purpose of diagnosis, it can be considered to have been involved if confirmed by pathology.
Involvement of the lacrimal glands and the major salivary glands in IgG4-related disease (IgG4-RD) is bilateral (but can be asymmetric). Involvement of the glands can be determined by either a clinical examination or a radiological study (e.g., positron emission tomography scan or CT scan).
Chest
Peribronchovascular and septal thickening in the lung must be determined by a cross- sectional imaging study of the chest.
The paravertebral band-like soft tissue in the thorax is usually right-sided, located between T8 and T11, and does not encase the aorta.
Pancreas and biliary tree
Diffuse pancreas enlargement usually encompasses more than two-thirds of the pancreas.
The type of biliary involvement that is highly consistent with IgG4-related sclerosing cholangitis involves the proximal biliary tract (i.e., intrahepatic and extrapancreatic portions of the extrahepatic bile ducts). The bile duct walls often have smooth thickening.
Kidney
Hypocomplementemia pertains to low serum levels of C3, C4 or both.
Renal pelvic wall thickening can be either unilateral or bilateral, usually without severe stenosis or luminal irregularity.
Low-density areas in both renal cortices can be seen only on contrast-enhanced CT and are usually patchy or round- shaped in appearance.
Retroperitoneum
The location of IgG4-related retroperitoneal fibrosis or periaortitis is typically circumferential or on the anterolateral sides of the aorta. The segment of aorta involved tends to be the infrarenal aorta, often extending to include the iliac vessels.

Table 4. The 2019 American College of Rheumatology/European League Against Rheumatism classification criteria for IgG4-RD (Wallace ZS., 2020)

Step	Categorical assessment or numerical weight
Step 1. Entry criteria	
Characteristic* clinical or radiological involvement of a typical organ (e.g., pancreas, salivary glands, bile ducts, orbits, kidney, lung, aorta, retroperitoneum, pachymeninges or thyroid gland (Riedel's thyroiditis)) OR pathological evidence of an inflammatory process accompanied by a lymphoplasmacytic infiltrate of uncertain aetiology in one of these same organs	**Yes†** or No

Step	Categorical assessment or numerical weight
***Step 2. Exclusion criteria: domains and items*‡**	Yes or **No**§
Clinical	
Fever	
No objective response to glucocorticoids	
Serological	
Leucopenia and thrombocytopenia with no explanation	
Peripheral eosinophilia	
Positive antineutrophil cytoplasmic antibody (specifically against proteinase 3 or myeloperoxidase)	
Positive SSA/Ro or SSB/La antibody	
Positive double-stranded DNA, RNP or Sm antibody	
Other disease-specific autoantibody	
Cryoglobulinemia	
Radiological	
Known radiological findings suspicious for malignancy or infection that have not been sufficiently investigated	
Rapid radiological progression	
Long bone abnormalities consistent with Erdheim-Chester disease	
Splenomegaly	
Pathological	
Cellular infiltrates suggesting malignancy that have not been sufficiently evaluated	
Markers consistent with inflammatory myofibroblastic tumour	
Prominent neutrophilic inflammation	
Necrotizing vasculitis	
Prominent necrosis	
Primarily granulomatous inflammation	
Pathologic features of macrophage/histiocytic disorder	
Known diagnosis of the following:	
Multicentric Castleman's disease	
Crohn's disease or ulcerative colitis (if only pancreatobiliary disease is present)	
Hashimoto thyroiditis (if only the thyroid is affected)	
If case meets entry criteria and does not meet any exclusion criteria, proceed to step 3.	
Step 3. Inclusion criteria: domains and items	
Histopathology	
Uninformative biopsy	0
Dense lymphocytic infiltrate	+4
Dense lymphocytic infiltrate and obliterative phlebitis	+6
Dense lymphocytic infiltrate and storiform fibrosis with or without obliterative phlebitis	+13

Table 4. (Continued)

Step	Categorical assessment or numerical weight
Immunostaining**	0–16, as follows:
	Assigned weight is 0 if the IgG4+:IgG+ ratio is 0%–40% or indeterminate and the number of IgG4+ cells/hpf is 0–9.‡‡ Assigned weight is 7 if: (1) the IgG4+:IgG+ ratio is ≥41% and the number of IgG4+cells/hpf is 0–9 or indeterminate or (2) the IgG4+:IgG+ ratio is 0–40% or indeterminate and the number of IgG4+ cells/hpf is ≥10 or indeterminate. Assigned weight is 14 if: (1) the IgG4+:IgG+ ratio is 41%–70% and the number of IgG4+ cells/hpf is ≥10 or (2) the IgG4+:IgG+ ratio is ≥71% and the number of IgG4+ cells/hpf is 10–50. Assigned weight is 16 if the IgG4+:IgG+ ratio is ≥71% and the number of IgG4+ cells/hpf is ≥51.
Serum IgG_4 concentration	
Normal or not checked	0
>Normal but <2× upper limit of normal	+4
2–5× upper limit of normal	+6
≥>5× upper limit of normal	+11
Bilateral lacrimal, parotid, sublingual and submandibular glands	
No set of glands involved	0
One set of glands involved	+6
Two or more sets of glands involved	+14
Chest	
Not checked or neither of the items listed is present	0
Peribronchovascular and septal thickening	+4
Paravertebral band-like soft tissue in the thorax	+10
Pancreas and biliary tree	

Step	Categorical assessment or numerical weight
Not checked or none of the items listed is present	0
Diffuse pancreas enlargement (loss of lobulations)	+8
Diffuse pancreas enlargement and capsule-like rim with decreased enhancement	+11
Pancreas (either of above) and biliary tree involvement	+19
Kidney	
Not checked or none of the items listed is present	0
Hypocomplementemia	+6
Renal pelvis thickening/soft tissue	+8
Bilateral renal cortex low-density areas	+10
Retroperitoneum	
Not checked or neither of the items listed is present	0
Diffuse thickening of the abdominal aortic wall	+4
Circumferential or anterolateral soft tissue around the infrarenal aorta or iliac arteries	+8
Step 4: Total inclusion points	
A case meets the classification criteria for IgG4-RD if the entry criteria are met, no exclusion criteria are present, and the total points is ≥20	

*Refers to enlargement or tumour-like mass in an affected organ except in (1) the bile ducts, where narrowing tends to occur, (2) the aorta, where wall thickening or aneurysmal dilatation is typical and (3) the lungs, where thickening of the bronchovascular bundles is common.

†If entry criteria are not fulfilled, the patient cannot be further considered for classification as having IgG4-RD.

‡Assessment for the presence of exclusion criteria should be individualised depending on a patient's clinical scenario.

§If exclusion criteria are met, the patient cannot be further considered for classification as having IgG4-RD.

¶Only the highest weighted item in each domain is scored.

**Biopsies from lymph nodes, mucosal surfaces of the gastrointestinal tract and skin are not acceptable for use in weighting the immunostaining domain.

††'Indeterminate' refers to a situation in which the pathologist is unable to clearly quantify the number of positively staining cells within an infiltrate, yet can still ascertain that the number of cells is at least 10/hpf. For a number of reasons, most often pertaining to the quality of the immunostain, pathologists are sometimes unable to count the number of IgG4+ plasma cells with precision yet even so, can be confident in grouping cases into the appropriate immunostaining result category.

hpf, high-power field; IgG4-RD, IgG4-related disease.

DIFFERENTIAL DIAGNOSIS

IgG4-related disease needs exclusion of cancer, malignant lymphoma, granulomatosis with polyangiitis (GPA), sarcoidosis, eosinophilic granulomatosis with polyangiitis (EGPA), etc., but particularly important to distinguish it from malignant tumors.

The Activity Evaluation Scales for Monitoring Treatment Response

The IgG4-RD Responder Index (RI) is a scale that evaluates the activity and severity of IgG4-related diseases, and is also evaluated internationally as one of the activity evaluation scales for monitoring treatment response (Wallace ZS.., 2018).

Treatment

Not all patients with IgG4-related disease require treatment, and some patients may be followed up without treatment (Stone JH., 2012).

Induction Therapy

Glucocorticoids

Oral glucocorticoids are the first-line treatment in patients with active IgG4-related disease or patients with significant organ involvement.

Maintenance Therapy

After induction therapy, maintenance therapy may be given if the condition of the patient with IgG4-related disease becomes stable (Masamune A, 2017).

Immunomodulators

Several immunomodulators have been applied as alternatives or steroid sparing agents to IgG4-related disease, but there is little evidence to support the efficacy of these drugs (Hart PA, 2013).

B Cell Targeting Therapy

Rituximab (RTX)

B cell depletion with rituximab (RTX) has been effective in patients whose IgG4-related disease is resistant to or contraindicated for glucocorticoids and conventional immunomodulators (Khosroshahi A, 2015) (Hart PA, 2013).

It has also been reported that removal of CD20 + plasmablast-precursors by rituximab reduced the number of plasmablasts involved in disease activity (Mattoo H, 2014).

Long-Term Prognosis of IgG4-Related Disease

IgG4-related disease has long been considered a reversible condition with a good prognosis. However, recent studies have shown that long-term prognosis can be a progressive condition with organ damage or a course of malignancy.

References

Hart P. A., T. M. (2013). Treatment of relapsing autoimmune pancreatitis with immunomodulators and rituximab: the Mayo Clinic experience. *Gut, 62*, 1607-15.

Khosroshahi A. W. Z. (2015). International Consensus Guidance Statement on the Management and Treatment of IgG4-Related Disease. *Arthritis Rheumatol, 67*, 1688-99.

Kikuchi Y., Koarada S. et al. *Arthritis Rheum* 2002.

Kikuchi Y., Koarada S., et al. *Ann Rheum Dis*. 2001.

Kikuchi Y., Koarada S., et al. *Clin Exp Rheumatol*. 2008.

Koarada S. et al. *Ann Rheum Dis*. 2015,

Koarada S. et al. *Arthritis Rheum* 1999.

Koarada S. et al. *Clin Dev Immunol*. 2012;2012-1.

Koarada S. et al. *Clin Dev Immunol*. 2012;2012-2.

Koarada S. et al. *Open Rheumatol J*. 2013.

Koarada S. et al. *Rheumatology* (Oxford). 2001.

Koarada S, et al. *World J. Rheumatol*. 2016.

Koarada S. *Rheumatology* (Oxford). 2010.

Masamune A., N. I. (2017). Randomised controlled trial of long-term maintenance corticosteroid therapy in patients with autoimmune pancreatitis. *Gut, 66*, 487-94.

Mattoo H., M. V. T. (2014). De novo oligoclonal expansions of circulating plasmablasts in active and relapsing IgG4-related disease. *J Allergy Clin Immunol, 134*, 679-87.

Stone J. H., K. A. (2012). Recommendations for the nomenclature of IgG4-related disease and its individual organ system manifestations. *Arthritis Rheum, 64*, 3061.

Wallace Z. S., N. R. (2020). The 2019 American College of Rheumatology/European League Against Rheumatism classification criteria for IgG4-related disease. *Ann Rheum Dis, 79*, 77-87.

Wallace Z. S., K. A. (2018). An international, multi-specialty validation study of the IgG4-related disease responder index. *Arthritis Care Res*, Feb [cited. 2018 Feb 18].

Yamashita Y. et al. *J Exp Med*. 1996.

About the Editor

Syuichi Koarada
Associated Professor
Division of Rheumatology, Faculty of Medicine, Saga University

Dr. Koarada is a doctorate (PhD and MD) in Immunology from Saga University, Saga, Japan. He worked at UPMC (University of Pittsburgh Medical Center) (1999-2001) as an Associated Professor. Currently, Dr. Koarada is an Associated Professor of Saga University. His specialty is rheumatology and clinical immunology. He has published more than 100 scientific papers and 11 books. He has published the book series about imaging and clinical immunology in rheumatology every year regularly. He is certified as a specialist by Board Certified, Japanese Board of Internal Medicine, The Japanese college of Rheumatology, and Board certified, Sonography of Rheumatology. He received the Award of Japan Society for Clinical Immunology for his work on RP105 in B cells in 2011.

INDEX

β

A

B

C

D

E

F

G

S

T

U

W